T0339577

Personalized Predictive Modeling in Type 1 Diabetes

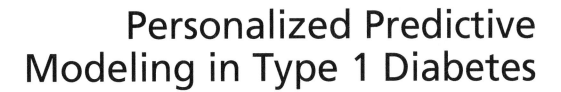

Personalized Predictive Modeling in Type 1 Diabetes

Eleni I. Georga
Unit of Medical Technology and Intelligent Information Systems, Department of Materials Science and Engineering, University of Ioannina, Ioannina, Greece

Dimitrios I. Fotiadis
Unit of Medical Technology and Intelligent Information Systems, Department of Materials Science and Engineering, University of Ioannina, Ioannina, Greece
and
Department of Biomedical Research, Institute of Molecular Biology and Biotechnology, Foundation for Research and Technology - Hellas (FORTH), Ioannina, Greece

Stelios K. Tigas
Department of Endocrinology, School of Medicine, University of Ioannina, Ioannina, Greece

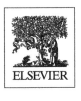

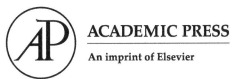

ACADEMIC PRESS
An imprint of Elsevier

Academic Press is an imprint of Elsevier
125 London Wall, London EC2Y 5AS, United Kingdom
525 B Street, Suite 1800, San Diego, CA 92101-4495, United States
50 Hampshire Street, 5th Floor, Cambridge, MA 02139, United States
The Boulevard, Langford Lane, Kidlington, Oxford OX5 1GB, United Kingdom

Notices

Knowledge and best practice in this field are constantly changing. As new research and experience broaden our
understanding, changes in research methods, professional practices, or medical treatment may become necessary.

Practitioners and researchers must always rely on their own experience and knowledge in evaluating and using any
information, methods, compounds, or experiments described herein. In using such information or methods they
should be mindful of their own safety and the safety of others, including parties for whom they have a professional
responsibility.

To the fullest extent of the law, neither the Publisher nor the authors, contributors, or editors, assume any liability
for any injury and/or damage to persons or property as a matter of products liability, negligence or otherwise, or
from any use or operation of any methods, products, instructions, or ideas contained in the material herein.

Library of Congress Cataloging-in-Publication Data
A catalog record for this book is available from the Library of Congress

British Library Cataloguing-in-Publication Data
A catalogue record for this book is available from the British Library

ISBN: 978-0-12-804831-3

For Information on all Academic Press publications
visit our website at https://www.elsevier.com/books-and-journals

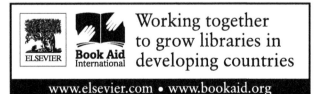

Working together
to grow libraries in
developing countries

www.elsevier.com • www.bookaid.org

Publisher: Mara Conner
Acquisition Editor: Fiona Geraghty
Editorial Project Manager: Thomas Van Der Ploeg
Production Project Manager: Anusha Sambamoorthy
Cover Designer: Maria Inez Cruz

Typeset by MPS Limited, Chennai, India

Contents

Preface

Diabetes care has evolved considerably over the years with the development of advanced medical technologies and therapeutics. Prognosis and prevention of critical hypoglycemic or hyperglycemic excursions may improve the quality of life of patients with type 1 diabetes. On this basis, extensive research has been performed toward the construction of intelligent personalized predictive models of blood glucose concentration by employing physiological models of the glucose–insulin system and advanced time-series and machine-learning regression models of health and lifestyle information.

This book provides a unified, comprehensive coverage of the state-of-the-art methods and algorithmic approaches which have been applied to predictive modeling of blood glucose concentration in type 1 diabetes, aiming at supporting the transfer of knowledge in the field as well as the development of innovative personalized predictive, and eventually, preventive diabetes management solutions. Simple autoregressive models of the continuous glucose monitoring (CGM) time series as well as multivariate nonlinear machine learning–based regression models are featured, analyzed, and contrasted with respect to the (i) feature set (univariate or multivariate), (ii) regression technique (linear or nonlinear), (iii) learning mechanism (batch or sequential), and (iv, v) model selection and model validation processes. The comparative assessment of modeling techniques along with the illustration of theory with examples based on real data are considered major assets of our book. More specifically:

- Chapter 1, Background and Preview, is an introductory chapter aiming at familiarizing the reader with the basic components of daily diabetes care and outlining the basic concepts of linear/nonlinear dynamic identification and short-term prediction of blood glucose concentration.
- Chapter 2, Pathophysiology and Management of Type 1 Diabetes, describes both normal physiology of glucose metabolism and pathophysiology of diabetes, placing special emphasis on the glucose counterregulatory system. Current approaches to glycemic control assessment and to intensive insulin therapy are also discussed.
- Chapter 3, Methodology for Developing a Glucose Prediction Model, provides a methodology toward developing a data-driven glucose prediction model, having approximated the underlying glucose system by a parameterized function of observed input–output data. The process of gathering, in a standardized way, the information upon which the model is going to be constructed is also delineated.
- Chapter 4, Physiological Models and Exogenous Input Modeling, focuses on mathematical models of the kinetics of exogenous materials (i.e., subcutaneously administered insulin, glucose ingestion) in the glucose–insulin system, ranging from

pure compartmental models to more complex mechanistic models. Extensions of system models, primarily of the minimal glucose model, to include the physiological effects of exercise are also presented.

- Chapter 5, Linear Time Series Models of Glucose Concentration, is the first one from a quartet of chapters devoted to data-driven modeling approaches of subcutaneous glucose concentration in type 1 diabetes. Basic definitions of linear time-invariant models are provided along with a description and comparative assessment of the findings of the most influential studies in the field. In addition, the results of a preliminary linear predictive analysis of the glucose dynamics of two individuals with type 1 diabetes are presented and discussed.
- Chapter 6, Nonlinear Models of Glucose Concentration, focuses on nonlinear glucose prediction schemes based on linearly parameterized or kernel-based regression models. A univariate linear (with respect to the parameters) regression analysis of the glucose dynamics in type 1 diabetes is also conducted, which complements the autoregressive analysis performed in Chapter 5, Linear Time Series Models of Glucose Concentration.
- Chapter 7, Prediction Models of Hypoglycemia, presents state-of-the-art approaches to hypoglycemia detection and prediction emphasizing on the definition of an event and, subsequently, a true positive prediction, and the evaluation of each method over CGM or blood glucose data. In addition, the results of a multivariate kernel-based approach are analyzed, aiming at presenting to the reader a fully featured example.
- Chapter 8, Adaptive Glucose Prediction Models, approaches the problem of glucose prediction in type 1 diabetes from the point of view of adaptive linear (least mean square and recursive least squares) or nonlinear (extended Kalman filters, real-time recurrent neural networks) models for regression. Sparse kernel adaptive filters are proposed as a learning scheme for the nonlinear dynamical system of glucose and their performance is evaluated and compared with that of time-invariant nonlinear regression models.
- Chapter 9, Existing and Potential Applications of Glucose Prediction Models, presents the individual modules of an artificial pancreas system, with emphasis on the employed control algorithms, and discusses the safety and efficacy of current paradigms in an outpatient setting. The incorporation of glucose models into upcoming mobile diabetes application, featuring cognitive capabilities, is also discussed.
- Chapter 10, Conclusions and Future Trends, summarizes the major outcomes of the literature on predictive modeling of glucose concentration in type 1 diabetes, and presents an integrative, with respect to the data and analysis methods, glucose model which takes advantage of genomics and multi-omics analytics.

The target audience of this book primarily comprises practitioners and researchers with specialties in data-driven predictive modeling of the glucose system in type 1 diabetes. This book is also intended to graduate and undergraduate students in the field of medicine and biomedical engineering. Finally, the book may be beneficial for professionals from various disciplines including, but not limited to, Health, Computer Science, Biomedical Engineering, and Information and Communication Technologies.

This work was carried out at the Unit of Medical Technology and Intelligent Information Systems (MEDLAB) at the University of Ioannina, whose research excellence in the field of biomedical engineering is internationally acknowledged.

We would like to thank our team in the Unit of Medical Technology and Intelligent Information Systems for their scientific and emotional support during the time of the writing of this book. We are also grateful to the Editorial Team for their valuable guidance throughout the publishing process. We also express our sincere gratitude to our families who contributed to the final realization of this work through the continuous motivation and inspiration they provided to us.

Eleni I. Georga, Dimitrios I. Fotiadis, Stelios K. Tigas
University of Ioannina, Ioannina, Greece

Terminology List

Eyglycemia: Eyglycemia is defined as normal blood-glucose concentration. The American Diabetes Association standards of diabetes care state that for nonpregnant adults with diabetes (1) the preprandial capillary plasma glucose concentration should range from 80 to 130 mg/dL and (2) the peak postprandial (1−2 hours after the beginning of the meal) capillary plasma glucose concentration should be <180 mg/dL.

Hypoglycemia: Hypoglycemia in diabetes is a complication of intensive insulin therapy characterized by a low blood-glucose concentration and accompanied by common autonomic or neuroglycopenic symptoms. The International Hypoglycemia Study Group recommends (1) a plasma-glucose concentration alert value of ≤70 mg/dL and (2) a plasma-glucose concentration of <54 mg/dL, detected by self-monitoring of plasma glucose, continuous glucose monitoring (for at least 20 minutes), or a laboratory measurement of plasma glucose, as clinically significant biochemical hypoglycemia which should be reported in clinical trials.

Intensive insulin therapy: It encompasses multiple-dose insulin injections (three to four injections per day) or continuous subcutaneous insulin infusion, aiming at replicating the pattern of physiologic insulin secretion and achieving targeted glycemic goals.

Randomized controlled clinical trial: Experimental study design in which a sample of participants is randomly assigned to two groups, i.e., the intervention and the control (usual care) group which are followed in parallel, and a rigorous comparison of the intervention efficacy on biomedical or health-related outcomes in the two groups is analyzed.

Observational cohort study: Observational study design in which a group of patients with defined characteristics or a common exposure (variables of interest), but who do not have the outcome of interest, is followed over time to determine whether they develop the outcome of interest.

Linear system modeling: Discrete time description of a linear dynamical system through the parameterized impulse response functions of its inputs and of an additive random output disturbance. A class of linear models (e.g., autoregressive moving average models, state-space models) is defined whose parameters are learnt by prediction error methods based on observed input−output data.

Nonlinear regression modeling: A parametric model which is typically postulated as a linear combination of nonlinear fixed or adaptive basis functions of the input. Model parameter learning relies on least squares or regularized least squares optimization methods using observed input−output data.

Neural networks: A class of nonlinear parametric models for regression employing a fixed number of parametric basis functions, which are nonlinear functions of linear combinations of the input and whose parameters are learned along with model parameters during training. They exhibit universal approximation properties, whereas they define a nonconvex optimization problem.

Kernel-based regression: A class of nonlinear nonparametric models for regression transforming the input space into a high-dimensional Reproducing Kernel Hilbert Space (RKHS), where their output lies in the span of the finite set of kernels centered at the training input vectors. A form of constraint is imposed on the error function to avoid overfitting. Classic paradigms of kernel-based regression are support vector machines, relevant vector machines, and Gaussian processes.

Adaptive learning: Sequential fitting of a linear or nonlinear model to new input—output data relying on least mean square or recursive least squares and aiming at adapting model parameters to the time-varying behavior of the examined system.

Kernel adaptive filters: A class of nonlinear nonparametric models for regression which apply linear adaptive filtering (recursive least squares, least mean square) in a high-dimensional RKHS, to which the input space is mapped. A sparse regularized solution is usually obtained by applying an online sparsification criterion.

Compartmental modeling: A class of dynamic mathematical models representing the examined biological system by a number of distinct interconnected compartments whose identification is based on the conservation of mass principle and using multiple tracer experimental data.

Closed-loop system of glucose control: Medical system aiming at emulating the feedback glucose-responsive functionality of beta-cells in normal physiology of glucose metabolism by combining continuous glucose monitoring and subcutaneous insulin infusion technologies with, primarily, model predictive control, proportional integral derivative control, or fuzzy-logic algorithms

Precision medicine: According to the National Institutes of Health definition, precision medicine advocates that prognosis, diagnosis, and therapeutics of a disease should be driven by precise knowledge on an individual's genetics, environment, and lifestyle.

List of Abbreviations

ACF	autocorrelation function
AGP	ambulatory glucose profile
AIC	Akaike information criterion
AICc	corrected Akaike information criterion
ALD	approximate linear dependency
AP	artificial pancreas
AR	autoregressive
ARMA	autoregressive moving average
ARMAX	autoregressive moving average with extra inputs
ARX	autoregressive with extra inputs
AUC	area under the receiver operating characteristic curve
BIC	Bayesian information criterion
BJ	Box–Jenkins
CC	correlation coefficient
CG-EGA	continuous glucose error grid analysis
CGM	continuous glucose monitoring
CSII	continuous subcutaneous insulin infusion
ECG	electrocardiogram
EEG	electroencephalogram
EGA	error grid analysis
EHR	electronic health record
EKF	extended Kalman filter
ELM	extreme learning machine
ESOD	energy of the second-order differences
EWMA	exponentially weighted moving average
FFA	free fatty acids
FFNN	feed-forward neural network
FPG	fasting plasma glucose
FPR	false positive rate
GP	Gaussian processes
GSR	galvanic skin response
GTFM	general transfer function model
HAAF	hypoglycemia-associated autonomic failure
HbA1c	glycated hemoglobin
HRV	heart rate variability
ICR	insulin-to-carbohydrate ratio
IFG	impaired fasting glucose
IGT	impaired glucose tolerance
IIT	intensive insulin therapy
IVGTT	intravenous glucose-tolerance test
KAF	kernel adaptive filters
KLMS	kernel least mean square

KRLS	kernel recursive least squares
LMS	least mean square
LV	latent variable
LVX	latent variable with extra inputs
MAE	mean absolute error
MARD	mean absolute relative difference
MDI	multiple daily injections
MDL	minimum description length
MET	metabolic equivalent of task
MIMO	multiple-input multiple-output
MISO	multiple-input single-output
MPC	model predictive control
MTT	mixed-meal tolerance test
NHGB	net hepatic glucose balance
NSSE	normalized sum of the squared error
OGTT	oral glucose tolerance test
P-EGA	point-error grid analysis
PEM	prediction error method
PHR	personal health record
PID	proportional integral derivative
PRED-EGA	prediction-error grid analysis
PSD	power spectral density
QKLMS	quantized kernel least mean square
RBF	radial basis function
R-EGA	rate-error grid analysis
RF	random forest
RKHS	reproducing kernel Hilbert space
RLS	recursive least squares
RMSE	root mean squared error
RNN	recurrent neural network
ROC	receiver operating characteristic
RTRL	real-time recurrent learning
s.c.	subcutaneous
SAP	sensor-augmented pump
SISO	single-input single-output
SMBG	self-monitoring of blood glucose
SNS	sensitivity
SOM	self-organizing map
SVM	support vector machines
SVR	support vector regression
TG	temporal gain
WFNN	wavelet fuzzy neural network
WRLS	weighted recursive least squares

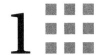

1

Background and Preview

1.1 Data-Driven Glucose Prediction Models and Clinical Impact

Diabetes is a group of metabolic disorders characterized by hyperglycaemia resulting from defects in insulin secretion, insulin action, or both [1]. Type 1 diabetes results from a cellular-mediated autoimmune destruction of the β-cells in the pancreas, leading to absolute insulin deficiency. On the other hand, type 2 diabetes is characterized by a progressive loss of insulin secretion on the background of insulin resistance [2]. According to the International Diabetes Federation, the number of people (adults 20–79 years) with diabetes worldwide is estimated to rise from 415 million in 2015 to 642 million in 2040, while type 1 diabetes is increasing by around 3% every year, particularly among children. Moreover, the long-term microvascular and macrovascular complications, associated with the chronic hyperglycaemia, render diabetes a major cause of early death in most countries.

The most vital and challenging issue for people with type 1 or advanced type 2 diabetes is the achievement and maintenance of euglycaemia overtime in a safe manner. The daily management of the disease can be seen as a feedback loop in which frequent self-monitoring of blood glucose (SMBG) is strongly associated with better glycaemic control. Intensive insulin therapy (IIT), implemented by either multiple daily injections (MDI) or continuous subcutaneous insulin infusion (CSII), could be the remedy for hyperglycaemia in type 1 diabetes, should it not increase the risk of hypoglycaemia, which is defined as a blood-glucose concentration below 70 mgdL^{-1}. The long-term benefits of IIT along with the increased frequency of hypoglycaemic events were first demonstrated by the Diabetes Control and Complications Trial [3]. Since then, despite the significant improvements in insulin analogues, hypoglycaemia has been recognized as the major barrier to the management of diabetes [4].

The reduction of the risk of hypoglycaemia is a matter of major interest in daily diabetes care. Hypoglycaemia in insulin-dependent diabetes patients is the aggregate of therapeutic hyperinsulinemia, as well as, attenuated sympathoadrenal response to falling plasma-glucose concentrations [5]. In addition, recent antecedent hypoglycaemia, prior exercise, and sleep further impair the physiological and behavioural defenses against a potential subsequent hypoglycaemia (i.e., hypoglycaemia-associated autonomic failure—HAAF) and, therefore, cause a vicious cycle of recurrent hypoglycaemia [4,6]. The awareness of these factors by individuals with diabetes may contribute to the prevention of hypoglycaemia on a daily basis. It is acknowledged that achieving and maintaining tight glycaemic control necessitates the proper consideration of extrinsic factors having a direct impact on subsequent glucose concentrations, such as nutrition, physical activity, patient's psychological status, and the overall lifestyle [2]. In addition to these, the endogenous processes involved in the regulation of glucose homeostasis, as well as the prominent intra- and interpatient variability in

Personalized Predictive Modeling in Type 1 Diabetes. DOI: http://dx.doi.org/10.1016/B978-0-12-804831-3.00001-7

response to insulin therapy [7−9], render glucose control in diabetes—a rather difficult procedure.

The technological advances in continuous glucose monitoring (CGM) and CSII have contributed to more efficient and safe therapeutic procedures, especially for insulin-treated diabetes [10]. The high temporal resolution of CGM offers the potential to gain a deeper insight into 24-h glucose dynamics in the subcutaneous space supporting a more informed and comprehensive decision-making in both clinical and self-monitoring conditions. The American Diabetes Association recommends, "CGM may be a supplemental tool to SMBG in those with hypoglycemia unawareness and/or frequent hypoglycemic episodes" [2]. The findings of numerous clinical trials have confirmed that CGM reduces HbA1c, an index of average glycaemic control over the preceding 2−3 months, in type 1 diabetes as compared to SMBG; however, they have not shown significant reductions in severe hypoglycaemia [11−13]. Modern CGM systems are able to provide customizable predictive alerts for upcoming critical events, which has been shown to improve hypoglyceamia detection [14,15]. Toward this direction, Facchinetti et al. [16] introduced the smart CGM sensor concept by adding three real-time signal processing algorithms for denoising, enhancement, and prediction to the Seven Plus CGM system (DexCom). In that way, the smoothness of the Seven Plus CGM time series improved by an average of 57%, the mean absolute relative difference (MARD) between blood-glucose measurements and CGM data reduced from 15.1% to 10.3%, and, finally, hypoglycaemic or hyperglycaemic events were predicted with an average horizon of 14 min. On the other hand, literature suggests that there are no significant differences in HbA1c or frequency of severe hypoglycaemia between CSII and MDI therapy [17,18]. Nevertheless, both CGM and CSII technologies form the basis for the development of more advanced technological solutions for controlling diabetes.

The effective integration of CGM and CSII technologies into one system, that is, sensor-augmented pump (SAP), allows improvements in glycemic control of type 1 diabetes when compared with MDI therapy or the individual components alone [1,19,20]; however, the problem of severe hypoglycaemia and, in particular, nocturnal hypoglycaemia is not solved. A far more promising approach to this problem is the automatic suspension of insulin delivery at a preset low-glucose threshold aiming at reducing basal insulinemia during the critical first few minutes of hypoglycaemia without causing rebound hyperglycaemia [21]. In particular, the so-called threshold-suspend feature available in the Medtronic Paradigm Veo pump was shown to significantly reduce the rate and the mean area under curve of nocturnal hypoglycaemic events by 31.8% and 37.5%, respectively, as compared to standard SAP therapy [22]. Moreover, the 24-h hypoglycaemic exposure was also reduced during the 3-month study, without significant changes in HbA1c levels. A following study did support that this technology has the potential to reduce the combined rate of severe and moderate hypoglycaemia in patients with type 1 diabetes [23]. Of great importance, the effectiveness of suspending the insulin pump delivery when the predicted risk of hypoglycaemia is high was demonstrated both by simulations and experiments [24−26]. It is acknowledged that SAP with threshold-suspend is the epitome of today's diabetes technology and that is the next step for an automated closed-loop artificial pancreas, the most promising therapeutic approach to β-cell replacement.

Lately, incremental steps have also been taken toward a portable closed-loop system for overnight glucose control suitable for outpatient use [27−30]. However, further research is needed to ensure the reliable, stable, and safe operation of the whole system given the limitations of existing subcutaneous glucose sensors and wireless communications. The control algorithm is currently implemented either with proportional−integral−derivative (PID) control or model-predictive control (MPC) [31,32]. PID control as a reactive feedback mechanism cannot effectively correct sudden hypoglycaemia or hyperglycaemia. On the other hand, MPC uses mathematical models of diabetes physiology or data-driven models to predict the short-term glucose dynamics. MPC not only allows for better regulation of glucose in both steady state (e.g., overnight) and dynamic conditions (e.g., postprandial, during exercise) but also mitigates the time lags imposed by the subcutaneous route in glucose sensing and insulin absorption. We should also emphasize the utility of low-glucose predictive alerts available in both CGM and closed-loop systems [14,15,24−26], which act as a safeguard mechanism against hypoglycaemia. A modular architectural approach to closed-loop control has been proposed in Refs. [2,31] that allows the hierarchical integration of diverse components starting from functionalities assuring patient's safety (i.e., insulin pump suspension if hypoglycaemia is anticipated) to customizable MPC of basal insulin rate in real time. Two following randomized crossover studies demonstrated the utility of that concept for designing and testing different closed-loop control configurations [33]. To this end, more proactive and sensitive to overall patient's context predictive algorithms may result in tighter glycaemic control minimizing the risk of hypoglycaemia, while setting the appropriate circumstances for closing the loop during the day.

The ever-increasing computational power of smartphones, the rise of mobile health devices, and the improved wireless communication technologies have contributed altogether to the development of remarkable mobile tools for diabetes self-management [10]. A number of mobile diabetes applications have been developed, either for research or commercial purposes, to support self-monitoring and decision-making on a daily basis [34−40]. Contemporary paradigms offer precise self-monitoring and indirect decision support through effective tools for data tracking and data visualization. The findings of mobile diabetes interventions suggest that well-designed mobile tools with decision-support features have the potential to enhance self-management outcomes. Daily self-monitoring information can be efficiently analysed, retrospectively or in real-time, to provide patients with supportive feedback related to diabetes management. The application of advanced data analytics can lead to more efficient treatment recommendations grounded entirely on the knowledge present in the data. For instance, data-mining techniques could further promote the individualization of daily care of diabetes facilitating the recognition of established patterns in self-monitoring data and, eventually, the interpretation a patient's status. The provision of real-time blood-glucose predictions on the mobile device is considered a challenging problem. For instance, the METABO [41] and DIAdvisor [42] type 1 diabetes management systems allowed efficient glucose prediction algorithms to be executed directly on mobile devices, which were used for patient self-monitoring. Undeniably, the plethora of measurement data in combination with existing large infrastructures on the cloud, machine-learning libraries, and web services could be all utilized for multiparametric and multiscale predictive analysis of patient's context.

Medical care in diabetes can be enhanced by the development of computational models of glucose metabolism, which offer the potential to predict the blood-glucose response to various stimuli. As has been discussed previously, predictive models of glucose concentration have the potential to further advance insulin-treated diabetes management either in open-loop conditions by providing advanced knowledge of abnormal glycaemic variations and facilitating the appropriate patient reaction in crucial situations, such as asymptomatic hypoglycaemia, or in closed-loop conditions as an integral component of the control algorithm [24,26,43,44]. Considerable research efforts have been reported toward the development of mathematical models suitable for simulating the physiology of healthy blood-glucose metabolism as well as the pathophysiology of type 1 diabetes [45,46]. Linear compartmental models, which are a class of dynamic models based on mass conservation principles, have been mainly used for studying the underlying processes involved in the regulation of glucose. Despite the fact that new important quantitative knowledge has been gained on glucose metabolism and control by insulin [47−49], the predictive capability of compartmental models is still limited due to the inherent complexity of the glucose-insulin system. On the other hand, data-driven modeling techniques are able to predict the glucose concentration by utilizing only the information hidden in the input−output data, without needing a-priori knowledge about the relationship between them. Initial machine-learning approaches to predict the time course of the blood-glucose concentration in subjects with type 1 diabetes were evaluated using discrete blood-glucose measurements, which were recorded three or more times daily [50−52]. CGM provided significant insight into daily glycaemic dynamics, giving rise to more accurate predictions of glucose concentration in the blood as well as in the subcutaneous interstitial fluid. In the latter case, the time lag between blood and subcutaneous glucose, which ranges from 5 to 15 min [53], can be mitigated using predictive models of sufficient long-term prediction horizon. It has been demonstrated that machine-learning techniques and time-series analysis can produce short-term predictions of high accuracy by utilizing information on CGM data, insulin dose administration, carbohydrates intake, and physical activity. In general, predictive algorithms should (1) learn the effect of therapy and patient's context (e.g., meals, physical activities, and stress) on subsequent glucose dynamics and (2) produce customizable solutions that explain the intra- and interpatient variability. Nevertheless, further experimental or well-designed observational clinical studies are needed to investigate the feasibility of such techniques in the daily self-management of diabetes.

The testing procedure of the glucose predictive models can be also greatly supported by employing realistic computer models of the human metabolic system. The University of Virginia/Padova type 1 diabetes simulator has been accepted by the Food and Drug Administration (FDA) as a substitute to animal trials in the preclinical testing of closed-loop control strategies [54]. Its main feature is that it includes 300 in-silico subjects validated against real clinical data and representing well the observed variability of key metabolic parameters in the general population with type 1 diabetes. The base of the mathematical model of the simulator is the glucose-insulin meal model of Dalla Man et al. [47,48], while in-silico glucose sensors and insulin pumps have also been implemented. In general, computer simulation testing of data-driven predictive or control algorithms is an important helper in this process.

1.2 Linear and Nonlinear Modeling Approaches

The prediction of the short-term course of glucose concentration, in the plasma or in the subcutaneous space, of individuals with type 1 diabetes is a research problem that has been widely studied, particularly, since the adoption of CGM and CSII in the daily management of the disease. From a data-driven perspective, the dynamic system of glucose metabolism is approximated by a parameterized model, describing the relation between the input and the system's output, with linear-system identification and linear regression being the two dominant modeling approaches.

The k-step-ahead prediction of glucose concentration at time t, that is, $y(t)$, is denoted by $\hat{y}(t|\theta)$ and is obtained by a function $\hat{y}(t|\theta) = f(Z^{t-kT}, \theta)$ of observations of previous input−output data up to time $t - kT$ (denoted by Z^{t-kT}), with T being the sampling interval of glucose concentration and $\theta \in R^m$ the parameters of the model. The function f might be linear or nonlinear with respect to the input Z^{t-kT}, and its parameters are learnt on a training set Z by (regularized) least squares implemented recursively or in a batch way (i.e., $\hat{\theta} = \mathrm{argmin}_{\theta \in R^m} E(\theta)$, where $E(\theta)$ is the error function). In general, the formulation of the input, the class of the model, and the parameter estimation method, along with the quality of the observed data, determine the generalization error of a glucose-predictive model.

Well-established representations of $\hat{y}(t|\theta) = f(Z^{t-kT}, \theta)$ from linear-system theory have been applied to glucose predictive modeling by assuming that the underlying system of glucose is linear and time invariant. The premise that near-future blood-glucose concentrations can be predicted by exploiting the recent history of CGM profile was initially suggested by Bremer and Gough [55]. The significant short-term statistical interdependence in blood-glucose dynamics, as was identified by the sample autocorrelation function (ACF) of frequently sampled (every 10 min) blood-glucose data of type 1 patients monitored over 2 days under ambulatory conditions, led to the successful identification of time-invariant linear autoregressive (AR) models of varying order. However, the error of k-step-ahead predictions ($k > 1$) was comparable to the error that would be incurred by assigning the mean value of past measurements as the estimate of future measurements. AR and AR moving average (ARMA) models of the CGM time series with constant parameters [56−59] were subsequently found to have sufficiently accurate, short-term (up to 30 min) predictive capacity. In Ref. [56], smoothing of raw stationary CGM glucose data using Tikhonov regularization and deriving AR models of order 30 through regularized least squares resulted in physiologically plausible AR coefficients, reflecting the temporal behaviour of the ACF of the glucose signal, and stable accurate 30-min-ahead predictions of the subcutaneous glucose concentration with negligible root-mean-squared errors and time lags. In a subsequent study [60], Gani et al. proved the feasibility of a universal, individual-independent AR predictive model of short-term (30 min or less) glucose concentration after removing high-frequency dynamics in the glucose signal. Using data collected from three different studies, involving subjects with both type 1 and 2 diabetes and employing three different CGM devices, they found that the frequency content in the glucose signals is conserved across different individuals. The latter observation in tandem with the invariance of the AR coefficients to a periodic signal's (as glucose concentration) amplitude and phase and sole dependency on its frequency explains the similarity of the derived AR models. This was also attributed to the regularization imposed on the fitting of the AR model [61].

The efficient development of AR predictive models is directly linked with the proper understanding of the predictive power of the spectrum of the examined signal itself. In an in-depth analysis of the frequency components of the subcutaneous glucose concentration signal, it was found that it retains the four major frequency bands of the blood-glucose signal, as suggested by Rahaghi and Gough [62], despite the time delays and signal attenuation from blood-to-interstitial transport [61]. Subband AR modeling of CGM signals of individuals with type 1 diabetes revealed that (1) the highest frequency band (with periods between 5 and 15 min), which is associated with rapid pulsatile insulin secretion in healthy individuals, has very low energy content and is noninformative with respect to glucose prediction in type 1 diabetes; (2) the power spectral densities estimated by the subband AR models were less resolved than those obtained from the reference glucose signal; however, they captured the frequency information present in the glucose signal sufficiently well; and (3) the frequency band accounting for the intrinsic glycaemic response to food and insulin intake was essential for the accurate prediction of glucose concentration up to 50 min ahead, matching those obtained by the reference model consisting of all three bands.

Because of the intrinsic nonlinearity and nonstationarity of the glucose regulatory system [46], nonlinear dynamical models of glucose prediction in type 1 diabetes have been efficiently applied. Moreover, a model that is able to represent and infer the response of the glucose metabolism to the exogenous inputs (e.g., carbohydrates intake, subcutaneous insulin administration, and exercise) may allow predictions for longer horizons compared with AR models.

A thorough analysis of ambulatory blood-glucose data from one subject [58] demonstrated the need for nonlinear predictive modeling of blood-glucose dynamics. Compartmental modeling of the glucose and insulin fluxes formed the main exogenous inputs to the system. Linear model identification and prediction through ARMA, ARMA with extra inputs (ARMAX) and subspace-based models resulted in highly correlated residuals. The separation of the dynamics in the system by a general transfer function model (GTFM) did reduce the autocorrelation of the residuals but the predictive capacity degraded as prediction horizon increased. To this end, the spectral coherence between the input and the output variables supported the presence of nonlinear dynamics in the glucose system. Among a number of input−output nonlinear transformations, a Wiener model with a Chebychev polynomial nonlinearity extended the GTFM and resulted in a slight improvement in performance. Authors concluded that the accurate modeling and prediction of the glucose concentration is mainly hindered by (1) the existence of unrepresented inputs and unmeasured disturbances that have a significant impact on the glucose concentration and (2) the identifiability issues arising from the almost concurrent and, more importantly, in a specified ratio delivery of insulin and carbohydrates.

The effect of input excitation, concerning subcutaneous insulin boluses and carbohydrate content of meals, on the predictive capability of linear dynamic AR models with extra inputs (ARX), ARMAX, and Box−Jenkins (BJ) models have been investigated by Finan et al. in a simulation study [63]. Quantifying the degree of linear dependence between the input vectors by the condition number of the respective input matrix, they demonstrated that the performance of the ARMAX and BJ models in the case of 1-h ahead predictions is strongly and negatively correlated with the condition number, whereas these correlations are slightly weaker for 2-h ahead predictions. On the other hand, the performance of the ARX models, which is inferior compared with the other two models, is correlated with the condition number to a significantly lesser extent.

Nonlinearity is typically incorporated into the glucose model by black-box parameterizations and, particularly, neural networks and kernel-based regression models, which rely on batch learning algorithms (e.g., back-propagation and quadratic programing). In order to address the nonlinear behaviour of the subcutaneous glucose time series, Pérez-Gandía et al. [64] developed a neural network model based on the CGM values during the preceding 20 min, which, however, showed limited performance. More accurate predictions were achieved by applying a recurrent neural network (RNN) on a wider (200-min) CGM history [65]. The development of predictive models incorporating more comprehensive information is supported by the fact that (i) the auto-correlation function of the subcutaneous glucose measurements vanishes at about 30 min [66] and, (ii) a number of exogenous inputs play a vital role in glucose regulation. More specifically, multivariate nonlinear, with respect to the input, regression techniques of machine learning, such as feed-forward [67–69] and RNNs [70,71], and support vector regression (SVR) [72] were efficiently used for this purpose demonstrating the effect of additional inputs on short- and long-term predictions. The results of these studies are highly dependent on the input which is used, which, in all cases, includes the past continuous measurements of the subcutaneous glucose concentration and quantitative information concerning the carbohydrates intake and/or the exogenous insulin administration. The combination of a RNN with compartmental models of plasma-insulin concentration and carbohydrates absorption was proposed in Refs. [70,71]. Zecchin et al. demonstrated that feed-forward [68] as well as jump neural networks [69] exploiting not only the past CGM data but also meal information allow for improved accuracy when compared to Refs. [64,73] over a 30-min horizon. A more comprehensive feature set has been considered in Ref. [67] which encompassed qualitative descriptors of the lifestyle and the emotional status of the patient. In addition, the inclusion of real physical activity data, recorded continuously throughout the observation days, in glucose predictive models has recently emerged, which is very important considering the prominent effect of exercise on glucose concentration. In Ref. [72], Georga et al. proposed an individualized predictive model relying on SVR of multiple input variables concerning the recent subcutaneous glucose profile, the effect of food and insulin intake, the energy expenditure due to physical activities, and the time of the day (as a predictor of the 24-h variations of glucose). By utilizing different input cases, the effect of each input to the prediction accuracy was quantified, and it was demonstrated that both short-term and mostly long-term (i.e., for 60 and 120 min) predictions become significantly more accurate and safe when all the available information is used.

Although hypoglycaemia is the limiting factor in the glycaemic management of insulin-treated diabetes, there have been only a few studies that went one step further by addressing the problem of hypoglycaemic event prediction. This problem involves the successful prediction of the beginning of the event and, therefore, differs from predicting single hypoglycaemic values [74,75]. On this basis, statistical and time-series methods were evaluated on CGM recordings of patients with type 1 diabetes who underwent an insulin-induced hypoglycaemia test during their admission in clinical research centers and for hypoglycaemic thresholds ranging from 60 to 90 mgdL^{-1} [76−78]. The results obtained are promising with sensitivity reaching 100% and lead times close to the examined prediction horizons (up to 55 min) [78]. With the view to embedding these new models eventually into CGM systems or into diabetes advisory mobile systems, the need to test them under free-living conditions in daily life is evident. The SVR-based model presented in Ref. [72] was extended to predict hypoglycaemic events 30 and 60 min in advance based on real-life data. It was shown that the prediction of nocturnal hypoglycaemic events, which are potentially fatal if untreated, becomes more accurate when HAAF-related inputs are additionally considered [79].

1.3 The Stationarity Hypothesis in Glucose Prediction Problem

The analysis of the short-term subcutaneous glucose dynamics in the frequency domain has verified that a universal or global AR glucose prediction model in type 1 diabetes is feasible in different frequency ranges, which characterize different physiological mechanisms exemplified by the periodicity of their oscillations [60,80]. However, the high inter- and intrapatient variability of glucose dynamics in response to exogenous inputs supports the individualization of the predictive models and their continuous adaptation to both biological (e.g., variations in insulin sensitivity or body mass) and environmental changes (e.g., variations in the level of physical activity) as well. For instance, the slow decaying of the sample ACF of frequently sampled glucose data from subjects with type 1 diabetes under ambulatory conditions over 2 days as well as their nonconstant mean and variance evidenced a nonstationary process, which effect on AR modeling for each patient was ameliorated by taking the first difference of the glucose measurements [55]. The need for capturing the variations in the system dynamics can be partially met by performing a periodic patient-specific reestimation of model parameters. Nevertheless, sequential (or recursive) learning algorithms with the inherent ability to represent the time-varying behaviour of the glucose regulatory system would allow for a better representation of spatial and temporal input−output dependencies.

The feasibility of a recursive in time solution to predict the short-term subcutaneous glucose dynamics in type 2 diabetes has been demonstrated in Refs. [74,81]. In particular, weighted recursive least squares (WRLS) with an adjustable forgetting factor, according to the variation of model parameters, was used to identify both ARMA and ARMAX models of subcutaneous glucose concentration. It was shown that a multivariate ARMAX model including physiological signals related to a subject's physical activity and emotional condition outperforms a univariate model as applied to type 2 patients. Similarly, constrained WRLS with a time-varying forgetting factor provided a stable 30-min-ahead ARMAX prediction model of glucose concentration in patients with type 1 diabetes, which parameters related to the insulin on-board and physical activity conform to physiological constraints [82]. Its incorporation into a generalized predictive insulin controller allowed the accurate prediction of hypoglycaemic events and led to the prevention of postexercise hypoglycaemia [83]. The fusion of real-time adaptive models (RNN and AR) resulted in 100% prediction accuracy of hypoglycaemic events for patients under SAP therapy during everyday living conditions [84,85].

A discrete-time nonlinear dynamic system of glucose in type 1 diabetes which state as well as time-varying coefficients were estimated by an extended Kalman filter (EKF) and, in which the effect of food intake and subcutaneous insulin delivery were modeled through normalized finite impulse response filter functions, was found to outperform a recursively identified ARX having a similar configuration [86]. However, EKF-identified state-space models provide a solution to nonlinear problems that is nonoptimal. In this context, novel nonlinear recursive frameworks to the online identification and prediction of the dynamic glucose system in type 1 diabetes, taking advantage of kernel adaptive filters (KAF), can be evaluated. KAF combine the universal approximation property of neural networks (for universal kernels) with the convexity of least squares problems [87]. More specifically, they are capable of handling nonlinearities by expressing all operations in terms of inner products in the Reproducing Kernel Hilbert Space (RKHS) sparsifying, in parallel, the solution online to confine the structure of the underlying radial basis function network and, consequently, accomplish regularization. Targeting at a real-time AR or multivariate model that can be eventually embedded in a portable computing device, special emphasis should be placed at their time and space complexity in combination with their convergence behavior and generalization capacity.

An alternative approach to the problem of glucose prediction than that of recursive model identification and purely subject-dependent solutions has been proposed by Naumova et al. [88]. They presented a metalearning subject-independent optimization procedure for adjusting the hyperparameters of an iterated Tikhonov regularization learning algorithm (i.e., the regularization parameter and the parameters of the kernel generating the associated RKHS) to each new input. Both 30- and 60-min predictions of that regularized scheme, with input previous, but not necessarily equi-sampled, CGM measurements were significantly better compared to two state-of-the-art glucose prediction methods [57,67]. Zhao et al. utilized the concept of model migration; a base ARX model is first built from a representative subject and, then, proper customization of the parameters concerning only the exogenous inputs (i.e., food and insulin) is performed for a new subject using a small amount of data [89]. Results are reported for in-silico subjects and show that model migration presents better generalization ability than individualized models when training and testing conditions differ.

A complementary procedure to adaptive learning can be considered the individualized evaluation of the short-term predictors of glucose concentration and the subsequent refinement of the model's input [90]. In Ref. [91], Georga et al. proposed feature ranking as a preprocessing step in the construction of patient-specific glucose predictive models prompted by the substantial interpatient deviations in SVR model's hyperparameters. Two feature-evaluation algorithms suitable for regression problems (i.e., random forest and RReliefF) produced rational, robust results revealing not only the global importance of features concerning the subcutaneous glucose profile, time of prediction, and plasma-insulin concentration but also the different role of food intake and physical activity among patients; the generality and effectiveness of which results was demonstrated with respect to the performance of kernel-based regression modeling.

Moving toward a more precise daily care of diabetes, the focus of this book is modeling practices that lead to personalized, adaptive, real-time, predictive data-driven solutions of blood glucose, which are highly accurate as well as computationally efficient.

References

[1] American Diabetes Association. Diagnosis and classification of diabetes mellitus. Diabetes Care 2014;37 (Suppl. 1):S81−90.

[2] American Diabetes Association. Standards of medical care in diabetes—2016 abridged for primary care providers. Clin Diabetes 2016;34(1):3−21.

[3] DCCT. The effect of intensive treatment of diabetes on the development and progression of long-term complications in insulin-dependent diabetes mellitus. The Diabetes Control and Complications Trial Research Group. N Engl J Med 1993;329(14):977−86.

[4] Cryer PE. The barrier of hypoglycemia in diabetes. Diabetes 2008;57(12):3169−76.

[5] Cryer PE, Davis SN, Shamoon H. Hypoglycemia in diabetes. Diabetes Care 2003;26(6):1902−12.

[6] Cryer PE. Exercise-related hypoglycemia-associated autonomic failure in diabetes. Diabetes 2009;58 (9):1951−2.

[7] Soeborg T, et al. Absorption kinetics of insulin after subcutaneous administration. Eur J Pharm Sci 2009;36(1):78−90.

[8] Guerci B, Sauvanet JP. Subcutaneous insulin: pharmacokinetic variability and glycemic variability. Diabetes Metab 2005;31(4 Pt 2). p. 4S7−4S24.

[9] Heinemann L. Variability of insulin absorption and insulin action. Diabetes Technol Ther 2002;4 (5):673−82.

[10] Georga E, et al. Wearable systems and mobile applications for diabetes disease management. Health Technol 2014;4:101−12.

[11] Juvenile Diabetes Research Foundation Continuous Glucose Monitoring Study Group, et al. Continuous glucose monitoring and intensive treatment of type 1 diabetes. N Engl J Med 2008;359(14):1464−76.

[12] Phillip M, et al. Use of continuous glucose monitoring in children and adolescents (*). Pediatr Diabetes 2012;13(3):215−28.

[13] Pickup JC, Freeman SC, Sutton AJ. Glycaemic control in type 1 diabetes during real time continuous glucose monitoring compared with self-monitoring of blood glucose: meta-analysis of randomised controlled trials using individual patient data. BMJ 2011;343. p. d3805.

[14] Keenan DB, Cartaya R, Mastrototaro JJ. Accuracy of a new real-time continuous glucose monitoring algorithm. J Diabetes Sci Technol 2010;4(1):111−18.

[15] McGarraugh G, Bergenstal R. Detection of hypoglycemia with continuous interstitial and traditional blood glucose monitoring using the FreeStyle Navigator Continuous Glucose Monitoring System. Diabetes Technol Ther 2009;11(3):145−50.

[16] Facchinetti A, et al. Real-time improvement of continuous glucose monitoring accuracy: the smart sensor concept. Diabetes Care 2013;36(4):793−800.

[17] Pickup JC, Sutton AJ. Severe hypoglycaemia and glycaemic control in type 1 diabetes: meta-analysis of multiple daily insulin injections compared with continuous subcutaneous insulin infusion. Diabet Med 2008;25(7):765−74.

[18] Yeh HC, et al. Comparative effectiveness and safety of methods of insulin delivery and glucose monitoring for diabetes mellitus: a systematic review and meta-analysis. Ann Intern Med 2012;157(5):336−47.

[19] Norgaard K, et al. Routine sensor-augmented pump therapy in type 1 diabetes: the INTERPRET study. Diabetes Technol Ther 2013;15(4):273−80.

[20] Bergenstal RM, et al. Effectiveness of sensor-augmented insulin-pump therapy in type 1 diabetes. N Engl J Med 2010;363(4):311−20.

[21] Hirsch IB. Reducing hypoglycemia in type 1 diabetes: an incremental step forward. Diabetes Technol Ther 2013;15(7):531−2.

[22] Bergenstal RM, et al. Threshold-based insulin-pump interruption for reduction of hypoglycemia. N Engl J Med 2013;369(3):224−32.

[23] Ly TT, et al. Effect of sensor-augmented insulin pump therapy and automated insulin suspension vs standard insulin pump therapy on hypoglycemia in patients with type 1 diabetes: a randomized clinical trial. JAMA 2013;310(12):1240−7.

[24] Buckingham B, et al. Outpatient safety assessment of an in-home predictive low-glucose suspend system with type 1 diabetes subjects at elevated risk of nocturnal hypoglycemia. Diabetes Technol Ther 2013;15(8):622−7.

[25] Buckingham B, et al. Prevention of nocturnal hypoglycemia using predictive alarm algorithms and insulin pump suspension. Diabetes Care 2010;33(5):1013−17.

[26] Hughes CS, et al. Hypoglycemia prevention via pump attenuation and red-yellow-green "traffic" lights using continuous glucose monitoring and insulin pump data. J Diabetes Sci Technol 2010;4(5):1146−55.

[27] Elleri D, et al. Evaluation of a portable ambulatory prototype for automated overnight closed-loop insulin delivery in young people with type 1 diabetes. Pediatr Diabetes 2012;13(6):449−53.

[28] Kovatchev B, et al. Feasibility of outpatient fully integrated closed-loop control: first studies of wearable artificial pancreas. Diabetes Care 2013;36(7):1851−8.

[29] O'Grady MJ, et al. The use of an automated, portable glucose control system for overnight glucose control in adolescents and young adults with type 1 diabetes. Diabetes Care 2012;35(11):2182−7.

[30] Phillip M, et al. Nocturnal glucose control with an artificial pancreas at a diabetes camp. N Engl J Med 2013;368(9):824−33.

[31] Cobelli C, Renard E, Kovatchev B. Artificial pancreas: past, present, future. Diabetes 2011;60(11):2672−82.

[32] Kovatchev B. Diabetes technology: markers, monitoring, assessment, and control of blood glucose fluctuations in diabetes. Scientifica 2012;2012:14.

[33] Breton M, et al. Fully integrated artificial pancreas in type 1 diabetes: modular closed-loop glucose control maintains near normoglycemia. Diabetes 2012;61(9):2230−7.

[34] Klonoff DC. Continuous glucose monitoring: roadmap for 21st century diabetes therapy. Diabetes Care 2005;28(5):1231−9.

[35] El-Gayar O, et al. Mobile applications for diabetes self-management: status and potential. J Diabetes Sci Technol 2013;7(1):247−62.

[36] Baron J, McBain H, Newman S. The impact of mobile monitoring technologies on glycosylated hemoglobin in diabetes: a systematic review. J Diabetes Sci Technol 2012;6(5):1185−96.

[37] Eng DS, Lee JM. The promise and peril of mobile health applications for diabetes and endocrinology. Pediatr Diabetes 2013;14(4):231−8.

[38] Holtz B, Lauckner C. Diabetes management via mobile phones: a systematic review. Telemed J E Health 2012;18(3):175−84.

[39] Liang X, et al. Effect of mobile phone intervention for diabetes on glycaemic control: a meta-analysis. Diabet Med 2011;28(4):455−63.

[40] Tran J, Tran R, White JR. Smartphone-based glucose monitors and applications in the management of diabetes: an overview of 10 salient "Apps" and a novel smartphone-connected blood glucose monitor. Clin Diabetes 2012;30(4):173−8.

[41] Georga E, et al. Data mining for blood glucose prediction and knowledge discovery in diabetic patients: the METABO diabetes modeling and management system. Conf Proc IEEE Eng Med Biol Soc 2009;2009:5633−6.

[42] Poulsen JU, et al. A diabetes management system empowering patients to reach optimised glucose control: from monitor to advisor. Conf Proc IEEE Eng Med Biol Soc 2010;2010:5270−1.

[43] Zecchin C, et al. Reduction of number and duration of hypoglycemic events by glucose prediction methods: a proof-of-concept in silico study. Diabetes Technol Ther 2013;15(1):66−77.

[44] Dua P, Doyle 3rd FJ, Pistikopoulos EN. Multi-objective blood glucose control for type 1 diabetes. Med Biol Eng Comput 2009;47(3):343−52.

[45] Makroglou A, Li J, Kuang Y. Mathematical models and software tools for the glucose−insulin regulatory system and diabetes: an overview. Appl Numer Math 2006;56(3−4):559−73.

[46] Caumo A, Simeoni M, Cobelli C. Chapter 12—glucose modelling. Modeling methodology for physiology and medicine. San Diego: Academic Press; 2001. p. 337−72.

[47] Dalla Man C, Camilleri M, Cobelli C. A system model of oral glucose absorption: validation on gold standard data. IEEE Trans Biomed Eng 2006;53(12 Pt 1):2472−8.

[48] Dalla Man C, Rizza RA, Cobelli C. Meal simulation model of the glucose−insulin system. IEEE Trans Biomed Eng 2007;54(10):1740−9.

[49] Mitsis GD, Markakis MG, Marmarelis VZ. Nonlinear modeling of the dynamic effects of infused insulin on glucose: comparison of compartmental with Volterra models. IEEE Trans Biomed Eng 2009;56 (10):2347−58.

[50] Robertson G, et al. Blood glucose prediction using artificial neural networks trained with the AIDA diabetes simulator: a proof-of-concept pilot study. JECE 2011;2011. p. 2−2.

[51] Tresp V, Briegel T, Moody J. Neural-network models for the blood glucose metabolism of a diabetic. IEEE Trans Neural Netw 1999;10(5):1204−13.

[52] Liszka-Hackzell JJ. Prediction of blood glucose levels in diabetic patients using a hybrid AI technique. Comput Biomed Res 1999;32(2):132−44.

[53] Kovatchev BP, Shields D, Breton M. Graphical and numerical evaluation of continuous glucose sensing time lag. Diabetes Technol Ther 2009;11(3):139−43.

[54] American Diabetes Association. Professional practice committee for the standards of medical care in diabetes-2016. Diabetes Care 2016;39(Suppl 1):S107−8.

[55] Bremer T, Gough DA. Is blood glucose predictable from previous values? A solicitation for data. Diabetes 1999;48(3):445−51.

[56] Gani A, et al. Predicting subcutaneous glucose concentration in humans: data-driven glucose modeling. IEEE Trans Biomed Eng 2009;56(2):246−54.

[57] Reifman J, et al. Predictive monitoring for improved management of glucose levels. J Diabetes Sci Technol 2007;1(4):478−86.

[58] Stahl F, Johansson R. Diabetes mellitus modeling and short-term prediction based on blood glucose measurements. Math Biosci 2009;217(2):101−17.

[59] Cescon M, Johansson R. Linear modeling and prediction in diabetes physiology. In: Marmarelis V, Mitsis G, editors. Data-driven modeling for diabetes. Springer Berlin Heidelberg; 2014. p. 187–222.

[60] Gani A, et al. Universal glucose models for predicting subcutaneous glucose concentration in humans. IEEE Trans Inf Technol Biomed 2010;14(1):157–65.

[61] Lu Y, et al. The importance of different frequency bands in predicting subcutaneous glucose concentration in type 1 diabetic patients. IEEE Trans Biomed Eng 2010;57(8):1839–46.

[62] Rahaghi FN, Gough DA. Blood glucose dynamics. Diabetes Technol Ther 2008;10(2):81–94.

[63] Finan DA, et al. Effect of input excitation on the quality of empirical dynamic models for type 1 diabetes. AIChE J 2009;55(5):1135–46.

[64] Pérez-Gandía C, et al. Artificial neural network algorithm for online glucose prediction from continuous glucose monitoring. Diabetes Technol Ther 2010;12(1):81–8.

[65] Allam F, et al. A recurrent neural network approach for predicting glucose concentration in type-1 diabetic patients. In: Iliadis L, Jayne C, editors. Engineering applications of neural networks: 12th INNS EANN-SIG international conference, EANN 2011 and 7th IFIP WG 12.5 international conference, AIAI 2011, Corfu, Greece, September 15–18, 2011, Proceedings Part I. Berlin, Heidelberg: Springer Berlin Heidelberg; 2011. . 254–259.

[66] Kovatchev B, Clarke W. Peculiarities of the continuous glucose monitoring data stream and their impact on developing closed-loop control technology. J Diabetes Sci Technol 2008;2(1):158–63.

[67] Pappada SM, et al. Neural network-based real-time prediction of glucose in patients with insulin-dependent diabetes. Diabetes Technol Ther 2011;13(2):135–41.

[68] Zecchin C, et al. Neural network incorporating meal information improves accuracy of short-time prediction of glucose concentration. IEEE Trans Biomed Eng 2012;59(6):1550–60.

[69] Zecchin C, et al. Jump neural network for online short-time prediction of blood glucose from continuous monitoring sensors and meal information. Comput Methods Programs Biomed 2014;113(1):144–52.

[70] Mougiakakou SG, et al. SMARTDIAB: a communication and information technology approach for the intelligent monitoring, management and follow-up of type 1 diabetes patients. IEEE Trans Inf Technol Biomed 2010;14(3):622–33.

[71] Zarkogianni K, et al. An insulin infusion advisory system based on autotuning nonlinear model-predictive control. IEEE Trans Biomed Eng 2011;58(9):2467–77.

[72] Georga E, et al. Multivariate prediction of subcutaneous glucose concentration in type 1 diabetes patients based on support vector regression. IEEE J Biomed Health Inform 2012;17(1):71–81.

[73] Sparacino G, et al. Glucose concentration can be predicted ahead in time from continuous glucose monitoring sensor time-series. IEEE Trans Biomed Eng 2007;54(5):931–7.

[74] Eren-Oruklu M, et al. Adaptive system identification for estimating future glucose concentrations and hypoglycemia alarms. Automatica (Oxford) 2012;48(8):1892–7.

[75] Palerm CC, Bequette BW. Hypoglycemia detection and prediction using continuous glucose monitoring—a study on hypoglycemic clamp data. J Diabetes Sci Technol (Online) 2007;1(5):624–9.

[76] Eren-Oruklu M, Cinar A, Quinn L. Hypoglycemia prediction with subject-specific recursive time-series models. J Diabetes Sci Technol 2010;4(1):25–33.

[77] Cameron F, et al. Statistical hypoglycemia prediction. J Diabetes Sci Technol 2008;2(4):612–21.

[78] Dassau E, et al. Real-time hypoglycemia prediction suite using continuous glucose monitoring: a safety net for the artificial pancreas. Diabetes Care 2010;33(6):1249–54.

[79] Georga EI, et al. A glucose model based on support vector regression for the prediction of hypoglycemic events under free-living conditions. Diabetes Technol Ther 2013;15(8):634–43.

[80] Zhao C, Sun Y, Zhao L. Interindividual glucose dynamics in different frequency bands for online prediction of subcutaneous glucose concentration in type 1 diabetic subjects. AIChE J 2013;59(11):4228–40.

[81] Eren-Oruklu M, et al. Estimation of future glucose concentrations with subject-specific recursive linear models. Diabetes Technol Ther 2009;11(4):243–53.

[82] Turksoy K, et al. Hypoglycemia early alarm systems based on multivariable models. Ind Eng Chem Res 2013;52(35)1–19.

[83] Turksoy K, et al. Multivariable adaptive identification and control for artificial pancreas systems. IEEE Trans Biomed Eng 2014;61(3):883–91.

[84] Daskalaki E, et al. An early warning system for hypoglycemic/hyperglycemic events based on fusion of adaptive prediction models. J Diabetes Sci Technol 2013;7(3):689–98.

[85] Daskalaki E, Diem P, Mougiakakou S. Adaptive algorithms for personalized diabetes treatment. In: Marmarelis V, Mitsis G, editors. Data-driven modeling for diabetes: diagnosis and treatment. Berlin, Heidelberg: Springer Berlin Heidelberg; 2014. p. 91–116.

[86] Wang Q, et al. Personalized state-space modeling of glucose dynamics for type 1 diabetes using continuously monitored glucose, insulin dose, and meal intake: an extended Kalman filter approach. J Diabetes Sci Technol 2014;8(2):331–45.

[87] Liu W, Principe JC, Haykin S. Kernel adaptive filtering: a comprehensive introduction. Wiley Publishing; 2010. p. 209.

[88] Naumova V, Pereverzyev SV, Sivananthan S. A meta-learning approach to the regularized learning-case study: blood glucose prediction. Neural Netw 2012;33:181–93.

[89] Zhao C, Yu C. Rapid model identification for online subcutaneous glucose concentration prediction for new subjects with type I diabetes. IEEE Trans Biomed Eng 2015;62(5):1333–44.

[90] Yamaguchi M, et al. Prediction of blood glucose level of type 1 diabetics using response surface methodology and data mining. Med Biol Eng Comput 2006;44(6):451–7.

[91] Georga EI, et al. Evaluation of short-term predictors of glucose concentration in type 1 diabetes combining feature ranking with regression models. Med Biol Eng Comput 2015;53(12):1305–18.

Pathophysiology and Management of Type 1 Diabetes

2.1 Normal Physiology of Glucose Metabolism

Glucose is an obligate metabolic fuel for the brain, whereas it competes with free fatty acids (FFAs) as a fuel regarding the other tissues. Euglycemia, defined as a plasma-glucose concentration within a relatively narrow range (70-140 mg/dL), is the result of an effective balance between the rates of glucose influx and efflux from the circulation [1,2]. Blood glucose is derived from three sources: (1) the intestinal absorption following the ingestion of a meal, (2) the breakdown of glycogen in liver and muscles (i.e., glycogenolysis), and (3) the formation of glucose in liver and kidney from other noncarbohydrate carbon compounds (i.e., gluconeogenesis). As is shown in Fig. 2.1, the pathways of glucose disposal include glycolysis and direct storage as glycogen; the glucose undergoing glycolysis can be either oxidized or converted to gluconeogenic precursors and the newly formed glucose is either released into plasma or incorporated in hepatic glycogen [3]. The major gluconeogenic precursors include lactate, glycerol, glutamine, and alanine and, additionally, amino acids from proteolysis (i.e., the breakdown of proteins into smaller polypeptides or amino acids) are converted to alanine and glutamine.

2.1.1 Glucoregulatory Factors

Glucose homeostasis is tightly regulated by a number of hormonal, neural, and substrate glucoregulatory factors. The maintenance of the plasma-glucose level within a certain range under various physiologic conditions such as fasting, exercise, and feeding depends on the supply of sufficient amounts of substrates, on the actions of hormones regulating carbohydrate and intermediary metabolism as well as on the function of enzymes regulating the utilization and storage of glucose glycolysis, gluconeogenesis, and glycogen synthesis and breakdown.

More specifically, the key glucoregulatory hormones include:

- Insulin which is secreted from the β-cells of the pancreatic islets and exerts its action through binding to its receptors in insulin-sensitive tissues (e.g., skeletal muscle, adipose tissue, liver). Insulin is the main hormone which lowers the plasma-glucose concentration by (1) suppressing hepatic as well as renal glucose production, (2) promoting glucose uptake by insulin-sensitive tissues, and (3) reducing circulating FFA level. The rate of insulin secretion from the β-cells of the pancreatic islets is itself regulated in response to circulating glucose concentration; it is secreted in increasing amounts as glucose concentration increases above ∼60 mg/dL [4,5]. In the

Personalized Predictive Modeling in Type 1 Diabetes. DOI: http://dx.doi.org/10.1016/B978-0-12-804831-3.00002-3

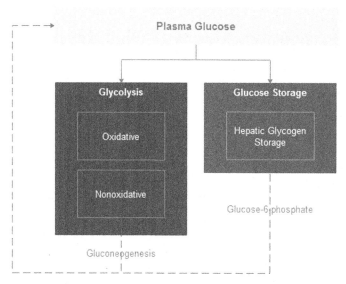

FIGURE 2.1 Metabolic fate of plasma glucose.

postabsorptive state (i.e., the period between meals when all of the last meal has been absorbed), basal insulin secretion ($\sim 5-10\ \mu U/mL$) regulates glucose primarily by inhibiting glucose and FFA release, while tissue glucose uptake is augmented during postprandial conditions ($\sim 40-50\ \mu U/mL$) [1,5].

- Glucagon which is secreted from the α-cells of the pancreatic islets in response to low plasma-glucose levels. Its glucose-raising (counterregulatory) action consists in enhancing hepatic glucose production through hepatic glycogenolysis. The subsequent glucose-induced insulin secretion and insulin's direct effect on the liver suppresses the glycogenolytic response of glucagon.

- Epinephrine which is secreted from the chromaffin cells of the adrenal medulla in response to a low plasma-glucose concentration and its metabolic actions are, mostly, mediated through $\beta2$-adrenergic receptors. It increases hepatic glycogenolysis and, indirectly, hepatic as well as renal gluconeogenesis by increasing gluconeogenic precursors availability and plasma FFAs. In addition, epinephrine reduces glucose uptake in skeletal muscle. The effect of epinephrine on glucose production, similarly to that of glucagon, is temporary; however, epinephrine is a potent hyperglycemic factor due to its sustained effect on glucose uptake.

- Growth hormone and cortisol are glucose counterregulatory hormones, which increase the synthesis of gluconeogenic enzymes and reduce glucose transport. In addition, cortisol can impair insulin secretion. Unlike glucagon and epinephrine, their effect appears after several hours and they act synergistically to regulate plasma glucose concentration.

- Gastrointestinal inhibitory polypeptide (GIP) and glucagon-like peptide-1 (GLP-1) incretin hormones which are effectively stimulated by meal ingestion. Both GIP and

GLP-1 enhance insulin secretion, which explains the greater increase in plasma-insulin levels in response to an oral glucose load compared with an isoglycemic amount of intravenously infused glucose. GLP-1 potentiates insulin secretion according to plasma-glucose concentration, and, also, suppresses postprandial glucagon secretion and gastric emptying, and promotes satiety reducing food intake and body weight.

In addition, elevated plasma levels of FFAs stimulate hepatic and renal gluconeogenesis and inhibit glucose transport into skeletal muscle. The hormones that induce lipolysis, insulin, and plasma-glucose concentration constitute the major regulators of circulating FFAs.

2.1.2 The Postabsorptive State

The mechanisms associated with endogenous glucose production (i.e., glycogenolysis and gluconeogenesis) and glucose disposal into tissues differ between the postabsorptive and the postprandial state. The postabsorptive state can be considered a steady state since the rates of endogenous glucose production and utilization are equal (2.2 mg/kg/min on average) [2,6]. As is portrayed in Fig. 2.2, in the postabsorptive state, ∼50% of endogenous glucose production derives from glycogenolysis and the remainder from gluconeogenesis, with the liver accounting for 80% of total glucose influx [1,7,8]. Moreover, the disposal of glucose occurs primarily via the glycolytic pathway; glucose taken up by tissues is increasingly released back into the circulation in the form of gluconeogenic precursors [1,9]. In particular, insulin-independent glucose utilization in the brain, the splanchnic tissues, the kidney, and the blood cells accounts for approximately 50%, 10%, 10%, and 5%, respectively, of basal glucose uptake, whereas insulin-dependent glucose utilization, primarily in the skeletal muscle and secondarily in the adipose tissue, accounts for the remaining 25% [1]. The amount of glucose entering the circulation due to glycogenolysis diminishes with the duration of fasting, as the hepatic glycogen content is reduced, and gluconeogenesis becomes the

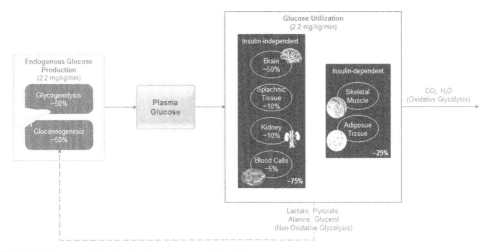

FIGURE 2.2 Glucose metabolism in the postabsorptive state.

predominant or sole source of glucose production. Under prolonged fasting conditions, renal gluconeogenesis is substantially stimulated and the kidney contributes equally to the systemic gluconeogenesis. In addition, the insulin/glucagon ratio decreases, glucose uptake by most tissues is progressively reduced and their energy supply increasingly derives from lipolysis (i.e., the breakdown of triglycerides into FFAs and glycerol), fatty acid oxidation, and ketogenesis (i.e., the breakdown of fatty acids and ketogenic amino acids into ketone bodies). Nevertheless, despite the increase in plasma levels of FFAs, glycerol, and counterregulatory hormones, the rate of gluconeogenesis is limited due to the reduced plasma availability of lactate and amino acids. The rate of glucose utilization temporarily exceeds that of glucose production yielding to a decrease in plasma-glucose concentration, which eventually stabilizes to 55−65 mg/dL [10].

2.1.3 The Postprandial State

In the postprandial state, the increase of plasma glucose concentration and the subsequent increase of insulin secretion from the pancreatic β-cells result in (1) suppression of endogenous glucose production and (2) stimulation of the hepatic and posthepatic glucose disposal; these two processes are key determinants of the assimilation of exogenous glucose and, therefore, postprandial glucose homeostasis. Fig. 2.3 illustrates the time course of plasma concentrations of glucose, insulin, and glucagon following the ingestion of 75 g of glucose in healthy subjects [1]. Plasma-glucose concentration reaches its peak in 30−60 minutes and returns to its postabsorptive levels within 3−4 hours. Plasma-insulin concentration exhibits a similar behavior to that of plasma glucose being three to fourfold higher than its basal levels,

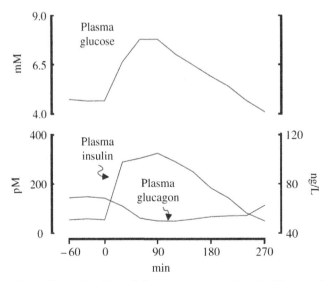

FIGURE 2.3 Changes in plasma glucose, insulin, and glucagon after ingestion of a 75-g oral glucose load in normal volunteers. *Principles of Diabetes Mellitus, Normal Glucose Homeostasis, 2004, 39−56, John E. Gerich, Steven D. Wittlin, Christian Meyer, (©Springer Science + Business Media New York 2004) With permission of Springer.*

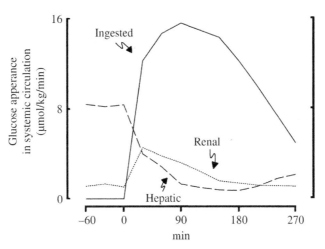

FIGURE 2.4 Changes in rates of entry of glucose into the circulation from ingested glucose, liver, and kidney. *Principles of Diabetes Mellitus, Normal Glucose Homeostasis, 2004, 39–56, John E. Gerich, Steven D. Wittlin, Christian Meyer, (©Springer Science + Business Media New York 2004) With permission of Springer.*

whereas plasma-glucagon concentration is suppressed by ∼50%. Correspondingly, as is shown in Fig. 2.4, the rate of glucose appearance into the systemic circulation reaches its peak in 60–80 minutes and gradually declines thereafter [1]. During this interval, the hepatic glucose production, unlike renal glucose production, is suppressed by 80%. In particular, the rate of glucose appearance into the circulation after the ingestion of a meal depends on (1) the composition of the meal and, mainly, its carbohydrate content, (2) the rate of gastric emptying, (3) the digestion within the lumen of the small intestine, and (4) the rate of absorption into the portal vein [11]. Fig. 2.5 illustrates a summary of the routes and sites of postprandial glucose disposal [3]. In contrast to the postabsorptive state, a smaller proportion of the plasma glucose is disposed of through the glycolytic pathway (∼66% of overall glucose disposal), whereas a significant amount is stored as glycogen through the direct (glucose from the small intestine to liver glycogen) and indirect (from glucose forming lactate in peripheral tissues which is then converted to glucose-6-phosphate and glycogen in the liver) pathway of glycogen deposition.

2.1.4 Glucose Counterregulation

Glucose counterregulation concerns those processes that prevent or rapidly correct hypoglycemia i.e., a plasma-glucose concentration value below 70 mg/dL [6]. Fig. 2.6 depicts the arterialized venous glycemic thresholds for the activation of the main counterregulatory factors in healthy subjects [2]. First, the suppression of endogenous insulin secretion, as glucose concentration declines below 80–85 mg/dL, promotes endogenous glucose production and reduces insulin-stimulated glucose uptake. Second, a further reduction of glucose concentration marginally below the hypoglycemic threshold (65–70 mg/dL) induces the activation of

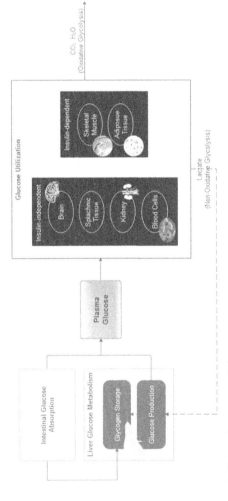

FIGURE 2.5 Glucose metabolism in the postprandial state.

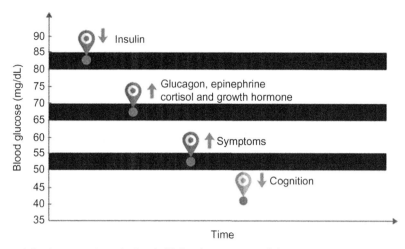

FIGURE 2.6 Arterialized venous glycemic thresholds for the activation of the main counterregulatory mechanisms during decreasing plasma-glucose concentrations in healthy subjects. The red (black in print versions) dots represent discrete blood-glucose measurements.

counterregulatory hormones: (1) glucagon constitutes the primary defense against hypoglycemia, primarily by increasing hepatic glucose production, initially via breakdown of glycogen and later by gluconeogenesis, (2) epinephrine response to hypoglycemia becomes critical in the case of glucagon deficiency, and (3) cortisol and growth hormones, whose counterregulatory effects are delayed, are involved in prolonged hypoglycemia. Lower glucose concentrations, below 50−55 mg/dL, cause neurogenic and neuroglycopenic hypoglycemic symptoms, and ultimately, decrements in cognitive functions at levels below 50 mg/dL.

2.1.5 Classification of Diabetes

Diabetes mellitus is a group of metabolic diseases characterized by hyperglycemia resulting from defects in insulin secretion, insulin action, or both [12]. The chronic hyperglycemia of diabetes is associated with long-term microvascular (diabetic neuropathy, nephropathy, and retinopathy) and macrovascular (coronary artery disease, peripheral arterial disease, and stroke) complications. The vast majority of patients with diabetes fall into two major categories, namely, type 1 and type 2 diabetes. Type 1 diabetes, which accounts for 5%−10% of all patients with diabetes, is characterized by an absolute deficiency of insulin secretion. On the other hand, type 2 diabetes is a more prevalent category (accounting for ∼90%−95% of those with diabetes) and is characterized by a combination of resistance to insulin action and an inadequate compensatory insulin secretory response. Gestational diabetes is defined as diabetes diagnosed in the second or third trimester of pregnancy, that is not clearly either preexisting type 1 or type 2 diabetes, and similar to type 2 diabetes its main underlying pathophysiological abnormality is insulin resistance. Other specific types of diabetes are associated with genetic defects in the pancreatic β-cell function, genetic defects in insulin action, diseases of the exocrine pancreas, endocrinopathies, drug- or chemical-induced diabetes, infections, uncommon forms of immune-mediated disorders, or other genetic syndromes sometimes associated with diabetes.

2.1.5.1 Type 1 Diabetes

Immune-mediated diabetes is caused by a cellular-mediated autoimmune destruction of the β-cells in the pancreatic islets usually leading to an absolute deficiency of insulin secretion [12]. The course of development of autoimmune type 1 diabetes is typically divided into a series of stages, beginning with genetic susceptibility and ending with complete loss of the β-cells of the pancreatic islets (Fig. 2.7) [13]. Autoimmune markers, which are present in 85%–90% of individuals diagnosed with fasting hyperglycemia, include islet cell autoantibodies, autoantibodies to insulin, autoantibodies to glutamic acid decarboxylase (GAD65) and autoantibodies to the tyrosine phosphatases IA-2, IA-2β and ZnT8 [12,14]. This form of diabetes exhibits multiple genetic predispositions; for instance, the expression of two or more autoantibodies in first degree relatives of patients with immune-mediated type 1 diabetes indicates an increased risk (>90%) over the next 10 years [15]. In addition, the disease has strong, either predisposing or protective, human leukocyte antigen (HLA) associations with linkage to the DQA and DQB genes. Immune-mediated diabetes commonly occurs in childhood and adolescence; nevertheless, it can develop at any age. The levels of insulin autoantibodies are strongly correlated with the age of onset, being higher in infants and children (<5 years old). In contrast, adults are mostly positive to GAD65 autoantibodies. The rate of β-cell destruction varies also with age, being typically rapid in infants and children and slow

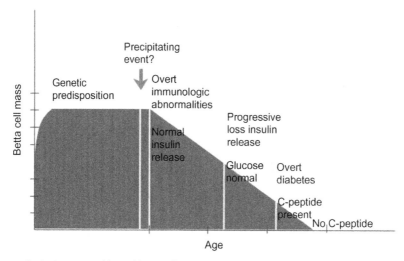

FIGURE 2.7 Hypothetical stages and loss of beta cells in an individual progressing to type 1A diabetes (from Teaching Slides at www.barbaradaviscenter.org). *Reproduced with permission from Eisenbarth, GS. Reprinted from Journal of Allergy and Clinical Immunology, 125 (2 Suppl 2), Aaron W. Michels, George S. Eisenbarth, Immunologic endocrine disorders, S226–S237, © 2010 American Academy of Allergy, Asthma & Immunology. Published by Mosby, Inc. All rights reserved. (2010), with permission from Elsevier.*

in adults, which in turn, coincides with the presence of ketoacidosis as the first manifestation of the disease in younger individuals who develop the disease. C-peptide concentration decreases with the loss of insulin secretory capacity and, therefore, can provide insight into disease progression. We should note that these patients are also prone to other autoimmune disorders such as Graves' disease, Hashimoto's thyroiditis, Addison's disease, vitiligo, celiac disease, autoimmune hepatitis, myasthenia gravis, and pernicious anemia.

Idiopathic type 1 diabetes is characterized by episodic ketoacidosis and varying degrees of insulin deficiency between episodes [14,16]. The specific etiology of this rare form of type 1 diabetes is not known; it is strongly inherited, lacks immunological evidence of β-cell deficiency and is not HLA associated.

2.1.5.2 Type 2 Diabetes

Type 2 diabetes is characterized by a predominant resistance to insulin action and a relative deficiency of insulin secretion [12,14]. Hyperglycemia develops gradually and remains asymptomatic for many years, which hinders the prompt diagnosis of the disease. Plasma-insulin concentration in patients with type 2 diabetes appears normal or elevated; nevertheless, it is insufficient to compensate for insulin resistance and correct hyperglycemia. The insulin secretory deficiency often worsens in the long-run and absolute insulin replacement therapy is needed. In contrast to immune-mediated type 1 diabetes, type 2 diabetes is not caused by immune-mediated destruction of pancreatic β-cells, with its etiology being unidentified. The risk of developing this form of diabetes increases with age and obesity, particularly intraabdominal obesity, and it is more prevalent in women with prior gestational diabetes mellitus and in individuals with hypertension or dyslipidemia. Types 2 diabetes is also associated with a greater genetic predisposition as compared to the autoimmune form of type 1 diabetes, although its genetics are complex and not well defined.

2.1.6 Diagnosis of Diabetes

The diagnosis of diabetes is based on plasma-glucose criteria, either the fasting plasma glucose (FPG) or the 2-hour plasma glucose after a 75-g oral glucose tolerance test (OGTT), or the glycated hemoglobin (HbA1c) criterion [12]. Additionally, a random plasma-glucose concentration value of ≥ 200 mg/dL accompanied with classic hyperglycemic symptoms or a hyperglycemic crisis constitutes a widely used diagnostic criterion for diabetes. The current diagnostic criteria for diabetes are summarized in Table 2.1 [12]. The concordance between FPG and OGTT as well as between HbA1c and either plasma-glucose criterion is imperfect, with the HbA1c designated cut point presenting the lower sensitivity. More specifically, the HbA1c cut point of $\geq 6.5\%$ has been found to identify one-third fewer cases of undiagnosed diabetes than an FPG cut point of ≥ 126 mg/dL, which is partially offset by the HbA1c test's greater applicability (fasting is not required). In addition, HbA1c, as a biomarker of chronic glycemia, exhibits less interday variability and greater preanalytical stability compared with FPG and OGTT. However, age, race/ethnicity, and anemia/hemoglobinopathies should be also taken into consideration when using HbA1c to diagnose diabetes.

Table 2.1 Criteria for the Diagnosis of Diabetes

HbA1C ≥6.5%. The test should be performed in a laboratory using a method that is NGSP certified and standardized to the Diabetes Control and Complications Trial (DCCT) assay[a]

OR

FPG ≥126 mg/dL (7.0 mmol/L). Fasting is defined as no caloric intake for at least 8 h[a]

OR

Two-hour plasma glucose ≥200 mg/dL (11.1 mmol/L) during an OGTT. The test should be performed as described by the World Health Organization, using a glucose load containing the equivalent of 75 g anhydrous glucose dissolved in water[a]

OR

In a patient with classic symptoms of hyperglycemia or hyperglycemic crisis, a random plasma glucose ≥200 mg/dL (11.1 mmol/L)

[a]In the absence of unequivocal hyperglycemia, criteria 1−3 should be confirmed by repeat testing.

Those individuals whose glycemic status does not meet the diagnostic criteria for diabetes but it tends toward hyperglycemia have been referred to as having prediabetes, an intermediate stage associated with an increased risk of diabetes, as well as cardiovascular disease development in the future. Prediabetes is formally defined as impaired fasting glucose (IFG), i.e., 100 mg/dL ≤ FPG ≤ 125 mg/dL, or impaired glucose tolerance (IGT), i.e., 140 mg/dL ≤2-hour plasma glucose during an OGTT ≤199 mg/dL, or an HbA1c range of 5.7%−6.4%. In particular, there is a continuous and curvilinear increase in the risk of diabetes with increasing IFG or IGT or HbA1c. Literature findings suggest that individuals with a low first-phase insulin secretory response (<100 μU/mL), assessed by the intravenous glucose tolerance test, who concurrently express pancreatic autoantibodies are at high risk of developing immune-mediated type 1 diabetes.

2.1.7 Pathophysiology of Hypoglycemia

2.1.7.1 Definition and Classification of Hypoglycemia

The American Diabetes Association and Endocrine Society Workgroup on Hypoglycemia and Diabetes defined iatrogenic hypoglycemia in patients with diabetes as "all episodes of an abnormally low plasma-glucose concentration that expose the individual to potential harm" [17]. A self-monitored plasma or subcutaneous glucose concentration of 70 mg/dL was suggested as a cut-off point at which individuals with diabetes should be concerned about the possibility of developing hypoglycemia. The cut-off point of 70 mg/dL approximates (1) the lower limit of the normal postabsorptive plasma-glucose concentration, (2) the glycemic threshold for activation of glucose counterregulatory systems in nondiabetic individuals, and (3) the upper limit of plasma-glucose level reported to reduce counterregulatory responses to subsequent hypoglycemia [17]. Symptoms of hypoglycemia are either mediated by neuroglycopenia (e.g., cognitive impairment, behavioral changes, confusion, weakness, blurred vision, difficulty speaking, seizure, coma, or, if untreated, death) or the increased release of norepinephrine (e.g., anxiety, palpitation, tremor) or acetylcholine neurotransmitters (e.g.,

Table 2.2 The American Diabetes Association and Endocrine Society Classification of Hypoglycemia on Diabetes

Severe hypoglycemia	An event requiring assistance of another person to actively administer carbohydrates, glucagon, or take other corrective actions. Plasma-glucose concentrations may not be available during an event, but neurological recovery following the return of plasma glucose to normal is considered sufficient evidence that the event was induced by a low plasma-glucose concentration
Documented symptomatic hypoglycemia	An event during which typical symptoms of hypoglycemia are accompanied by a measured plasma-glucose concentration ≤ 70 mg/dL
Asymptomatic hypoglycemia	An event not accompanied by typical symptoms of hypoglycemia but with a measured plasma-glucose concentration ≤ 70 mg/dL
Probable symptomatic hypoglycemia	An event during which symptoms typical of hypoglycemia are not accompanied by a plasma-glucose determination but that was presumably caused by a plasma-glucose concentration ≤ 70 mg/dL
Pseudo-hypoglycemia	An event during which the person with diabetes reports any of the typical symptoms of hypoglycemia with a measured plasma-glucose concentration > 70 mg/dL but approaching that level

sweating, hunger) from the sympathetic nervous system. Nevertheless, the diagnosis of hypoglycemia relies on the concurrent presence of three criteria, called Wripple's triad, which involve (1) low plasma-glucose concentration, (2) symptoms consistent with hypoglycemia, and (3) relief of symptoms when plasma-glucose concentration is raised within the physiological range. Table 2.2 presents the classification of hypoglycemia according to the American Diabetes Association and Endocrine Society Workgroup [17]. Recently, the International Hypoglycaemia Study Group recommended that a glucose threshold < 54 mg/dL should be used to define "clinically significant biochemical hypoglycemia" and should be reported in relevant clinical studies [18].

2.1.7.2 Glucose Counterregulatory Pathophysiology in Diabetes

Hypoglycemia in individuals with type 1 or insulin-deficient type 2 diabetes is the result of therapeutic hyperinsulinemia and attenuated physiological and behavioral response to falling plasma-glucose concentrations [2,19−21]. The former factor is primarily related to patient's actions leading to relative (with respect to the rates of glucose influx and efflux out of the circulation) or absolute excess of circulating insulin (e.g., incorrect insulin dosing, type, or timing), low plasma-glucose availability (e.g., missed meal, overnight fast, exercise, alcohol consumption), while the latter one is inextricably linked to the pathophysiology of diabetes and, more specifically, to the clinical syndromes of defective glucose counterregulation and hypoglycemia unawareness. In type 1 diabetes or insulin-deficient type 2 diabetes, the counterregulatory system fails to prevent or restore hypoglycemia: (1) plasma-insulin concentration, as a function of the clearance of administered insulin, is not necessarily reduced, (2) the primary defense against hypoglycemia, i.e., increase of glucagon secretion, is lacking, and (3) epinephrine response to hypoglycemia is attenuated. The attenuated adrenomedullary epinephrine

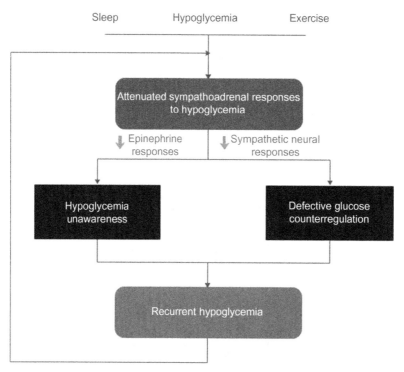

FIGURE 2.8 Schematic diagram of HAAF in type 1 or advanced type 2 diabetes. *Modified from Cryer, P.E., The barrier of hypoglycemia in diabetes. Diabetes, 2008. 57(12): p. 3169—3176.*

response to hypoglycemia on the background of absent insulin and glucagon responses comprises the clinical syndrome of defective glucose counterregulation. On the other hand, an attenuated sympathetic neural response results in hypoglycemia unawareness. According to the concept of Hypoglycemia-Associated Autonomic Failure (HAAF) in diabetes, recent antecedent hypoglycemia as well as prior exercise or sleep further impair the sympathoadrenal (sympathetic neural and adrenomedullary) responses to a potential subsequent hypoglycemia and, therefore, cause a "vicious cycle" of recurrent hypoglycemia [2,22]. More specifically, as is illustrated in Fig. 2.8, recent hypoglycemic events (even asymptomatic ones), exercise and sleep, intensify both defective glucose counterregulation and hypoglycemia unawareness by reducing epinephrine and neurogenic symptom responses, respectively, during subsequent hypoglycemia. To this end, the short-term avoidance of hypoglycemia has been demonstrated to improve glucose counterregulation and hypoglycemia awareness in most patients [19].

2.2 Glucose Monitoring

2.2.1 Self-monitoring of Blood Glucose

Self-monitoring of blood glucose (SMBG) constitutes an integral component of effective diabetes management allowing patients to assess their instant glycemic status and adjust accordingly treatment decisions. Contemporary blood-glucose meters have evolved in terms of accuracy, usability, and functionality rendering SMBG more convenient for end-users. Increased daily frequency of SMBG in type 1 diabetes is associated with better long-term glycemic control and, more specifically, with lower HbA1c levels (−0.2% per additional test per day) and fewer acute complications [23,24]. The American Diabetes Association recommends that most patients on intensive insulin regimen (multiple-dose insulin or insulin pump therapy) should consider SMBG prior to meals and snacks, occasionally postprandially, at bedtime, prior to exercise, when they suspect low blood glucose, after treating low blood glucose until they are normoglycemic, and prior to critical tasks such as driving, which corresponds to 6−10 (or more) measurements daily [14]. The clinical utility of SMBG in patients who use basal insulin or oral agents is less well established and subject to the extent of integration of that information into self-management, and, potentially, clinical management plans. Nevertheless, the temporal resolution of SMBG is not sufficient to describe the daily glucose dynamics, especially during the night when blood glucose is seldom measured [25,26].

2.2.2 Continuous Glucose Monitoring

Minimally invasive CGM technologies rely on a subcutaneously implantable sensor that measures the glucose concentration in the interstitial fluid, which correlates well with the glucose concentration of plasma, at intervals of 1−5 minutes. CGM systems, such as Guardian REAL Time (Medtronic) and FreeStyle Navigator II (Abbot Diabetes Care), inform patients in real-time on their subcutaneous glucose levels, trends and rate of change including customizable predictive alerts for hypo- and hyperglycemic excursions [27−33]. CGM is considered a supplemental tool to SMBG, in particular for those with hypoglycemia unawareness or frequent hypoglycemic episodes. The retrospective evaluation of CGM data by healthcare providers may be of benefit in detecting crucial glycemic patterns (e.g., dawn phenomenon, postprandial hyperglycemia, asymptomatic, and nocturnal hypoglycemia) that are not evident during standard SMBG, and in assessing the effects of modifications in treatment [26]. CGM systems operating in a blinded mode are employed for this purpose (e.g., IPro2 Professional CGM Evaluation by Medtronic).

CGM requires calibration with SMBG, and its accuracy is highly dependent on the calibration algorithm applied for estimating blood glucose from the subcutaneous one as well as on the filtering technique used for enhancing the signal-to-noise ratio [34,35]. The accuracy and reliability of commercially available CGM devices has been evaluated in several clinical trials [36−39]. A comparative effectiveness analysis showed that the FreeStyle Navigator (Abbot Diabetes Care) had the best accuracy as compared to the Seven Plus (DexCom) and the Guardian REAL Time (Medtronic) systems, with the aggregate mean absolute relative difference of all paired reference blood-glucose points being 11.8% ± 11%, 16.5% ± 17.8%, and 20.3% ± 18.0%, respectively [36]. In addition, the percentage of total sensor glucose values, a measure of reliability, was 100% for the Guardian and the Navigator, and 76% for the Seven Plus.

The findings of numerous clinical trials confirm that CGM reduces HbA1c in type 1 diabetes as compared to SMBG; however, they have not shown consistent reductions in severe hypoglycemia [26,30,40]. Equally important, baseline glycemic control and frequency of CGM sensor usage are determinants of its HbA1c-lowering effect on type 1 diabetes for all age groups, while age ($\geq$25 years) correlates with CGM success [30]. A meta-analysis of randomized control trials in adults with type 1 diabetes demonstrated that (1) CGM results in lower HbA1c levels by 0.30% on average as compared to SMBG, (2) every one day increase of sensor usage per week increased the effect of CGM on HbA1c by 0.15%, and (3) every 1% increase in baseline HbA1c increased the effect by 0.126% [40]. On the other hand, there is no evidence of the usefulness of the CGM technology in pediatric and adolescent population with type 1 patients [26]. It has been also demonstrated that CGM can be of considerable benefit to individuals with type 1 diabetes who already have tight control (HbA1c 7.0%−7.5%), especially as regards hypoglycemia occurrence [27,29]. The increased adherence to sensor use and the ongoing education on its proper use are considered of paramount importance in order to realize the full potential of this therapeutic tool. The continuously improved accuracy of CGM effected its approval for making therapeutic decisions in Europe [41,42]. In this direction, standardization of the presentation and analysis of CGM data is considered crucial to optimizing decision making in both clinical and self-monitoring conditions [25,43].

2.2.3 HbA1c Testing

HbA1c is a laboratory test used to screen for diagnose and monitor diabetes. It reflects the average plasma-glucose concentration over the preceding 2−3 months and serves as a biomarker primarily of long-term glycemic control and, secondarily, of treatment adequacy. The strong positive correlation ($r = 0.92$) between HbA1c and average plasma-glucose concentration has led the estimation of the average glucose (eAG) corresponding to each HbA1c value (Table 2.3) [44]. HbA1c is definitely a strong predictor of microvascular and, to a lesser extent, macrovascular complications of the disease [45−47] and, therefore, the American Diabetes Association recommends its routine (at least twice per year in patients who are meeting glycemic goals) testing as part of continuing diabetes care. Current glycemic targets recommended by the American Diabetes Association for nonpregnant adults with diabetes are (1) HbA1c < 7%, (2) preprandial capillary plasma glucose in the range of 80−130 mg/dL, and (3) peak postprandial capillary plasma glucose (measured 1−2 hours after the beginning

Table 2.3 Mean Glucose Levels for Specified HbA1c Levels

HbA1c %	Mean Plasma-Glucose Concentration	
	mg/dL	mmol/L
6	126	7.0
7	154	8.6
8	183	10.2
9	212	11.8
10	240	13.4
11	269	14.9
12	298	16.5

of the meal) less than 180 mg/dL. The recommendations concerning preprandial and post-prandial plasma-glucose levels have been shown to correlate with an HbA1c of <7%. It is acknowledged that each target should not be applied rigidly and must be individualized to the needs of each patient and his or her disease factors [14]. A further reduction of HbA1c cut-off point from 7% to 6% has been demonstrated to be associated with a substantially increased risk of hypoglycemia, which outweighs its potential benefits.

2.3 Insulin Delivery

2.3.1 Insulin Analogs

Recombinant DNA technology allowed the development and production of regular human insulin as well as of analogs to human insulin with desirable pharmacokinetic/pharmacody-namic properties [15,48]. Available insulin preparations differ in the time to onset of action, time of peak action and duration of action, and are classified according to their pharmacodynamics as rapid-acting, short-acting, intermediate-acting, and long-acting insulins. Table 2.4 presents the pharmacodynamic characteristic of currently available insulins; however, these can vary considerably among individuals [49]. The gradual dissociation (30−60 minutes) of regular insulin hexamers into dimers and monomers, which are the forms of insulin which are absorbed into the bloodstream, determines its onset time and time course of insulin action. Rapid-acting insulin analogs (e.g., Lispro, Aspart, Glulisine) result from changes in the amino acid sequence of human insulin, which leads to a more rapid dissociation rate of the hexamer into dimeric and monomeric forms in comparison with regular insulin when injected into the subcutaneous tissue. This, in turn, leads to a more rapid onset of 15−30 minutes, a peak in 30−90 minutes and a shorter duration of action of 4−6 hours. The addition of either excess

Table 2.4 Pharmacodynamics of Currently Available Insulin Preparations

Insulin Preparation	Onset of Action (h)	Peak Action (h)	Effective Duration of Action (h)	Maximum Duration (h)
Rapid-Acting Analogues				
Insulin lispo	0.25−0.5	0.5−1.5	3−4	4−6
Insulin aspart	0.25−0.5	0.5−1.25	3−4	4−6
Insulin glulisine	0.25−0.5	0.5−1.25	3−4	4−6
Short-Acting				
Regular	0.5−1	2−3	3−6	6−8
Intermediate-Acting Analogues				
NPH	2−4	6−10	10−16	14−16
Long-Acting Analogues				
Insulin glargine	0.5−1.5	8−16	18−20	20−24
Insulin detemir	0.5−1.5	6−8	14	~20
Insulin degludec	0.5−1.5	None	24	40

zinc or the protein protamine (e.g., Neutral Protamine Hagedorn—NPH) into regular insulin or rapidly acting insulin formulations reduces the absorption rate from the subcutaneous tissue into the bloodstream and, therefore, prolongs their action curves. NPH insulin exhibits an intermediate-acting profile with an onset of action of 2−4 hours, peak action from 6 to 10 hours and duration of action up to 16 hours. Glargine insulin is a long-acting insulin which has no pronounced peak and which does provide 24-hour of basal insulin supply. To mention that higher doses, particularly of regular or NPH insulin, prolong the duration of action.

The absorption of subcutaneously injected insulin into the bloodstream shows substantial intrapatient and interpatient variability, with the time for 50% of insulin to disappear from the injection site T50% varying approximately by 25% within the same individual and up to 50% among individuals [48,49]. Of note, the pharmacokinetic profile of rapid-acting insulin analogs, insulin glargine and insulin detemir is more reproducible. The variability of the rate of insulin absorption is explained by the following factors, with most of them being associated with the blood flow differences at the site of injection [48,49]:

1. Site of injection: Abdominal injection results in the fastest absorption, arm injection results in a faster absorption than thigh or hip injection.
2. Insulin concentration: Smaller concentrations result in a faster absorption.
3. Exercise: Exercising the injection area within 1 hour of injection increases the rate of insulin absorption.
4. Heat application or local massage: Heating as well as massaging of the injection site increases the rate of insulin absorption.

2.3.2 Principles of Intensive Insulin Therapy

The degree of hyperglycemia in diabetes, which depends on the severity of the underlying pathogenic processes, determines the need for insulin replacement therapy as well as the intensity of the therapy. Individuals with type 1 diabetes require exogenous insulin administration for survival at a rate of 0.5−1.0 U/kg of body weight per day. Intensive insulin therapy, defined as multiple-dose insulin injections (MDI) (three to four injections per day) or CSII, aims to replicate the pattern of physiologic insulin secretion and achieve desired glycemic goals [14]. In particular, a basal-bolus injection regimen is the commonest approach to MDI therapy in type 1 diabetes; long-acting insulin is used to cover basal insulin needs, and rapid- or short-acting insulin before each meal is used to control postprandial glucose excursions or correct hyperglycemia during the day. The American Diabetes Association recommends that patients match the timing and dose of prandial (bolus) insulin to the premeal blood-glucose concentration, carbohydrate intake, and anticipated activity.

CSII therapy relies on an insulin pump that is designed to supply a continuous flow of rapid-acting insulin which is infused subcutaneously at a customizable rate, allowing, in parallel, the on-demand administration of supplementary bolus doses (i.e., prandially, hyperglycemia) [49]. The insulin pump consists of (1) a wearable device holding the insulin reservoir and the interface for programming the insulin, (2) an infusion set that includes a thin tube that delivers insulin from the reservoir to the infusion site and a cannula inserted subcutaneously to deliver insulin, and (3) an infusion set insertion device. Moreover, available insulin pumps offer additional functionality (e.g., bolus calculator, insulin-on-board calculator, reminders on bolus insulin, direct connection with blood-glucose meter, personal therapy management software) that facilitates the administration of insulin therapy. In view of ambulatory use, insulin pumps have already improved a lot in terms of safety and miniaturization. A key safety issue of CSII is the risk of insulin under-delivery due to the gradually altered absorption of insulin at the subcutaneous delivery site.

Despite improvements in insulin analogues after the Diabetes Control and Complications Trial (DCCT) [45], hypoglycemia remains the main side effect of intensive insulin therapy. The advantages of insulin pump therapy over MDI therapy include greater flexibility and more precise administration [50,51]. A systematic meta-analysis concluded that there are minimal differences in HbA1c and frequency of severe hypoglycemia between the two forms of intensive insulin therapy in type 1 adults and children [50,51]. On the other hand, sensor-augmented pump (SAP) therapy with the threshold-based or predictive low-glucose insulin suspend feature has been shown to reduce the incidence and duration of hypoglycaemia in patients with type 1 diabetes, when compared with MDI therapy or the individual components alone [52–60].

2.3.3 Artificial Pancreas Approaches

A closed-loop artificial pancreas should ideally provide 24-hour automatic control of insulin delivery with the aim of achieving tight glucose control and minimizing the risk of hypoglycemia. The realization of this idea is predictably gradual starting from overnight closed-loop insulin delivery. Closed-loop systems of glucose control in type 1 diabetes consist of a CGM sensor, an insulin pump and a control algorithm of insulin infusion rate primarily driven by recent CGM measurements [61,62], with proper integration of those components being of paramount importance toward ambulatory use. To this end, the advances in smartphone technology have enabled the realization of an automated, portable closed-loop artificial pancreas. The superiority of overnight closed-loop delivery of insulin in children and adults with type 1 diabetes over conventional insulin pump therapy has been demonstrated in clinical settings [63–69]; moreover, the safety and efficacy of such a system in settings outside the hospital i.e., at a diabetes camp has been shown [58]. Current multicenter, long-term, large-scale trials examine the safety and efficacy of 24 hours closed-loop control for children, adolescents, and adults under free-living conditions [56,70–75]. The primary challenge is the control algorithm whose functionality should replicate that of a physiologic pancreas and which is currently implemented either with proportional–integral–derivative control or model predictive control [61,62]. The individual components of closed-loop insulin control will be covered in-depth in Chapter 9, Existing and Potential Applications of Glucose Prediction Models.

References

[1] Shrayyef MZ, Gerich JE. Normal glucose homeostasis. In: Poretsky L, editor. Principles of diabetes mellitus. Boston, MA: Springer US; 2010. p. 19−35.

[2] Cryer PE. Chapter 34—Hypoglycemia A2—Melmed, Shlomo. In: Polonsky KS, Larsen PR, Kronenberg HM, editors. Williams textbook of endocrinology. 13th ed. Philadelphia: Content Repository Only!; 2016. p. 1582−607.

[3] Woerle HJ, et al. Pathways for glucose disposal after meal ingestion in humans. Am J Physiol Endocrinol Metab 2003;284(4):E716−25.

[4] Aronoff SL, et al. Glucose metabolism and regulation: beyond insulin and glucagon. Diabetes Spectrum 2004;17(3):183−90.

[5] Gerich JE. Control of glycaemia. Baillieres Clin Endocrinol Metab 1993;7(3):551−86.

[6] Cryer PE. The prevention and correction of hypoglycemia. Comprehensive physiology. John Wiley & Sons, Inc; 2010.

[7] Landau BR, et al. Contributions of gluconeogenesis to glucose production in the fasted state. J Clin Invest 1996;98(2):378−85.

[8] Stumvoll M, et al. Renal glucose production and utilization: new aspects in humans. Diabetologia 1997;40(7):749−57.

[9] Perriello G, et al. Estimation of glucose−alanine−lactate−glutamine cycles in postabsorptive humans: role of skeletal muscle. Am J Physiol 1995;269(3 Pt 1):E443−50.

[10] Ekberg K, et al. Contributions by kidney and liver to glucose production in the postabsorptive state and after 60 h of fasting. Diabetes 1999;48(2):292−8.

[11] Dinneen S, Gerich J, Rizza R. Carbohydrate metabolism in non-insulin-dependent diabetes mellitus. N Engl J Med 1992;327(10):707−13.

[12] American Diabetes, A. Diagnosis and classification of diabetes mellitus. Diabetes Care 2014;37(Suppl 1): S81−90.

[13] Michels AW, Eisenbarth GS. Immunologic endocrine disorders. J Allergy Clin Immunol 2010;125 (2Suppl 2):S226−37.

[14] American Diabetes, A. Standards of medical care in diabetes—2016 abridged for primary care providers. ClinDiabetes 2016;34(1):3−21.

[15] Atkinson MA. Chapter 32—Type 1 diabetes mellitus A2—Melmed, Shlomo. In: Polonsky KS, Larsen PR, Kronenberg HM, editors. Williams textbook of endocrinology. 13th ed. Philadelphia: Content Repository Only! 2016. p. 1451−83.

[16] Association AD. Diagnosis and classification of diabetes mellitus. Diabetes Care 2014;37(Supplement 1): S81−90.

[17] Seaquist ER, et al. Hypoglycemia and diabetes: a report of a workgroup of the American Diabetes Association and the Endocrine Society. J Clin Endocrinol Metab 2013;98(5):1845−59.

[18] *Glucose concentrations of less than 3.0 mmol/l (54 mg/dl) should be reported in clinical trials: a joint position statement of the american diabetes association and the european association for the study of diabetes.* Diabetes Care, 2017. 40(1): p. 155-157.

[19] Cryer PE. The barrier of hypoglycemia in diabetes. Diabetes 2008;57(12):3169−76.

[20] Cryer PE, Davis SN, Shamoon H. Hypoglycemia in diabetes. Diabetes Care 2003;26(6):1902−12.

[21] Cryer P. Hypoglycemia during therapy of diabetes. In: De Groot LJ, et al., editors. Endotext. MA: South Dartmouth; 2000.

[22] Cryer PE. Exercise-related hypoglycemia-associated autonomic failure in diabetes. Diabetes 2009;58 (9):1951−2.

[23] Miller KM, et al. Evidence of a strong association between frequency of self-monitoring of blood glucose and hemoglobin A1c levels in T1D exchange clinic registry participants. Diabetes Care 2013;36 (7):2009−14.

[24] Ziegler R, et al. Frequency of SMBG correlates with HbA1c and acute complications in children and adolescents with type 1 diabetes. Pediatr Diabetes 2011;12(1):11−17.

[25] Bergenstal RM, et al. Recommendations for standardizing glucose reporting and analysis to optimize clinical decision making in diabetes: the Ambulatory Glucose Profile (AGP). Diabetes Technol Ther 2013;15(3):198−211.

[26] Phillip M, et al. Use of continuous glucose monitoring in children and adolescents (*). Pediatr Diabetes 2012;13(3):215−28.

[27] Battelino T, et al. Effect of continuous glucose monitoring on hypoglycemia in type 1 diabetes. Diabetes Care 2011;34(4):795−800.

[28] Garg S, et al. Improvement in glycemic excursions with a transcutaneous, real-time continuous glucose sensor: a randomized controlled trial. Diabetes Care 2006;29(1):44−50.

[29] Juvenile Diabetes Research Foundation Continuous Glucose Monitoring Study, G., et al. The effect of continuous glucose monitoring in well-controlled type 1 diabetes. Diabetes Care 2009;32(8):1378−83.

[30] Juvenile Diabetes Research Foundation Continuous Glucose Monitoring Study, G., et al. Continuous glucose monitoring and intensive treatment of type 1 diabetes. N Engl J Med 2008;359(14):1464−76.

[31] Vigersky RA, et al. Short- and long-term effects of real-time continuous glucose monitoring in patients with type 2 diabetes. Diabetes Care 2012;35(1):32−8.

[32] Keenan DB, Cartaya R, Mastrototaro JJ. Accuracy of a new real-time continuous glucose monitoring algorithm. J Diabetes Sci Technol 2010;4(1):111−18.

[33] McGarraugh G, Bergenstal R. Detection of hypoglycemia with continuous interstitial and traditional blood glucose monitoring using the FreeStyle Navigator Continuous Glucose Monitoring System. Diabetes Technol Ther 2009;11(3):145−50.

[34] Rossetti P, et al. Estimating plasma glucose from interstitial glucose: the issue of calibration algorithms in commercial continuous glucose monitoring devices. Sensors (Basel) 2010;10(12):10936−52.

[35] Sparacino G, Facchinetti A, Cobelli C. "Smart" continuous glucose monitoring sensors: on-line signal processing issues. Sensors 2010;10(7):6751−72.

[36] Damiano ER, et al. A comparative effectiveness analysis of three continuous glucose monitors. Diabetes Care 2013;36(2):251−9.

[37] Freckmann G, et al. Performance evaluation of three continuous glucose monitoring systems: comparison of six sensors per subject in parallel. J Diabetes Sci Technol 2013;7(4):842−53.

[38] Garg SK, et al. Comparison of accuracy and safety of the SEVEN and the Navigator continuous glucose monitoring systems. Diabetes Technol Ther 2009;11(2):65−72.

[39] Kovatchev B, et al. Comparison of the numerical and clinical accuracy of four continuous glucose monitors. Diabetes Care 2008;31(6):1160−4.

[40] Pickup JC, Freeman SC, Sutton AJ. Glycaemic control in type 1 diabetes during real time continuous glucose monitoring compared with self monitoring of blood glucose: meta-analysis of randomised controlled trials using individual patient data. BMJ 2011;343:d3805.

[41] Rodbard D. Continuous glucose monitoring: a review of successes, challenges, and opportunities. Diabetes Technol Ther 2016;18(Suppl. 2):S3−13.

[42] Facchinetti A. *Continuous glucose monitoring sensors: past, present and future algorithmic challenges*. Sensors (Basel) 2016;16:12.

[43] Fonseca VA, et al. *Continuous glucose monitoring: a consensus conference of the american association of clinical endocrinologists and american college of endocrinology*. Endocrine Practice 2016;22(8):1008−21.

[44] Nathan DM, et al. Translating the A1C assay into estimated average glucose values. Diabetes Care 2008;31(8):1473–8.

[45] DCCT. The effect of intensive treatment of diabetes on the development and progression of long-term complications in insulin-dependent diabetes mellitus. The Diabetes Control and Complications Trial Research Group. N Engl J Med 1993;329(14):977–86.

[46] UK Prospective Diabetes Study (UKPDS) Group. Effect of intensive blood-glucose control with metformin on complications in overweight patients with type 2 diabetes (UKPDS 34). Lancet 1998;352 (9131):854–65.

[47] Skyler JS, et al. Intensive glycemic control and the prevention of cardiovascular events: implications of the ACCORD, ADVANCE, and VA diabetes trials: a position statement of the American Diabetes Association and a scientific statement of the American College of Cardiology Foundation and the American Heart Association. Diabetes Care 2009;32(1):187–92.

[48] Donner T. Insulin-pharmacology, therapeutic regimens and principles of intensive insulin therapy. In: De Groot LJ, et al., editors. Endotext. MA: South Dartmouth; 2000.

[49] Hirsch IB, Skyler JS. The management of type 1 diabetes. In: De Groot LJ, et al., editors. Endotext. MA: South Dartmouth; 2000.

[50] Pickup JC, Sutton AJ. Severe hypoglycaemia and glycaemic control in type 1 diabetes: meta-analysis of multiple daily insulin injections compared with continuous subcutaneous insulin infusion. Diabet Med 2008;25(7):765–74.

[51] Yeh HC, et al. Comparative effectiveness and safety of methods of insulin delivery and glucose monitoring for diabetes mellitus: a systematic review and meta-analysis. Ann Intern Med 2012;157(5):336–47.

[52] Bergenstal RM, et al. Threshold-based insulin-pump interruption for reduction of hypoglycemia. N Engl J Med 2013;369(3):224–32.

[53] Ly TT, et al. Effect of sensor-augmented insulin pump therapy and automated insulin suspension vs standard insulin pump therapy on hypoglycemia in patients with type 1 diabetes: a randomized clinical trial. JAMA 2013;310(12):1240–7.

[54] Norgaard K, et al. Routine sensor-augmented pump therapy in type 1 diabetes: the INTERPRET study. Diabetes Technol Ther 2013;15(4):273–80.

[55] Bergenstal RM, et al. Effectiveness of sensor-augmented insulin-pump therapy in type 1 diabetes. N Engl J Med 2010;363(4):311–20.

[56] Thabit H, Hovorka R. Coming of age: the artificial pancreas for type 1 diabetes. Diabetologia 2016;59 (9):1795–805.

[57] Bequette BW. Hypoglycemia prevention using low glucose suspend systems. In: Marmarelis V, Mitsis G, editors. Data-driven modeling for diabetes: diagnosis and treatment. Berlin, Heidelberg: Springer Berlin Heidelberg; 2014. p. 73–89.

[58] Howsmon D, Bequette BW. Hypo- and hyperglycemic alarms: devices and algorithms. J Diabetes Sci Technol 2015;9(5):1126–37.

[59] Kropff J, DeVries JH. Continuous glucose monitoring, future products, and update on worldwide artificial pancreas projects. Diabetes Technol Ther 2016;18(Suppl. 2):S253–63.

[60] Buckingham BA, et al. Predictive low-glucose insulin suspension reduces duration of nocturnal hypoglycemia in children without increasing ketosis. Diabetes Care 2015;38(7):1197–204.

[61] Cobelli C, Renard E, Kovatchev B. Artificial pancreas: past, present, future. Diabetes 2011;60 (11):2672–82.

[62] Kovatchev B. Diabetes technology: markers, monitoring, assessment, and control of blood glucose fluctuations in diabetes. Scientifica 2012;2012:14.

[63] Atlas E, et al. MD-logic artificial pancreas system: a pilot study in adults with type 1 diabetes. Diabetes Care 2010;33(5):1072−6.

[64] Breton M, et al. Fully integrated artificial pancreas in type 1 diabetes: modular closed-loop glucose control maintains near normoglycemia. Diabetes 2012;61(9):2230−7.

[65] Hovorka R, et al. Manual closed-loop insulin delivery in children and adolescents with type 1 diabetes: a phase 2 randomised crossover trial. Lancet 2010;375(9716):743−51.

[66] Hovorka R, et al. Overnight closed loop insulin delivery (artificial pancreas) in adults with type 1 diabetes: crossover randomised controlled studies. BMJ 2011;342:d1855.

[67] Kovatchev B, et al. Multinational study of subcutaneous model-predictive closed-loop control in type 1 diabetes mellitus: summary of the results. J Diabetes Sci Technol 2010;4(6):1374−81.

[68] Weinzimer SA, et al. Fully automated closed-loop insulin delivery versus semiautomated hybrid control in pediatric patients with type 1 diabetes using an artificial pancreas. Diabetes Care 2008;31(5):934−9.

[69] Phillip M, et al. Nocturnal glucose control with an artificial pancreas at a diabetes camp. N Engl J Med 2013;368(9):824−33.

[70] Nimri R, et al. Closing the loop. Diabetes Technol Ther 2017;19(S1). p. S27-s41.

[71] Rodbard D. Continuous glucose monitoring: a review of recent studies demonstrating improved glycemic outcomes. Diabetes Technol Ther 2017;19(S3). p. S25-s37.

[72] Bally L, Thabit H, Hovorka R. Closed-loop for type 1 diabetes − an introduction and appraisal for the generalist. BMC Med 2017;15:14.

[73] Christiansen SC, et al. A review of the current challenges associated with the development of an artificial pancreas by a double subcutaneous approach. Diabetes Ther 2017;8(3):489−506.

[74] Weisman A, et al. Effect of artificial pancreas systems on glycaemic control in patients with type 1 diabetes: a systematic review and meta-analysis of outpatient randomised controlled trials. Lancet Diabetes Endocrinol 2017;5(7):501−12.

[75] Bergenstal RM, et al. Safety of a hybrid closed-loop insulin delivery system in patients with type 1 diabetes. JAMA 2016;316(13):1407−8.

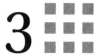
Methodology for Developing a Glucose Prediction Model

3.1 Experimental Design and Data Collection

A sufficiently informative dataset about the system to be modeled is required prior to any decision about the data driven prediction method. The observed data along with any prior information for the properties or the behavior of the examined system form the base for obtaining an accurate approximation of it.

The collection of data should be performed within the framework of experimental or well-designed observational clinical studies which are able to derive high-quality information. According to evidence-based medicine, these study designs have a high potential to evidence cause and effect (causal) relationships and identify associations between the observed quantities [1]. The differentiating characteristic between experimental and observational studies is that the former are specifically tailored to evaluate the impact of a type of intervention on biomedical or health-related outcomes; whereas, in the latter, no intervention is carried out by the investigator. The foremost experimental design in clinical research is the randomized controlled clinical trial, in which the initial sample of participants is randomly assigned to two groups, i.e., the intervention and the control (usual care) group which are followed in parallel, and a rigorous comparison of the intervention efficacy in the two groups is analyzed [2].

Observational studies are classified as cohort, case-control and cross-sectional studies [3]. In cohort studies, a group of patients with defined characteristics or a common exposure (variables of interest), but who do not have the outcome of interest, are followed over time to determine whether they develop the outcome of interest. Cohorts allow the calculation of relative risks for each variable and may distinguish causes from effects since they establish the temporal sequence of events. Of note, cohort studies can identify multiple groups according to the extent of exposure and can be implemented prospectively or retrospectively. In case-control studies, people with the outcome of interest are retrospectively compared with a control group (people without the outcome) and the relative risk for each predictor variable is approximated by odds ratios. Finally, in cross-sectional studies, a group of subjects is assessed at one point in time to determine whether they were exposed to a relevant factor and whether they have the outcome of interest. In opposite to other observational studies where reference to either exposure and/or outcome is explicitly made, in cross-sectional studies, some of the subjects will not have been exposed nor have the outcome of interest. Existing recommendations for reporting of clinical trials and observational studies facilitate their complete and transparent reporting and aid their critical appraisal and interpretation [4—7].

Personalized Predictive Modeling in Type 1 Diabetes. DOI: http://dx.doi.org/10.1016/B978-0-12-804831-3.00003-0

Glucose predictive models can be constructed on the basis of real-life or experimental data. The collection of real-life data is designed as an observational study where a group of patients is monitored/observed over a period of time (2−4 weeks) in real-life conditions [8,9]. On the other hand, the collection of experimental data is performed in a controlled environment (e.g., clinical center, camp) under strict clinical supervision [4,10−14]. In any case, the study should resemble the situation under which the prediction model is to be used. In addition, the generalizability (applicability) of the model largely depends on the source of the sample and the eligibility criteria used to select the participants of the study. To mention that the eligibility criteria are typically defined according to the following variables: (1) gender, (2) age, (3) diabetes type following American Diabetes Association criteria, (4) body mass index, (5) glycated hemoglobin, (6) absence of significant micro- and macro-vascular complications, (7) absence of a severe, chronic concomitant diseases that are invalidating or life-threatening, and (8) high level of compliance with investigator's instructions (as judged by the investigators).

The choice of predictor variables (input variables) and their manipulation during the study has a substantial influence on the observed glucose concentration (output variable). The most significant data types considered for analysis as well as the details of respective indicative methods of measurement are given below:

1. Capillary glucose data: They are assessed using a glucometer. The patient usually performs a measurement of capillary glucose values before and 2 hours after every meal (breakfast, lunch, and dinner), before sleep as well as in case of symptoms/signs compatible with hypoglycemia or hyperglycemia. All capillary glucose measurements are recorded by the patient using a specially designed diary and are reported annotating information such as: (1) time, (2) glucose values, (3) consequent insulin dose information, if appropriate, (4) previous and subsequent event (meal, exercise, sleep), if appropriate.

2. Continuous glucose monitoring (CGM): Measurement of interstitial glucose values in a continuous way is performed using a CGM system (CGMS) e.g., Medtronic iPro2. The information recorded by the CGMS is downloaded with the frequency required using proprietary software applications.

3. Food intake data: Patients are provided with a diary and are asked to record all eaten items during the study period, including the weight of the food with the highest possible precision. The nutritional content of each meal is postanalyzed by certified dieticians or is automatically computed using approved nutrient analysis software.

4. Insulin intake data: Patients are asked to fill, usually in the same diary used for capillary glucose measurements reporting, the time of insulin injection, the insulin type and units, and the injection site.

5. Physical activity data: The information on the performed physical activity can be collected either from a patient's diary or from a wearable activity monitoring device. The patient is asked to report in the diary a description of the exercise event, the intensity of the exercise on a subjective scale (e.g., mild, moderate, intense, very intense), and the start

and end time of the event. In addition, the patient can wear a monitoring device, e.g., SenseWear Armband, to assess energy expenditure and other relevant parameters related to physical activity including: caloric consumption, metabolic equivalents, resting time, lying time, sleeping time, and derived parameters. Data from the device are collected by the investigator using proprietary software.

6. Hypoglycemic event data: In case of a hypoglycemic event, the patient should record on his/her diary the following information: the time of the measurement (and, therefore, time of the event, which is considered to start together with the first glucose assessment), the glucose value, the need for external assistance which is a feature of severe hypoglycemia and the action taken to counteract the low glucose value.

A dataset obtained from an observational study may reveal associations between the input and the output but, in general, cannot infer causality owing to the high intercorrelation among the input variables as well as the influences of unmeasured variables which are independently associated with both the input and the output (i.e., confounding factors). On the other hand, in the context of an experimental study, the investigator manipulates the input so as to stimulate the glucose system, minimizing, in parallel, the effect of confounding factors. However, models built upon datasets from experimental studies have the potential of low generalizability due to the carefully controlled experimental conditions.

3.2 Predictive Modeling of Glucose Concentration in Type 1 Diabetes

The prediction of the short-term course of glucose concentration in the subcutaneous space constitutes a system identification problem where the ultimate objective is the construction of a mathematical model M of the underlying glucose dynamics based on observed input−output data. As is shown in Fig. 3.1, the output y of the examined system is the

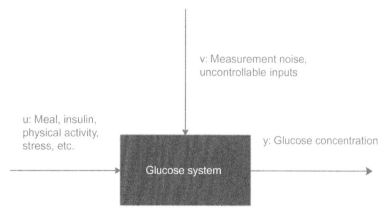

FIGURE 3.1 The system of glucose metabolism where u represents the input to the system, y represents the output of the system and v represents output disturbances.

glucose concentration, the input u to the system comprises measured quantities with a direct or indirect effect on glucose concentration (e.g., information on meals, insulin medication, physical activity, or stress), and v describes unmeasured output disturbances (e.g., measurement noise or other uncontrollable inputs). In the sequel, we will denote the input and the output of the system at time t by $u(t)$ and $y(t)$, respectively.

At the core of system identification lies (1) the learning of the parameters $\theta \in R^m$ of a parameterized model $M(\theta)$ using a particular set of observations Z and (2) the validation of the performance of $M(\theta)$ on other datasets through suitable measures of goodness of fit. In this context, the model $M(\theta)$ is used to provide k-step-ahead predictions of $y(t)$, which is denoted by $\hat{y}(t|\theta)$ to express the dependency on θ, and its general structure is given by

$$\hat{y}(t|\theta) = f(Z^{t-kT}, \theta), \tag{3.1}$$

where T is the sampling interval of glucose concentration and Z^{t-kT} comprises previous input−output data up to time $t - kT$. The function $\hat{y}(t|\theta) = f(Z^{t-kT}, \theta)$ might be linear or nonlinear with respect to Z^{t-kT}. Well-established representations of $\hat{y}(t|\theta) = f(Z^{t-kT}, \theta)$ from linear systems theory can be employed by assuming that the examined system of glucose is linear and time-invariant. Nonlinearity might be incorporated into the model either by exploiting a priori knowledge on the system's properties or by resorting to black-box parameterizations and, particularly, to linear, with respect to θ, regression models.

Let us assume a sequence of input−output samples $Z = \{(x^i, y_i)|i = 1, \ldots, N_Z\}$, where $(x^i, y_i) \in Z = X \times Y$, $X \subseteq R^d$ and $Y \subseteq R$, and a parametric class of functions $F = \{f_\theta : X \rightarrow Y, \; \theta \in R^m\}$. Each sample associates the input vector x^i corresponding to time $t_{i-k} = (i - k)T$ with the observed glucose concentration y_i at time $t_i = iT$, where k is the prediction step and T the sampling interval. Therefore, our objective is to infer a parametric approximation $f : X \rightarrow Y$ of the true mapping based on the given dataset Z to minimize a certain error function $E(\theta)$ [15]. The parameter vector $\theta \in R^m$ minimizing the error function $E(\theta)$ is denoted by

$$\hat{\theta} = \arg\min E(\theta). \tag{3.2}$$

The dataset which is used to estimate θ is called training set and it is denoted by Z_{train}, whereas the dataset on which the generalization ability of the model is assessed is called test set and it is denoted by Z_{test}. As we will see later in this chapter, $E(\theta)$ should account for the error of $M(\theta)$ over Z_{train} (i.e., $e_i = y(t_i) - \hat{y}(t_i|\theta)$ for $i = 1, \ldots, N_{Z_{\text{train}}}$) as well as for the complexity of the model in order to obtain a model which performs well on the test set Z_{test}.

In the following subsections, we will elaborate on (1) the formulation of the input of a glucose predictive model, (2) the basic principles of models of linear systems and linear models for regression, which constitute the basis of the literature on data driven glucose predictive modeling, and (3) the estimation methods for the parameters of the model.

3.2.1 Input Determination

Consider a set of variables $U = \{u_i|i = 1, \ldots, N_U\}$ including the dependent (output) variable (i.e., glucose concentration) and the independent (input) variables. The input $x \in R^d$ of the glucose predictive model is defined with respect to the time for which the prediction is made (i.e., t) and the prediction step k, and it consists of lagged values of each variable u_i in order to model the time delays in glucose regulation process [16]. In particular, the lagged values associated with variable u_i are defined as $\{u_i(t' - n_{u_i} T_{u_i}), \ldots, u_i(t' - T_{u_i}), u_i(t')\}$ and describe its values within the time window $[t' - n_{u_i} T_{u_i}, \ t']$, where $t' = t - kT$ and T_{u_i} denotes the sampling interval of u_i. The value of the parameter n_{u_i}, which physically shows the temporal effect of the input u_i on glucose, can be determined experimentally or based on theoretical results found in literature [17]. Thus, the input of the predictive model includes the following variables:

$$U' = \left\{ \underbrace{u_1\left(t' - n_{u_1} T_{u_1}\right), \ldots, u_1\left(t' - T_{u_1}\right), u_1(t')}_{u_1}, \ldots, \underbrace{u_{N_U}\left(t' - n_{u_{N_U}} T_{u_{N_U}}\right), \ldots, u_{N_U}\left(t' - T_{u_{N_U}}\right), u_{N_U}(t')}_{u_{N_U}} \right\}$$

(3.3)

and the size d of the input equals to

$$d = \sum_{i=1}^{N_U} \left(n_{u_i} + 1\right)$$

(3.4)

Consider that for each different variable we have obtained a time series $(u_i(t_1), \ldots, u_i(t_L))$ consisting of observations of variable u_i made over the time interval $[t_1, t_L]$ and with a sampling period T_{u_i}. The values of sampling periods should be such that they allow the synchronization of the time series. In the typical case, the output y is observed at the sampling instants $t_i = iT$, $i = 1, 2, \ldots$, where $T = 1$ or 5 minutes [3,18]. Accordingly, the input u is sampled concurrently with the output considering that it remains constant for $iT \leq t \leq (i+1)T$. A separate dataset $Z = \{(x^i, y_i)| i = 1, \ldots, N_Z\}$ is constructed for each subject such that each sample $(x^i, y_i) \in Z = X \times Y$, $X \subseteq R^d$, and $Y \subseteq R$, associates the input vector x^i corresponding to time $t_{i-k} = (i - k)T$ with the observed glucose concentration y_i at time $t_i = iT$. We define a one to one correspondence between sets $\{x_j | j = 1, \ldots, d\}$ and $\{u'_j | j = 1, \ldots, d\}$. A new sample is added into Z for each time instant in the glucose time series for which (1) all d variables $\{x_j | j = 1, \ldots, d\}$ can be defined and (2) the value of glucose concentration kT min ahead is available. The size of dataset (i.e., N_Z) depends mainly on the length of the observation period for each subject and, ideally, the time difference between two consecutive samples in Z is equal to the sampling period of the glucose time series, i.e., T. Nevertheless, the existence of gaps in the measured data reduces the value of N_Z. In addition, all samples (x^i, y_i) for which an event (e.g., food intake, insulin intake, intense exercise) exists within the time interval $[t_{i-k}, t_i]$ should be excluded from Z since they do not represent a rational mapping between the configured input and the output.

3.2.2 Models of Linear Systems

A time-invariant linear causal single-input–single-output system with input u and subject to additive random disturbance v can be described in discrete time by the parameterized impulse response functions g and h:

$$y(t) = \sum_{n=1}^{\infty} g_n(\theta)u(t-n) + \sum_{n=0}^{\infty} h_n(\theta)\varepsilon(t-n) = G(q,\theta)u(t) + H(q,\theta)\varepsilon(t), \quad t = 0, 1, 2, \ldots, \tag{3.5}$$

where $\{\varepsilon(t)\}$ is the white noise, i.e., a sequence of independent random variables with zero means and finite variances σ^2 [15]. The parameter vector θ ranges over a subset of R^m, i.e., $\theta \in \Theta \subset R^m$, where m is the dimension of θ. Note that, for ease of notation, the time interval T has been taken equal to one time unit. The terms $G(q,\theta)$ and $H(q,\theta)$ correspond to the transfer functions of the linear systems $y(t) = \sum_{n=1}^{\infty} g_n(\theta)u(t-n)$ and $v(t) = \sum_{n=0}^{\infty} h_n(\theta)\varepsilon(t-n)$, with $t = 0, 1, 2, \ldots$, and they are an expansion of the backward shift operator q^{-1} with $q^{-1}u(t) = u(t-1)$ and $q^{-1}\varepsilon(t) = \varepsilon(t-1)$:

$$G(q,\theta) = \sum_{n=1}^{\infty} g_n(\theta)q^{-n}, \tag{3.6}$$

$$H(q,\theta) = h_0(\theta) + \sum_{n=1}^{\infty} h_n(\theta)q^{-n}, \tag{3.7}$$

where $h_0(\theta) = 1$. Under the assumption that the filter $H(q,\theta)$ is inversely stable (i.e., $H^{-1}(q,\theta) = 1/H(q,\theta)$ and $H^{-1}(q,\theta) < \infty$) and considering that $y(s)$, $u(s)$ and, subsequently, $v(s)$ are known for $s \leq t-1$, the one-step-ahead prediction of $y(t)$ is given by

$$\hat{y}(t|\theta) = H^{-1}(q,\theta)G(q,\theta)u(t) + \left(1 - H^{-1}(q,\theta)\right)y(t). \tag{3.8}$$

Moreover, the corresponding k-step-ahead prediction of $y(t)$ is

$$\hat{y}(t|\theta) = \overline{H}_k(q,\theta)H^{-1}(q,\theta)G(q,\theta)u(t) + \left(1 - \overline{H}_k(q,\theta)H^{-1}(q,\theta)\right)y(t), \tag{3.9}$$

supposing that we have observed $y(s)$ for $s \leq t-k$ and $u(s')$ for $s' \leq t-1$, and defining $\overline{H}_k(q,\theta) = \sum_{n=0}^{k-1} h_n(\theta)q^{-n}$.

A common parameterization of the transfer functions $G(q,\theta)$ and $H(q,\theta)$ is to consider them rational in the backward shift operator q^{-1}. Therefore, (3.5) can now be written as

$$A(q)y(t) = \frac{B(q)}{F(q)}u(t) + \frac{C(q)}{D(q)}\varepsilon(t), \tag{3.10}$$

where $A(q)$, $B(q)$, $C(q)$, $D(q)$, and $F(q)$ are polynomials of q^{-1}. Eq. (3.10) defines a class of linear black-box models by setting a number of the polynomials equal to one. For instance, the Autoregressive with Extra Inputs model corresponds to the case where $C(q) = D(q) = F(q) = 1$:

$$y(t) = \frac{B(q)}{A(q)} u(t) + \frac{1}{A(q)} \varepsilon(t), \tag{3.11}$$

with $A(q) = 1 + a_1 q^{-1} + \cdots + a_{n_a} q^{-n_a}$ and $B(q) = b_1 q^{-1} + \cdots + b_{n_b} q^{-n_b}$. In accordance with (3.5) and (3.11), it holds that $G(q, \theta) = B(q)/A(q)$, $H(q, \theta) = 1/A(q)$ and the parameter vector is $\theta = [a_1, \ldots, a_{n_a}, b_1, \ldots, b_{n_b}]^T$. In the case where $A(q) = C(q) = D(q) = F(q) = 1$, $y(t)$ is modeled as a finite impulse response. Other common models of this type are the Autoregressive Moving Average with Extra Inputs for $D(q) = F(q) = 1$, $G(q, \theta) = B(q)/A(q)$, $H(q, \theta) = C(q)/A(q)$, and $\theta = [a_1, \ldots, a_{n_a}, b_1, \ldots, b_{n_b}, c_1, \ldots, c_{n_c}]^T$, and the Box−Jenkins models for $A(q) = 1$, $G(q, \theta) = B(q)/F(q)$, $H(q, \theta) = C(q)/D(q)$, and $\theta = [b_1, \ldots, b_{n_b}, c_1, \ldots, c_{n_c}, d_1, \ldots, d_{n_d}, f_1, \ldots, f_{n_f},]^T$.

State-space models of linear dynamical systems, unlike models defined by (3.10), have the potential to describe a priori knowledge on the physical mechanisms of the examined system, reducing, in that way, the number of adjustable parameters θ. The relationship between the input $u(t)$, noise $v(t)$, and output $y(t)$ is written as a system of first-order differential or difference equations using an auxiliary state vector $x(t)$, whose representation in discrete time is:

$$x(t + 1) = A(\theta)x(t) + B(\theta)u(t), \quad y(t) = C(\theta)x(t) + v(t), \tag{3.12}$$

where the transfer function $G(q, \theta)$ from $u(t)$ to $y(t)$ in (3.5) is given by $G(q, \theta) = C(\theta)(qI - A(\theta))^{-1}B(\theta)$.

Specific applications of linear models of the form of (3.5) to the prediction of glucose concentration will be described systematically in Chapter 5, Linear Time Series Models of Glucose Concentration [19−24], placing special emphasis on the properties of the models, their formulation for multivariable inputs, the estimation of parameters and the prediction error.

3.2.3 Linear Regression Models

In linear regression, the predictor $\hat{y}(t|\theta)$ is a linear model of the form:

$$f(x, \theta) = \sum_{j=0}^{m-1} \theta_j \phi_j(x) = \theta^T \phi(x), \tag{3.13}$$

in which $\theta = (\theta_0, \ldots, \theta_{m-1})^T$ is the vector of parameters and $\phi = (\phi_0, \ldots, \phi_{m-1})^T$ is the vector of nonlinear basis functions with θ_0 being the bias parameter and $\phi_0(x) = 1$. The function f maps the input vector $x = (x_1, \ldots, x_d)^T$, which describes input up to time $t - kT$, to the glucose concentration y at time t, with t being the time for which the prediction is made and k is the prediction step. The model defined by (3.13) is linear with respect to the parameters θ; however, it constitutes a nonlinear function of the input vector x as a result of the nonlinear functions $\phi_j(x)$ with $j = 1, \ldots, m - 1$.

Elaborate machine-learning algorithms are used to estimate the parameter vector θ. Neural networks employ a fixed number of parametric basis functions, which are nonlinear functions of linear combinations of the input and whose parameters are learned along with parameters θ during training [25]. Kernel methods transform the input space X into a high-dimensional Reproducing Kernel Hilbert Space H through the mapping $\phi : X \to H$ such that $\kappa(x, x') = \phi(x)^T \phi(x)$ with $\kappa : X \times X \to R$ a positive definite kernel function and $\phi(x) = \kappa(x, \cdot)$ $\forall x \in X$ [26−28]. The Representer Theorem ensures that the output of kernel methods lies in the span of the finite set of kernels centered at the training input vectors and is expressed by a nonparametric function of the form [27]:

$$f(x) = \sum_{j=1}^{N_{Z_{train}}} a_j \kappa(x^j, x), \tag{3.14}$$

where $a = (a_1, \ldots, a_N)^T$ is the coefficients vector. Since the number of adjustable parameters in (3.14) equals the size of the training dataset, some form of constraint should be imposed on the error function to avoid overfitting. Both neural network [29−33] and kernel methods [34−37] as they have been applied in the field of glucose predictive modeling are going to be described analytically in Chapter 6, Nonlinear Models of Glucose Concentration.

3.2.4 Parameter Estimation Methods

Given the training set Z_{train} of size $N_{Z_{train}}$, the error function $E(\theta)$ measures the error of the parametric prediction model $\hat{y}(t|\theta)$ on Z_{train}. The least squares method, which is the standard procedure for determining θ in linear regression, defines $E(\theta)$ in terms of the residual sum of squares:

$$E(\theta) = \sum_{i=1}^{N_{Z_{train}}} \left(y(t_i) - \hat{y}(t_i|\theta) \right)^2, \tag{3.15}$$

where $e_i = y(t_i) - \hat{y}(t_i|\theta)$, with $i = 1, \ldots, N_{Z_{train}}$, is the residual error associated with the ith sample in Z_{train}. Substituting (3.13) in (3.15), we obtain:

$$E(\theta) = \sum_{i=1}^{N_{Z_{train}}} \left(y_i - \theta^T \phi(x^i) \right)^2, \tag{3.16}$$

which is a quadratic function in θ. Therefore, should both the number and form of the non-linear basis functions were fixed, as is the case for linear models of the form (3.10), an analytical closed-form solution of (3.16) could be obtained by setting its gradient to zero and solving for θ [38]:

$$\nabla \sum_{i=1}^{N_{Z_{train}}} \left(y(t_i) - \hat{y}(t_i|\theta) \right)^2 = 0 \Rightarrow \nabla \sum_{i=1}^{N_{Z_{train}}} \left(y_i - \theta^T \phi(x^i) \right)^2 = 0 \Rightarrow \sum_{i=1}^{N_{Z_{train}}} \left(y_i - \theta^T \phi(x^i) \right) \phi(x^i)^T = 0$$

$$\Rightarrow \sum_{i=1}^{N_{Z_{train}}} y_i \phi(x^i)^T - \theta^T \sum_{i=1}^{N_{Z_{train}}} \phi(x^i) \phi(x^i)^T = 0 \Rightarrow \hat{\theta} = \left(\Phi^T \Phi \right)^{-1} \Phi^T Y, \tag{3.17}$$

where Φ is the $N_{Z_{train}} \times m$ matrix $\Phi : \Phi_{i,j} = \phi_j(x^i)$ and $\Phi^\dagger = (\Phi^T\Phi)^{-1}\Phi^T$ is the pseudo-inverse of Φ. We have implicitly assumed that the $m \times m$ matrix $\Phi^T\Phi$ is nonsingular; however, a regularized version of the least squares method is employed when $\Phi^T\Phi$ is singular or ill conditioned. Tikhonov regularization is of the most common forms of regularization which includes the L^2 norm of θ:

$$E(\theta) = \sum_{i=1}^{N_{Z_{train}}} \left(y^i - \theta^T\phi(x^i)\right)^2 + \frac{\lambda}{2}\|\theta\|^2, \tag{3.18}$$

where $\|\theta\|^2 = \theta_0^2 + \cdots + \theta_{m-1}^2$ and λ a positive scalar. Similarly, the solution to the regularized least squares problem (3.18) could be given by $\hat{\theta} = (\Phi^T\Phi + \lambda I)^{-1}\Phi^TY$, where I is the $m \times m$ identity matrix.

As we will discuss in Section 3.3, the prediction model resulting from the minimization of the error function, i.e., the solution of the least squares problem in the case of (3.15), should obtain good generalization ability on new data, which means that it should not overfit the training set. One technique that is usually applied in order to prevent overfitting is that of regularization, where the regularization term introduced to the error function controls model's complexity.

Provided that diabetes self-monitoring data arrive sequentially, sequential or recursive learning algorithms have also the potential to be applied to estimate the parameter vector θ. Given a sequence of training examples $Z = \{(x^1, y_1), (x^2, y_2), \ldots, (x^i, y_i)\}$ up to the time t_i, the estimator of $f : R^d \to R$ is built sequentially such that f_i (the estimate at iteration i) is updated on the basis of the last estimate f_{i-1} and the prediction error on the current example (x^i, y_i), i.e., $e_i = y_i - f_{i-1}(x^i, \theta)$. For instance, the least mean squares algorithm is derived by using, at each iteration i, the gradient of the instantaneous squared error, i.e., $-(y_i - \theta^T\phi(x^i))\phi(x^i)$ and, according to the method of stochastic gradient descent, it is formulated as follows:

$$\theta_i = \theta_{i-1} + \eta(y_i - \theta_{i-1}^T\phi(x^i))\phi(x^i), \tag{3.19}$$

where θ_i denotes the parameter vector at iteration i and η is the learning rate parameter. Various types of sequential methods for parameter estimation [15,39] and their predictive ability with respect to the short-term prediction of glucose are thoroughly discussed in Chapter 8, Adaptive Glucose Prediction Models [24,33,40−44].

3.2.4.1 A Bayesian Framework for Parameters Estimation

From a probabilistic perspective, the uncertainty over the output y can be modeled using a probability distribution function [15,38]. More specifically, following the framework given in [38], it is assumed that the output y for a new point $x \in R^d$ is estimated from a Gaussian distribution with mean value $\mu = f(x, \theta)$ and precision (inverse variance) $\beta = 1/\sigma^2$:

$$p(y|\theta) = \mathrm{N}(y|f(x, \theta), \beta^{-1}) = \frac{\sqrt{\beta}}{\sqrt{2\pi}}\exp\left\{-\frac{\beta}{2}(y - f(x, \theta))^2\right\}. \tag{3.20}$$

The additive noise ε on the observed values y is considered such that $y = f(x, \theta) + \varepsilon$, and it is further assumed to be Gaussian distributed with zero mean and constant precision β. The latter contributes to the total variance of the predictive distribution. The values of the unknown parameters θ are then obtained by assuming that y_i, with $i = 1, \ldots, N_{Z_{train}}$, are drawn independently from the distribution $p(y|\theta)$ and by maximizing the likelihood function:

$$p(Y|\theta) = \prod_{i=1}^{N_{Z_{train}}} N\left(y_i | f\left(x^i, \theta\right), \beta^{-1}\right), \tag{3.21}$$

with respect to θ on the basis of the data in Z_{train}. As is shown in (3.22), maximum likelihood is transformed to an equivalent problem, namely, the minimization of the negative logarithm of the likelihood. By using the standard form of the Gaussian distribution (3.20), we can observe that the minimization of the negative logarithm of the likelihood with respect to θ coincides with the minimization of the residual sum of squares error function (3.15).

$$\max_{\theta}\{p(Y|\theta)\} = \min_{\theta}\left\{-\ln p\left(Y|\theta\right)\right\} = \min_{\theta}\left\{-\sum_{i=1}^{N_{Z_{train}}} \ln N\left(y_i | f\left(x^i, \theta\right), \beta^{-1}\right)\right\}$$

$$= \min_{\theta}\left\{\frac{\beta}{2} \sum_{i=1}^{N_{Z_{train}}} \left(y_i - f\left(x^i, \theta\right)\right)^2 - \frac{N_{Z_{train}}}{2} \ln \beta + \frac{N_{Z_{train}}}{2} \ln(2\pi)\right\}. \tag{3.22}$$

Likewise, the value of β is obtained by maximizing (3.21) with respect to β, which gives:

$$\frac{1}{\hat{\beta}} = \frac{1}{N_{Z_{train}}} \sum_{i=1}^{N_{Z_{train}}} \left(y_i - f\left(x^i, \hat{\theta}\right)\right)^2, \tag{3.23}$$

with $\hat{\theta}$ and $\hat{\beta}$ denoting the maximum likelihood solution of the respective parameters.

In the case of maximum posterior approach, the optimization problem involves the maximization of the posterior probability $p(\theta|Y) = p(Y|\theta)p(\theta)/p(Y)$ with respect to θ. By assuming a Gaussian prior distribution on the parameters θ, i.e., $p(\theta) = N(\theta|0, \alpha^{-1}I)$, where α is the noise precision of the distribution, we find that

$$\max_{\theta}\{p(\theta|Y)\} = \max_{\theta}\{p(Y|\theta)p(\theta)\} = \min_{\theta}\left\{-\ln(p(Y|\theta)p(\theta))\right\} = \min_{\theta}\left\{\frac{\beta}{2} \sum_{i=1}^{N_{Z_{train}}} \left(y_i - f\left(x^i, \theta\right)\right)^2 + \frac{\alpha}{2}\|\theta\|^2\right\}, \tag{3.24}$$

which is a regularized version of (3.16). Therefore, least squares minimization and regularized least squares represent special cases of maximum likelihood and maximum posterior methods, respectively, under the assumption of a zero-mean Gaussian noise model.

3.3 Training and Evaluation of Glucose Prediction Models

3.3.1 Learning and Generalization

The construction of a glucose predictive model comprises two phases: (1) the training phase and (2) the validation phase. Given a dataset $Z = \{(x^i, y_i) | i = 1, \ldots, N_Z\}$ with $x^i \in R^d$ and $y_i \in R$, training means learning the $m \times 1$ parameter vector $\hat{\theta}$ of the parametric model $f(x, \theta)$ minimizing an error function $E(\theta)$ defined on Z. The ultimate objective of training is to obtain a predictive model with good generalization error, which is a measure of the expected loss of the prediction model on previously unseen data samples. The generalization error is decomposed into the sum of a squared bias, a variance and a constant noise term [38]:

$$generalization_error = (bias)^2 + variance + noise, \qquad (3.25)$$

where the *squared bias* term is proportional to the training error and reflects the model's ability to fit the data, the *variance* term measures a model's dependence on the particular training set, i.e., whether small perturbations to the training set lead to a significantly different solution, and the *noise* term models the intrinsic noise of the data. There is a trade-off between bias and variance with simple models having high bias and low variance and complex models having low bias and high variance. For instance, maximum likelihood or, equivalently, least squares can lead to overfitting for large values of m, especially for training sets of limited size. According to Occam's razor principle the simplest hypothesis (i.e., model) that fits the data should be preferred [45]. In what follows, we review some indicative approaches to balance the bias and the variance of a prediction model.

3.3.1.1 Regularization

Regularization obtains a smoother mapping by controlling the values of the parameters θ through the addition of a penalty term $\lambda\Omega$ to the objective function to be minimized:

$$\tilde{E}(\theta) = E(\theta) + \lambda\Omega, \qquad (3.26)$$

where the regularization coefficient λ determines the extent to which regularization constraints are imposed. Therefore, training involves the minimization of $\tilde{E}(\theta)$ with respect to θ. Tikhonov regularization is the simplest case of regularization which, as has been previously, mentioned includes the L^2 norm of θ:

$$\tilde{E}(\theta) = E(\theta) + \frac{\lambda}{2} \|\theta\|^2. \qquad (3.27)$$

3.3.1.2 Early Stopping

Early stopping is applied to batch learning algorithms where the minimization of the error function $E(\theta)$ constitutes an iterative procedure over the entire dataset, e.g., gradient descent. A validation set is used to determine the point at which the iterative learning procedure should stop and, similarly to regularization, overfitting is prevented by actually constraining the values of θ. At each iteration, both the training ($E(\theta)$) and the validation error are measured. Apparently, the error function $E(\theta)$ decreases gradually toward a local or global minimum. On the other hand, the error on the validation set decreases until the model starts to fit the noise in the dataset and, then, it shows an increasing trend. The increase in the validation error signifies the end of the training.

3.3.1.3 Ensemble of Models

A model combining multiple prediction models has the potential to produce significantly better predictions as compared with the individual ones. Bagging is one approach toward this direction according to which given the set Z and a model $f(x, \theta)$: (1) a number of datasets $Z_1, \ldots, Z_K$ is created by uniform sampling with replacement from Z, (2) $f(x, \theta)$ is trained on $Z_1, \ldots, Z_K$ resulting in K models $f_i(x, \theta)$ with $i = 1, \ldots, K$, and (3) the output of the final model for a new input x is computed by averaging the predictions of the individual models, i.e.,

$$f_{\text{average}}(x, \theta) = \frac{1}{K} \sum_{i=1}^{K} f_i(x, \theta). \tag{3.28}$$

Averaging the output of multiple models trained on different versions of the same dataset Z has been shown to reduce the variance in the generalization error, i.e., the sensitivity of a predictive model on the training set Z. In particular, the generalization error of the average model in (3.28) will not exceed the average of the errors of the individual models [38]. For instance, Random Forest is an ensemble of low correlated regression trees, where each tree is constructed using an independent set of random vectors generated from a fixed probability distribution [46]. Randomness is usually incorporated into the tree growing process by bootstrap resampling the original training set and randomly selecting d' out of d features to split a node.

Boosting is a much more powerful approach which differs from bagging since the individual models are trained sequentially with each dataset Z_i containing those samples that are not correctly learned until iteration i. The predictions of the individual models are combined using weighted averaging with weights reflecting the performance of f_i on Z_i and being computed as a function of the residuals errors. The generic gradient-based boosting method for regression computes the so-called pseudo-residuals equal to the negative gradient of the loss function and fits a base learner f_i to pseudo-residuals, i.e., the training set becomes $\{(x^n, r_n^{(i)}) | n = 1, \ldots, N_{Z_i}\}$, where $r_n^{(i)}$ is the residual associated with the nth sample at ith iteration [47].

3.3.2 Estimation of the Generalization Error

The generalization error is estimated on a representative subset of Z. The holdout and the crossvalidation methods are most commonly used to evaluate the performance of a predictive model.

In the holdout method, the original dataset Z is partitioned into two disjoint sets, called the training and the test set, i.e., Z_{train} and Z_{test}, respectively, where the test set should follow the same probability distribution as the training set. The error function $E(\theta)$ is optimized on the training set and, next, the generalization ability of the resulting model f is evaluated on the test set. The reliability of the holdout method depends on the partition of Z, i.e., both training and test set should be representative subsets of Z.

Repartitioning of Z with the same ratio of data for training and testing could result in a different generalization error, especially in the case where N_Z is small. K-fold crossvalidation overcomes this limitation by using each sample (x^i, y_i), with $i = 1, \ldots, N_Z$, exactly once for testing. In particular, K-fold crossvalidation partitions the dataset Z into K representative disjoint folds $Z_1, \ldots, Z_K$ of approximately equal size (i.e., $\approx N_z / K$). Then, a model f_i is trained on the dataset $Z - Z_i$ and tested on the dataset Z_i for $i = 1, \ldots, K$. The final generalization error of the predictive model is the average error over all K-folds, i.e., $error = \frac{1}{K} \sum_{i=1}^{K} error_i$, where $error_i$ is the error of f_i on the test set Z_i. Z can be partitioned in K-folds randomly or in a stratified way such that the mean response value (i.e., glucose concentration) is approximately equal in all folds. The variance of the estimated validation error increases with K, whereas the opposite holds for the bias.

3.3.2.1 Generalization Error in Online Learning

In online learning, the expected generalization performance of the model is represented as a function of the number of training examples in Z (i.e., learning curve), which, in addition, expresses the convergence behavior of the learning algorithm. The learning curve is a plot of the instantaneous squared error e_i^2 versus the number of iterations [45]. To alleviate the effect of noise, the mean squared error $E[e_i^2]$ over an ensemble of models trained on independent datasets can be represented along with the variance of the error [39]. In case the distribution from which data is generated remains the same (stationary distribution), the dataset can be partitioned into training and test sets and, the learning curve becomes a plot of the squared error of f_i averaged over the test set versus the number of iterations i. However, in the general nonstationary case, the terms training and test set cannot be applied.

3.4 Validation of Glucose Prediction Models

3.4.1 Goodness of Fit

Statistical measures estimating the accuracy of forecast methods applied to univariate time series data can be used to assess the goodness of the fit of a glucose prediction model $f(x, \theta)$. The prediction error is defined as $e_i = y_i - \hat{y}_i$, where y_i denotes the observation of glucose concentration at time t_i and $\hat{y}_i$ the corresponding prediction of y_i by the model $f(x, \theta)$. The following measures are expressed in terms of the sum of absolute error $\sum_{i=1}^{N} |e_i|$ or squared error $\sum_{i=1}^{N} e_i^2$ over N observations:

- Mean Absolute Error (MAE):

$$\text{MAE} = \frac{1}{N} \sum_{i=1}^{N} |e_i|. \tag{3.29}$$

- Root mean squared error (RMSE):

$$\text{RMSE} = \sqrt{\frac{1}{N} \sum_{i=1}^{N} e_i^2}. \tag{3.30}$$

- Mean absolute percentage error:

$$\text{MAPE} = \left(\frac{1}{N} \sum_{i=1}^{N} \left| \frac{e_i}{y_i} \right| \right) \times 100\%. \tag{3.31}$$

- Root Mean Square Percentage Error:

$$\text{RMSPE} = \sqrt{\frac{1}{N} \sum_{i=1}^{N} \left(\frac{e_i}{y_i} \right)^2} \times 100\%. \tag{3.32}$$

- Coefficient of Determination:

$$R^2 = \frac{\sum_{i=1}^{N} (\hat{y}_i - \bar{y})^2}{\sum_{i=1}^{N} (y_i - \bar{y})^2} = 1 - \frac{\sum_{i=1}^{N} e_i^2}{\sum_{i=1}^{N} (y_i - \bar{y})^2}, \tag{3.33}$$

where $\bar{y}$ is the average value of y and provided that $\sum_{i=1}^{N} (y_i - \bar{y})^2 = \sum_{i=1}^{N} e_i^2 + \sum_{i=1}^{N} (\hat{y}_i - \bar{y})^2$.

The RMSE assumes that the individual errors e_i are unbiased and follow a normal distribution, whereas the MAE is more compatible with uniformly distributed errors; nevertheless, the MAE is less sensitive to outliers as compared to the MSE or the RMSE. Measures based on percentage errors are dimensionless and, provided that $y_i > 0$ in the case of glucose prediction, they are well defined. The coefficient of determination R^2, $0 \leq R^2 \leq 1$, captures the proportion of variability of the response variable (i.e., glucose concentration) which can be explained by the prediction model.

The sample Pearson correlation coefficient r can also be used as a measure of the linear relationship between y and $\hat{y}$:

$$r = \frac{\text{cov}(y, \hat{y})}{\sigma_y \sigma_{\hat{y}}}, \tag{3.34}$$

where $\text{cov}(y, \hat{y})$ is the covariance of y and $\hat{y}$, and σ_y (or $\sigma_{\hat{y}}$) is the standard deviation of y (or $\hat{y}$), which are defined as follows:

$$\text{cov}(y, \hat{y}) = \frac{1}{N-1} \sum_{i=1}^{N} (y_i - \bar{y})(\hat{y}_i - \bar{\hat{y}}),$$

$$\sigma_y = \sqrt{\frac{1}{N-1} \sum_{i=1}^{N} (y_i - \bar{y})^2},$$

$$\sigma_{\hat{y}} = \sqrt{\frac{1}{N-1} \sum_{i=1}^{N} (\hat{y}_i - \bar{\hat{y}})^2},$$

$$\bar{y} = \frac{1}{N} \sum_{i=1}^{N} y_i, \, \bar{\hat{y}} = \frac{1}{N} \sum_{i=1}^{N} \hat{y}_i. \tag{3.35}$$

The value of r ranges from -1 to 1, with a value of 1 (-1) meaning that y and $\hat{y}$ have a perfect positive (negative) linear relationship. A value of 0 implies that there is no linear relationship between the two variables.

The above-mentioned statistical measures estimate the proximity between y and $\hat{y}$ in space (i.e., point-to-point error) and do not consider their relationship in time. Consequently, they do not measure the regularity of predictions neither the time lag of the predicted time series with respect to the actual one [48,49]. Temporal gain (TG) is a measure of the average time gained in the detection of a critical event, i.e., a hypo/hyperglycemic event. It is defined as

$$TG = PH - delay, \tag{3.36}$$

where $PH = kT$ is the prediction horizon (recall that k is the number of prediction steps and T the sampling period of glucose measurements) and delay is the temporal shift minimizing the square of the L^2 distance between prediction and target. The delay is given by

$$delay = \arg\min_{j \in [0,k]} \left\{ \frac{1}{N-k+1} \sum_{i=1}^{N-k} \left(y_i - \hat{y}_{i+j} \right)^2 \right\} T. \tag{3.37}$$

$ESOD_{norm}$ is a measure of the smoothness of the predicted time series and, thus, the lower the ESOD value, the more regular the predicted time series. It is defined as the energy of the second-order differences (ESOD) (i.e., the sum of the squared second-order differences) of the predicted time series $\hat{y}$, normalized by the ESOD of the target time series y:

$$ESOD_{norm} = \frac{ESOD(\hat{y})}{ESOD(y)}, \tag{3.38}$$

where the ESOD of a time series x of length N is given by $ESOD(x) = \sum_{i=3}^{N} (x(i) - 2x(i-1) + x(i-2))^2$.

These two components, i.e., TG and $ESOD_{norm}$, are often inversely related, i.e., the greater the TG, the lower the regularity of prediction, and vice versa. The J index is a measure that simultaneously takes into account both measures:

$$J = \frac{ESOD_{norm}}{(TG_{norm})^2}, \tag{3.39}$$

with lower values of J indicating better predictions [48,49]. TG_{norm} is the TG of the predicted time series divided by the prediction horizon PH.

3.4.2 Continuous Glucose Error Grid Analysis

Continuous glucose error grid analysis (CG-EGA) has been developed as a method for evaluating the clinical accuracy of CGM readings as compared to reference blood glucose values, utilizing both spatial and the temporal characteristics of the glucose time series [50,51].

CG-EGA is an extension of the original EGA analysis, which is the gold standard for determining the accuracy of blood glucose meters [52]. CG-EGA comprises (1) the point-error grid analysis (P-EGA) which estimates the point accuracy of CGM readings, and (2) the rate-error grid analysis (R-EGA) which estimates the accuracy in terms of the rate and direction of glucose change. More specifically, let RBG(t) be the time series of reference blood glucose measurements made at regular time intervals over a time period and EBG(t) the respective CGM time series measured at the same time points. The point accuracy evaluates the difference between the corresponding blood glucose and CGM values at time t_i, i.e., RBG(t_i) − EBG(t_i), whereas the rate accuracy evaluates the difference in the rate of change between successive blood glucose and sensor measurements, i.e., $\frac{\text{RBG}(t_{i+1}) - \text{RBG}(t_i)}{\Delta t} - \frac{\text{EBG}(t_{i+1}) - \text{EBG}(t_i)}{\Delta t}$.

P-EGA, like the original Clarke error grid analysis, uses a scatter plot of reference blood glucose values versus the estimated CGM values which is subdivided into 5 zones: A_P, B_P, C_P, D_P, and E_P (Fig. 3.2A). Briefly, points that fall within zones A_P and B_P represent sufficiently accurate or acceptable glucose results, points in zone C_P may result in unnecessary corrections, points in zone D_P could lead to incorrect treatments, and points in zone E_P represent erroneous treatment. P-EGA allows the dynamic adjustment of the boundaries of the error zones depending on the blood glucose rate of change in order to account for the inherent delays between the blood and the interstitial glucose. In particular, the boundaries of the error zones are identical to those of the original EGA in the case where the blood glucose rate of change is within −1 to 1 mg/dL/min. However, if blood glucose is falling at a rate of −2 to −1 mg/dL/min or faster than −2 mg/dL/min, the upper boundaries of upper A_P, B_P, and D_P zones are raised by 10 and 20 mg/dL, respectively. Similarly, when blood glucose is rising at a rate of 1 to 2 mg/dL/min or faster than 2 mg/dL/min, the lower limits of lower A_P, B_P, and D_P zones are expanded by 10 and 20 mg/dL, respectively.

R-EGA uses the scatter plot of the rate of change of reference blood glucose values versus the rate of change of estimated CGM readings, with the boundaries of both the x- and y-axes ranging from −4 to 4 mg/dL/min (Fig. 3.2B). In accordance with P-EGA, the scatter plot is divided into five zones, i.e., A_R, B_R, C_R, D_R, and E_R which have the same clinical meaning as the original EGA discussed earlier. In particular, (1) the A_R zone signifies an accurate fit with an error within ± 1 mg/dL/min; however, the boundaries of A_R zone are progressively expanded to ± 2 mg/dL/min for blood glucose rates greater than ± 2 mg/dL/min, (2) the B_R zone shows benign errors in estimating the reference blood glucose rate of change that do not cause inaccurate clinical interpretation or result in treatment that leads to a negative outcome, (3) the C_R zone represents the overestimation (upper C_R) or underestimation (lower C_R) of an insignificant reference rate (between −1 to 1 mg/dL/min) which could lead to overtreatment, (4) the D_R zone indicates the failure to detect a rapid decline (upper D_R) or rise (lower D_R) in blood glucose, and (5) the E_R zone indicates that the CGM rate of change is opposite to the reference one with the upper E_R erroneously estimating a blood glucose rise and the lower E_R erroneously estimating a blood glucose fall.

Finally, the results of P-EGA and R-EGA are combined into one matrix stratified by blood glucose levels. As is shown in Fig. 3.3, the combined error matrix is computed separately for

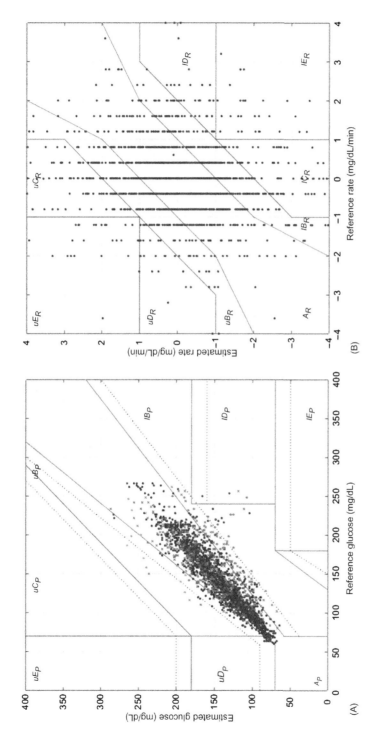

FIGURE 3.2 (A) P-EGA divided into upper (u) and lower (l) A_P, B_P, C_P, D_P, and E_P zones. Dark blue (marked with a dot symbol) points correspond to the case where the blood glucose rate of change is within −1 to 1 mg/dL/min. Dark red (lying at the lower zones and marked with an x symbol) and magenta (lying at the lower zones and marked with a diamond symbol) points correspond to the case where blood glucose is rising at a rate of 1 to 2 mg/dL/min or faster than 2 mg/dL/min, respectively. Dark green (lying at the upper zones and marked with an x symbol) and cyan points (lying at the upper zones and marked with a diamond symbol) correspond to the case where blood glucose is falling at a rate of −2 to −1 mg/dL/min or faster than −2 mg/dL/min, respectively. (B) R-EGA divided into upper (u) and lower (l) A_R, B_R, C_R, D_R, and E_R zones.

		P-EGA										
		Hypoglycemia			Euglycemia			Hyperglycemia				
		A	D	E	A	B	C	A	B	C	D	E
R-EGA	A	73.9	15.2	0.0	66.7	3.2	0.0	51.7	2.1	0.0	0.2	0.0
	B	6.5	4.3	0.0	17.2	1.3	0.0	18.8	0.2	0.0	0.0	0.0
	uC	0.0	0.0	0.6	2.8	0.5	0.0	6.4	0.9	0.0	0.3	0.0
	IC	0.0	0.0	0.0	2.0	0.4	0.0	5.5	0.7	0.0	0.0	0.0
	uD	0.0	0.0	0.0	1.3	0.0	0.0	4.1	0.2	0.0	0.0	0.0
	ID	0.0	0.0	0.0	3.5	0.1	0.0	4.1	1.0	0.0	0.0	0.0
	uE	0.0	0.0	0.0	0.0	0.0	0.0	0.2	0.2	0.0	0.0	0.0
	IE	0.0	0.0	0.0	0.9	0.1	0.0	2.2	1.0	0.0	0.2	0.0

Accurate readings
Benign errors
Erroneous readings

FIGURE 3.3 Error matrix combining R-EGA and P-EGA zones.

hypoglycemic ($\leq$70 mg/dL), euglycemic (71−180 mg/dL) and hyperglycemic ($>$180 mg/dL) glucose ranges. A clinical interpretation of the results is made through the definition of three types of prediction errors, i.e., Accurate Readings, Benign Errors, and Erroneous Readings, determining the clinical accuracy of treatment decisions. Sensor readings are considered clinically accurate when they fall into the A and B zones in both P-EGA and R-EGA. On the other hand, clinically benign errors are those with acceptable point accuracy (A_P or B_P zones) but significant errors in rate accuracy (C_R, D_R, or E_R), which are unlikely to have clinically negative therapeutic outcomes.

3.4.3 Prediction of Hypoglycemic Events

In accordance with the American Diabetes Association and the Endocrine Society recommendations, a plasma glucose concentration value below or equal to 70 mg/dL is considered as hypoglycemic [53]. A formal definition for the detection of hypoglycemic events in CGM data has not been provided yet; however, various heuristic approaches can be found in the literature. For instance, given a CGM system with a sampling period of $T = 5$ minutes, it is considered that (1) a hypoglycemic event starts when two at least successive subcutaneous glucose concentration values (i.e., 10 minutes or more) are $\leq$ 70 mg/dL, and (2) it ends when the glucose value rise above 70 mg/dL [34,40,54]. To treat potential oscillations either in the predicted or in the actual time series, consecutive hypoglycemic events that are $\leq$ 30 minutes away can typically be considered as the same event. Since hypoglycemia occurring during nocturnal sleep is important for diabetic patients, hypoglycemic events can

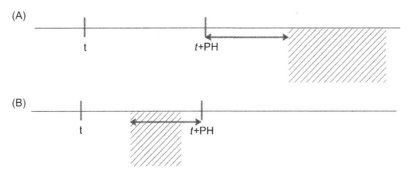

FIGURE 3.4 A true hypoglycemic event (denoted by the blue box) is predicted to happen at time t + PH, where PH is the prediction horizon (in minutes). The arrow line indicates the time distance between the start of the actual and the predicted event. The predicted event may (A) precede or (B) follow the actual one.

be separated into nocturnal and diurnal ones. In particular, nocturnal hypoglycemia is defined as each hypoglycemic event occurring at night when the individual is asleep, while all the other events are characterized as diurnal.

A prediction of a hypoglycemic event is considered true positive (TP) when the start of the actual hypoglycemic either precedes or follows the start of the predicted one by $\leq a$ minute, where a is usually bounded by the length of the prediction horizon. A typical example is illustrated in Fig. 3.4. Otherwise, when a true hypoglycemic event is not predicted or a false hypoglycemic event is predicted then a false-negative or a false-positive (FP) prediction, respectively, is identified. To note that the term true negative is not generally applied, which will mean to correctly identify a nonhypoglycemic region (i.e., euglycemia or hyperglycemia) as such.

The accuracy of a glucose prediction model with respect to the prediction of hypoglycemic events can be evaluated by computing measures such as sensitivity, precision and time lag. Sensitivity, defined as $TP/(TP + FN)$, relates to the method's ability to identify positive hypoglycemic events. On the other hand, precision, defined as $TP/(TP + FP)$, reflects the probability that a predicted event is true. Finally, *time_lag* is a highly crucial measure which reflects the TG in preventing the upcoming event and can be defined as the mean absolute temporal error between the start of the actual and the predicted hypoglycemic event.

Different approaches to hypoglycemia prediction, ranging from statistical methods to machine-learning techniques, will be presented analytically in Chapter 7, Prediction Models of Hypoglycemia.

3.5 Model Selection

Let us consider the training set Z_{train} and a set $\mathbf{M} = \{M_i(\theta_i)\}$ consisting of prediction models M_i of different type having parameters θ_i. Model selection finds the best model $\hat{M} \in \mathbf{M}$ for which a criterion relevant to the generalization error of the model is minimum. Moreover, given a predictive model $M(\theta)$ of a specific type, there exists a number of parameters which control its effective complexity and which are called hyperparameters. Typical examples of hyperparameters include (1) the order of polynomials of the backward shift operator q^{-1}, i.e., $A(q)$, $B(q)$, $C(q)$, $D(q)$, and $F(q)$ in linear models, (2) the number m of the nonlinear basis functions ϕ_j in linear regression, (3) the regularization coefficient λ in regularized least squares, as well as (4) the noise precision α of the prior distribution imposed on θ in maximum posterior. Fine tuning of these parameters is also a model selection problem, which is of paramount importance since, as we have previously stressed, the complexity of a prediction model defines to a great extent its generalization ability.

A structural approach toward model selection endorses the construction of several models with varying complexity and the selection of the best model according to their predictive performance on a subset of the training set Z_{train}, called the validation set. Nevertheless, if the training set is small, the estimation of hyperparameters, i.e., the model's complexity, based on the validation set would not be reliable. To this end, K-fold crossvalidation is usually applied where: (1) the training set Z_{train} is partitioned into K representative disjoint folds $V_1, \ldots, V_K$ of equal size, (2) for each combination of hyperparameters values, K models are trained on the dataset $Z_{\text{train}} - V_i$ and tested on the dataset V_i for $i = 1, \ldots, K$, and (3) the combination of values minimizing the average validation error over all K-folds, i.e., $\frac{1}{K} \sum_{i=1}^{K} \text{error}_i$ where error_i is the error on the validation set V_i, is subsequently selected. Note that after estimating the values of the hyperparameters, the prediction model $M(\theta)$ should be trained on the full training set Z_{train} to estimate the parameter vector θ. Although, crossvalidation is the most widely employed approach to model selection, it is computationally demanding especially when there are many hyperparameters and the training algorithm is intrinsically expensive.

An alternative approach to reduce the bias of more complex models supports the introduction of a relevant penalty term in the error function $E(\theta)$. Let m denote the number of adjustable parameters in the model M, i.e., the size of parameter vector θ, the Akaike information criterion (AIC) [55] selects the model which minimizes the following quantity:

$$\text{AIC} = -2 \ln p(Z_{\text{train}} | \theta_{\text{ML}}) + 2m, \tag{3.40}$$

where θ_{ML} is the value of θ maximizing the likelihood of Z_{train}. The corrected AIC (AICc) [56,57] applies to the case where the size of Z_{train} is small relative to the number of parameters and under the assumption that the model is univariate, linear, and with Gaussian error distribution:

$$\text{AICc} = \text{AIC} + \frac{2m(m + 1)}{N_{Z_{\text{train}}} - m - 1}. \tag{3.41}$$

Another variant of AIC, called the Bayesian information criterion (BIC) or minimum description length [58,59], is an approximation of the data distribution $\ln p(Z_{\text{train}} | M)$ and is defined by:

$$\text{BIC} = -2 \ln p(Z_{\text{train}} | \theta_{\text{MAP}}) + m \ln(N_{Z_{\text{train}}}), \tag{3.42}$$

where θ_{MAP} is the value of θ maximizing the posterior of Z_{train}. Information criteria such as AIC, AICc, and BIC have the advantage of being easily evaluated as compared to cross-validation; however, they could lead to misleading results if the underlying assumptions are not met.

Before proceeding to a detailed description of linear and nonlinear dynamical models of glucose prediction, we devote the next Chapter to the analysis of physiological models related to glucose regulation, which can complement the functionality of data driven ones or can be used for simulation purposes. Typical examples of them concern: (1) the absorptions kinetics of subcutaneously injected insulin, (2) the carbohydrate digestion and absorption, (3) the glucose dynamics during exercise, and (4) the glucose−insulin−glucagon physiology.

References

[1]   Burns PB, Rohrich RJ, Chung KC. The levels of evidence and their role in evidence-based medicine. Plast Reconstr Surg 2011;128(1):305−10.

[2]   Sibbald B, Roland M. Understanding controlled trials. Why are randomised controlled trials important? BMJ 1998;316(7126):201.

[3]   Langendam M, et al. Continuous glucose monitoring systems for type 1 diabetes mellitus. Cochrane Database Syst Rev 2012;1:CD008101.

[4]   Breton M, et al. Fully integrated artificial pancreas in type 1 diabetes: modular closed-loop glucose control maintains near normoglycemia. Diabetes 2012;61(9):2230−7.

[5]   Vandenbroucke JP, et al. Strengthening the reporting of observational studies in epidemiology (STROBE): explanation and elaboration. Int J Surg 2014;12(12):1500−24.

[6]   von Elm E, et al. The strengthening the reporting of observational studies in epidemiology (STROBE) statement: guidelines for reporting observational studies. Int J Surg 2014;12(12):1495−9.

[7]   Benchimol EI, et al. The reporting of studies conducted using observational routinely-collected health data (RECORD) statement. PLoS Med 2015;12(10):1−22.

[8]   Georga E, et al. Data mining for blood glucose prediction and knowledge discovery in diabetic patients: the METABO diabetes modeling and management system. Conf Proc IEEE Eng Med Biol Soc 2009;2009:5633−6.

[9]   Poulsen JU, et al. A diabetes management system empowering patients to reach optimised glucose control: from monitor to advisor. Conf Proc IEEE Eng Med Biol Soc 2010;2010:5270−1.

[10] Heinemann L, et al. HypoDE: research design and methods of a randomized controlled study evaluating the impact of real-time CGM usage on the frequency of CGM glucose values <55 mg/dl in patients with type 1 diabetes and problematic hypoglycemia treated with multiple daily injections. J Diabetes Sci Technol 2015;9(3):651−62.

[11] Juvenile Diabetes Research Foundation Continuous Glucose Monitoring Study, G., et al. Continuous glucose monitoring and intensive treatment of type 1 diabetes. N Engl J Med 2008;359(14):1464−76.

[12] Danne T, et al. The PILGRIM study: in silico modeling of a predictive low glucose management system and feasibility in youth with type 1 diabetes during exercise. Diabetes Technol Ther 2014;16(6):338−47.

[13] Phillip M, et al. Nocturnal glucose control with an artificial pancreas at a diabetes camp. N Engl J Med 2013;368(9):824−33.

[14] Cobelli C, et al. Pilot studies of wearable outpatient artificial pancreas in type 1 diabetes. Diabetes Care 2012;35(9):e65−7.

[15] Lennart L, editor. System identification: theory for the user. 2nd ed. Prentice Hall PTR, Upper Saddle River, New Jersey, USA; 1999.

[16] Ljung L. Perspectives on system identification. Annu Rev Control 2010;34(1):1−12.

[17] Kudva YC, et al. Closed-loop artificial pancreas systems: physiological input to enhance next-generation devices. Diabetes Care 2014;37(5):1184−90.

[18] Vashist S. Continuous glucose monitoring systems: a review. Diagnostics 2013;3(4):385.

[19] Cescon M, et al. Identification of individualised empirical models of carbohydrate and insulin effects on T1DM blood glucose dynamics. Int J Control 2014;87(7):1438−53.

[20] Cescon M, Johansson R, Renard E. Subspace-based linear multi-step predictors in type 1 diabetes mellitus. Biomed Signal Proc Control 2015;22:99−110.

[21] Finan DA, et al. Experimental evaluation of a recursive model identification technique for type 1 diabetes. J Diabetes Sci Technol 2009;3(5):1192−202.

[22] Gani A, et al. Predicting subcutaneous glucose concentration in humans: data-driven glucose modeling. IEEE Trans Biomed Eng 2009;56(2):246−54.

[23] Sparacino G, et al. Glucose concentration can be predicted ahead in time from continuous glucose monitoring sensor time-series. IEEE Trans Biomed Eng 2007;54(5):931−7.

[24] Wang Q, et al. Personalized state-space modeling of glucose dynamics for type 1 diabetes using continuously monitored glucose, insulin dose, and meal intake: an extended Kalman filter approach. J Diabetes Sci Technol 2014;8(2):331−45.

[25] Bishop CM. Neural networks for pattern recognition. New York, USA: Oxford University Press, Inc.; 1995. p. 482.

[26] Pillonetto G, et al. Kernel methods in system identification, machine learning and function estimation: a survey. Automatica 2014;50(3):657−82.

[27] Hofmann T, Scholkopf B, Smola AJ. Kernel methods in machine learning. Ann Stat 2008;36 (3):1171−220.

[28] Scholkopf B, Smola AJ. Learning with Kernels: support vector machines, regularization, optimization, and beyond. MIT Press, Cambridge, Massachusetts, USA; 2001. p. 632.

[29] Perez-Gandia C, et al. Artificial neural network algorithm for online glucose prediction from continuous glucose monitoring. Diabetes Technol Ther 2010;12(1):81−8.

[30] Zecchin C, et al. Jump neural network for online short-time prediction of blood glucose from continuous monitoring sensors and meal information. Comput Methods Programs Biomed 2014;113(1):144−52.

[31] Pappada SM, et al. Neural network-based real-time prediction of glucose in patients with insulin-dependent diabetes. Diabetes Technol Ther 2011;13(2):135−41.

[32] Zarkogianni K, et al. Comparative assessment of glucose prediction models for patients with type 1 diabetes mellitus applying sensors for glucose and physical activity monitoring. Med Biol Eng Comput 2015;53(12):1333−43.

[33] Daskalaki E, et al. Real-time adaptive models for the personalized prediction of glycemic profile in type 1 diabetes patients. Diabetes Technol Ther 2012;14(2):168−74.

[34] Georga EI, et al. A glucose model based on support vector regression for the prediction of hypoglycemic events under free-living conditions. Diabetes Technol Ther 2013;15(8):634−43.

[35] Georga E, et al. Multivariate prediction of subcutaneous glucose concentration in type 1 diabetes patients based on support vector regression. IEEE J Biomed Health Inform 2012;17(1):71−81.

[36] Wang Y, Wu X, Mo X. A novel adaptive-weighted-average framework for blood glucose prediction. Diabetes Technol Ther 2013;15(10):792−801.

[37] Naumova V, Pereverzyev SV, Sivananthan S. A meta-learning approach to the regularized learning-case study: blood glucose prediction. Neural Netw 2012;33:181—93.

[38] Bishop CM. Pattern recognition and machine learning (information science and statistics). Springer-Verlag New York, Inc. Secaucus, NJ, USA. Printed in Singapore.; 2006.

[39] Liu W, Principe JC, Haykin S. Kernel adaptive filtering: a comprehensive introduction. Published by John Wiley & Sons, Inc., Hoboken, New Jersey. Published simultaneously in Canada.; 2010. p. 209.

[40] Daskalaki E, et al. An early warning system for hypoglycemic/hyperglycemic events based on fusion of adaptive prediction models. J Diabetes Sci Technol 2013;7(3):689—98.

[41] Eren-Oruklu M, et al. Adaptive system identification for estimating future glucose concentrations and hypoglycemia alarms. Automatica (Oxf) 2012;48(8):1892—7.

[42] Eren-Oruklu M, et al. Estimation of future glucose concentrations with subject-specific recursive linear models. Diabetes Technol Ther 2009;11(4):243—53.

[43] Zhao C, Yu C. Rapid model identification for online subcutaneous glucose concentration prediction for new subjects with type I diabetes. IEEE Trans Biomed Eng 2015;62(5):1333—44.

[44] Bayrak ES, et al. Hypoglycemia early alarm systems based on recursive autoregressive partial least squares models. J Diabetes Sci Technol 2013;7(1):206—14.

[45] Sammut C, Webb GI. Encyclopedia of machine learning. Springer Publishing Company, Incorporated, New York, USA; 2011. p. 1058.

[46] Breiman L. Random forests. Mach Learn 2001;45(1):5—32.

[47] Duffy N, Helmbold D. Boosting methods for regression. Mach Learn 2002;47(2—3):153—200.

[48] Facchinetti A, et al. A new index to optimally design and compare continuous glucose monitoring glucose prediction algorithms. Diabetes Technol Ther 2011;13(2):111—19.

[49] Facchinetti A, et al. Real-time improvement of continuous glucose monitoring accuracy. Diabetes Care 2013;36(4):793—800.

[50] Clarke WL, Anderson S, Kovatchev B. Evaluating clinical accuracy of continuous glucose monitoring systems: continuous glucose-error grid analysis (CG-EGA). Curr Diabetes Rev 2008;4(3):193—9.

[51] Kovatchev BP, et al. Evaluating the accuracy of continuous glucose-monitoring sensors: continuous glucose-error grid analysis illustrated by TheraSense Freestyle Navigator data. Diabetes Care 2004;27(8):1922—8.

[52] Clarke WL. The original Clarke Error Grid Analysis (EGA). Diabetes Technol Ther 2005;7(5):776—9.

[53] Seaquist ER, et al. Hypoglycemia and diabetes: a report of a workgroup of the American Diabetes Association and the Endocrine Society. Diabetes Care 2013;36(5):1384—95.

[54] Eren-Oruklu M, Cinar A, Quinn L. Hypoglycemia prediction with subject-specific recursive time-series models. J Diabetes Sci Technol 2010;4(1):25—33.

[55] Akaike H. A new look at the statistical model identification. IEEE Trans Autom Control, 1974;19(6):716—23.

[56] Zucchini W. An introduction to model selection. J Math Psychol 2000;44(1):41—61.

[57] Hurvich CM, Tsai CL. Regression and time-series model selection in small samples. Biometrika 1989;76(2):297—307.

[58] Schwarz G. Estimating the dimension of a model. Ann Stat 1978;6(2):461—4.

[59] Rissanen J. Modeling by shortest data description. Automatica 1978;14(5):465—71.

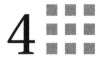

4

Physiological Models and Exogenous Input Modeling

4.1 Physiological Models of the Glucose−Insulin System

Modeling methodology of the glucose−insulin system applies general principles of modeling of biological and physiological systems. Having a model structure, mirroring the underlying physiology of the system, and a set of input−output data obtained from a particular experiment, a priori identifiability of model parameters, reasonable precision, physiological plausibility of the estimated parameters and model validity are essential desiderata of the system modeling process [1−5]. The increased complexity of the glucose−insulin system is reflected to the postulated structure of the model, which, in turn, is bidirectionally linked to the related problem of experimental design; though, simplifying assumptions are extensively adopted. Minimal, with respect to the number of parameters, models are, principally, used to quantify characteristic parameters related to glucose metabolism and can be identified from the transient response of one system variable [6]. On the other hand, maximal or large-scale simulation models provide a comprehensive representation of the glucose−insulin system; however, their identification needs more complex experimental protocols. In this section, we provide a concise overview of the classic minimal modeling approach [7] and, subsequently, we outline the components of a large-scale simulation model of the glucose metabolism in people with diabetes [8]. We consider this information particularly important toward a more coherent understanding of the physiological models presented in subsequent sections of this chapter. The interested reader is directed to outstanding reviews of the state-of-the-art in physiologically based modeling of the glucose−insulin dynamics [6,9].

4.1.1 Minimal Models of the Glucose−Insulin System

Bergman's glucose minimal model provides an estimation of glucose effectiveness (S_G) and insulin sensitivity (S_I) from an intravenous glucose−tolerance test (IVGTT) [6,7,10]. The glucose−insulin system is decomposed exactly into two subsystems, i.e., the glucose subsystem and the insulin one, which are linked via a negative feedback loop; the output of the glucose subsystem (i.e., plasma-glucose concentration) is fed back to the insulin subsystem and, similarly, the output of the insulin subsystem (i.e., plasma-insulin concentration) is fed back to the glucose subsystem. A single compartment is considered to represent glucose kinetics. In addition, insulin is assumed to regulate both glucose uptake by insulin-sensitive peripheral tissues and net hepatic glucose balance from a remote, with respect to plasma, compartment

Personalized Predictive Modeling in Type 1 Diabetes. DOI: http://dx.doi.org/10.1016/B978-0-12-804831-3.00004-2

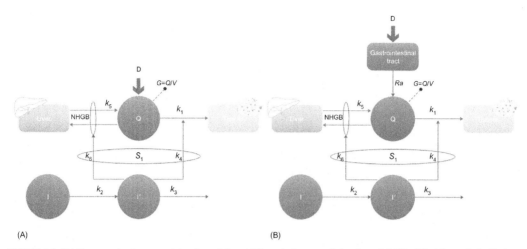

FIGURE 4.1 (A) Bergman's glucose minimal model and (B) oral glucose minimal model. *Modified from Cobelli, C., et al., Diabetes: models, signals, and control. IEEE Rev Biomed Eng, 2009, 2: 54–96.*

representing the interstitial fluid. The uniquely identifiable form of the glucose minimal model, corresponding to Fig. 4.1A, is given by:

$$\dot{Q}_1(t) = -(p_1 + X(t))Q(t) + p_1 Q_b + D\delta(t), \tag{4.1}$$

$$\dot{X}(t) = -p_2 X(t) + p_3(I(t) - I_b), \tag{4.2}$$

$$G(t) = \frac{Q(t)}{V}, \tag{4.3}$$

where Q (mg/kg) is plasma-glucose mass, I (μU/mL) is plasma-insulin concentration, $X(t) = (k_4 + k_6)I'(t)$ with I' denoting the above basal insulin concentration in the remote compartment, G (mg/dL) is plasma-glucose concentration, V (mL/kg) is the glucose distribution volume, and D (mg/kg) is the total amount of ingested glucose. Note that the subscript b denotes the basal steady-state value of the associated variable. The parameterization $p_1 = k_1 + k_5$ $p_2 = k_3$ and $p_3 = k_2(k_4 + k_6)$, with $k_i, i = 1,\ldots,5$ (min^{-1}) being rate parameters, ensures the a priori identifiability of the model. The initial conditions of (4.1) and (4.2) are $Q(0) = Q_b$ and $X(0) = 0$, respectively.

Indices of S_G (dL/kg/min) and S_I (dL/kg/min per (μU/mL)) are, then, estimated in terms of model parameters as follows:

$$S_G = -\frac{\partial \dot{Q}(t)}{\partial G(t)} = p_1 V, \tag{4.4}$$

$$S_I = -\frac{\partial^2 \dot{Q}(t)}{\partial I(t)\partial G(t)} = \frac{p_3}{p_2} V. \tag{4.5}$$

Model parameters are individually fitted to the *G* and *I* data obtained during an IVGTT glucose−insulin plasma concentration data by weighted nonlinear least squares, after deliberately omitting the first ∼10 minutes of the experiment. One-compartment modeling of glucose kinetics under nonsteady-state conditions (IVGTT) has been shown to contribute significantly to the observed overestimation of S_G and underestimation of S_I by Bergman's minimal model. Indeed, the accuracy of S_G and S_I estimates can be improved by considering a two-compartment model of glucose kinetics [11].

The oral minimal model [12−14] allows the estimation of S_G and S_I in a given individual from an oral glucose test, either a mixed-meal tolerance test (MTT) or an oral-glucose tolerance test (OGTT). MTT and OGTT not only constitute a more physiological route of perturbing the glucose−insulin system but also, through a smoother response of plasma-glucose and insulin than in the case of the IVGTT, enable the use of the one-compartment model of the glucose subsystem. The oral minimal model is built upon Bergman's minimal model (Fig. 4.1B), where the term $D\delta(t)$ in (4.1) is substituted by a parametric model (with respect to $a = [a_1, \ldots, a_8]^T$ and $a_0 = 0$) of the rate of oral glucose appearance into plasma (*Ra*):

$$Ra(a, t) = \begin{cases} a_{i-1} + \dfrac{a_i - a_{i-1}}{t_i - t_{i-1}}(t - t_{i-1}), & t_{i-1} \leq t \leq t_i, \ \ i = 1, \ldots, 8 \\ 0, & \text{otherwise} \end{cases}. \qquad (4.6)$$

Parameters V and p_1 are fixed to population values in order to ensure an a priori identifiable model and, additionally, a constraint is imposed on the total amount of the ingested glucose dose (*D*) that is actually absorbed into plasma [13]. Maximum a posteriori estimations are obtained for the remaining parameters imposing a Gaussian prior on p_2 [13]. At this point, we need to stress that the reference method for the reconstruction of the *Ra* time-course entails the implementation of multiple-tracer experiments; nonetheless, the oral minimal model has been shown to be a cost-effective solution as compared with the reference method.

4.1.2 Simulation Models of the Glucose−Insulin System

The quantitative knowledge gained on glucose−insulin metabolism, primarily by making use of multiple tracer experiments, enabled the development of a holistic simulation model of the glucose−insulin system in the postabsorptive state in normal human and people with type 2 diabetes [8]. Plasma-glucose *G* (mg/dL) and insulin *I* (pmol/*L*) concentrations are linked with (1) glucose fluxes, i.e., glucose rate of appearance *Ra*(mg/kg/min), endogenous glucose production EGP(mg/kg/min), insulin-dependent, and insulin-independent glucose utilization U_{id} and U_{ii}(mg/kg/min), respectively, and renal excretion *E*(mg/kg/min), and (2) insulin fluxes, i.e., insulin secretion *S*(pmol/kg/min) and insulin degradation *D*(pmol/kg/min). Herein, we focus on glucose and insulin subsystems, as well as, on the modeling of *Ra* and U_{id}, whereas the interested reader is directed particularly to the work of Dalla Man et al. [8] for clarifications and discussion of the remaining processes. Indeed, *Ra* modeling comprises an essential component of the overall model, which allows

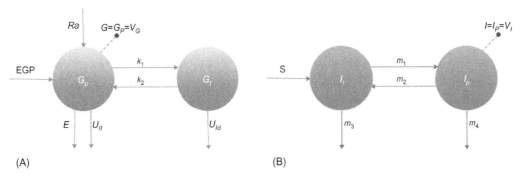

FIGURE 4.2 Schematic representation of the (A) glucose and (B) insulin subsystems of the glucose metabolism simulation model proposed by Dalla Man et al. *Modified from Dalla Man, C., R.A. Rizza, and C. Cobelli,* Meal simulation model of the glucose–insulin system. *IEEE Trans Biomed Eng, 2007. 54(10): p. 1740–1749.*

the description of the physiological changes following meal ingestion, and it will be extensively described in Section 4.3.

As is shown in Fig. 4.2, glucose and insulin kinetics are each described by a two-compartment model. In particular, G_p and G_t (mg/kg), which denote glucose masses in the plasma and rapidly equilibrating tissues, and in slowly equilibrating tissues, respectively, are given by

$$\dot{G}_p(t) = EGP(t) + Ra(t) - U_{ii}(t) - E(t) - k_1 G_p(t) + k_2 G_t(t), \qquad (4.7)$$

$$\dot{G}_t(t) = -U_{id}(t) + k_1 G_p(t) - k_2 G_t(t), \qquad (4.8)$$

where k_1 and k_2 (min^{-1}) are the corresponding rate parameters [15,16]. Let V_G (dL/kg) the distribution volume of glucose, G (mg/dL) is obtained as

$$G(t) = \frac{G_p(t)}{V_G}. \qquad (4.9)$$

Initially, at $t = 0$, it holds $G_p(0) = G_{pb}$, $G_t(0) = G_{tb}$, and $G(0) = G_b$ with subscript b denoting the basal steady-state. It is additionally considered that, in steady-state conditions (i.e., post-absorptive state), endogenous glucose production balances glucose utilization:

$$EGP_b = U_{id,b} + U_{ii,b} + E_b. \qquad (4.10)$$

Unlike insulin-independent glucose utilization [U_{ii}(mg/kg/min)] which is constant and equal to F_{cns}, insulin-dependent glucose utilization [U_{ii}(mg/kg/min)] depends nonlinearly on G_t and interstitial insulin concentration, X(pmol/L), using Michaelis–Menten kinetics:

$$U_{id}(t) = \frac{V_m(X(t))G_t(t)}{K_m(X(t)) + G_t(t)}, \qquad (4.11)$$

where $V_m(X(t)) = V_{m0} + V_{mx}X(t)$ and $K_m(X(t)) = K_{m0} + K_{mx}X(t)$. X is described by the following differential equation:

$$\dot{X}(t) = -p_{2U}X(t) + p_{2U}\left(I_p(t) - I_b\right), \tag{4.12}$$

with $X(0) = 0$ and p_{2U} (min^{-1}) being the rate constant. In the basal steady state, it holds:

$$G_{tb} = \frac{F_{cns} - EGP_b + k_1 G_{pb}}{k_2}, \tag{4.13}$$

$$U_b = U_{id,b} + U_{ii,b} = EGP_b = F_{cns} + \frac{V_{m0}G_{tb}}{K_{m0} + G_{tb}}. \tag{4.14}$$

Likewise, I_p and I_l(pmol/L), the insulin masses in the plasma and the liver, respectively, are given by

$$\dot{I}_l(t) = -(m_1 + m_3(t))I_l(t) + m_2 I_p(t) + S(t), \tag{4.15}$$

$$\dot{I}_p(t) = -(m_2 + m_4)I_p(t) + m_1 I_l(t), \tag{4.16}$$

$$I(t) = \frac{I_p(t)}{V_I}, \tag{4.17}$$

where m_1, m_2, and m_4 (min^{-1}) are the rate parameters and V_I (L/kg) is the distribution volume of insulin [17]. Degradation of insulin in the periphery, m_4 (min^{-1}) is assumed to be linear. On the contrary, a time-varying hepatic insulin degradation, $m_3(t)$ (min^{-1}), is considered:

$$m_3(t) = \frac{HE(t)m_1}{1 - HE(t)}. \tag{4.18}$$

HE concerns hepatic efflux of insulin (in particular, it is defined as the ratio of insulin flux which leaves the liver irreversibly to the total insulin flux leaving the liver), and it is assumed to be linearly related to $S(t)$:

$$HE(t) = -m_5 S(t) + m_6, \tag{4.19}$$

with $HE(0) = HE_b$ and, in the basal steady-state, the rate of insulin secretion is considered equal to that of insulin degradation:

$$S_b = m_3(0)I_{lb} + m_4 I_{pb} = D_b. \tag{4.20}$$

Parameter values are reported in Table 4.1 and, except for glucose and insulin subsystems, they have been estimated with precision from experimental data using nonlinear least squares, where the system identification is performed separately for each subsystem by using a forcing function strategy. Authors acknowledge the noninclusion in the model of diurnal variation of parameters as an important limitation.

Table 4.1 Parameters of Glucose–Insulin Simulation Models

Model #		Parameter	Unit	Value	
				Normal	*Type 2 Diabetes*
Dalla Man et al. [8]	*Glucose kinetics*	V_G	dL/kg	1.88	1.49
		k_1	min^{-1}	0.065	0.042
		k_2	min^{-1}	0.079	0.071
	Insulin kinetics	V_I	L/kg	0.05	0.04
		m_1	min^{-1}	0.190	0.379
		m_2	min^{-1}	0.484	0.673
		m_4	min^{-1}	0.194	0.269
		m_5	min kg/pmol	0.0304	0.0526
		m_6		0.6471	0.8118
		HE_b		0.6	0.6
	Glucose utilization	F_{cns}	mg/kg/min	1	1
		V_{m0}	mg/kg/min	2.50	4.65
		V_{mx}	(mg/kg/min)/pmol/L	0.047	0.034
		K_{m0}	mg/kg	225.59	466.21
		K_{mx}	mg/kg	≈ 0	≈ 0
		p_{2U}	min^{-1}	0.0331	0.0840

The glucose–insulin meal model by Dalla Man et al., after substituting the insulin secretion model with a model of subcutaneous insulin kinetics and increasing endogenous glucose production [18], formed the basis of the University of Virginia/Padova type 1 diabetes simulator, which has been accepted by the FDA as a substitute to animal trials in the preclinical testing of closed-loop control strategies [19]. Its main feature is that it includes 300 in silico subjects validated against real clinical data and representing well the observed variability of key metabolic parameters in the general type 1 diabetes population.

4.2 Subcutaneous Insulin Absorption

The absorption of subcutaneously administered insulin is governed by a number of mechanisms, including insulin self-assembly, subcutaneous (s.c.) diffusion, binding in the s.c. tissue, and appearance of insulin into plasma [20]. The rate of absorption of insulin into plasma, as described in Chapter 2, Pathophysiology and Management of Type 1 Diabetes, depends on the formulation of insulin, the injected volume, the concentration of insulin, the local subcutaneous blood flow and factors associated with blood flow differences at the site of injection (i.e., site of injection, exercise, heat application, or local massage), which synergistically contribute to an increased intra- and interpatient variability in absorption pharmacokinetics [21,22]. There is strong evidence supporting that the absorption rate of regular insulin is negatively correlated with insulin concentration and it is positively correlated with the injected volume. A strong determinant of the rate of insulin absorption is local s.c. blood flow, which under physiological conditions may vary more than $\pm 50\%$ from the normal flow (i.e., $4 - 6$ mL/min) [23]. One can find contradictory research findings on insulin degradation in the s.c. tissue; nevertheless, the imperfect systemic bioavailability of regular insulin and, to a much greater extent, of intermediate-acting analogues of insulin (i.e., Neutral Protamine Hagedorn—NPH) suggests s.c. degradation of insulin as a potential factor [23].

The absorption kinetics of insulin following s.c. administration is mathematically described by either pure compartmental models or mechanistic models, which parameters are identified from experimental data or are derived from the literature. Linear or nonlinear multicompartment models describing the delays imposed by the s.c. route of administration of different insulin formulations have been developed [24–30]. The landmark study by Mosekilde et al. [20] established the basic principles of mechanistic modeling of the s.c. kinetics of regular (soluble) insulin, which were adopted by several subsequent mechanistic models of the kinetics of regular insulin and insulin analogues [23,31–36]. Nucci and Cobelli, in a critical review of models of s.c. injected insulin kinetics, opined that a comprehensive quantitative description, with a sound mechanistic basis, of the underlying physicochemical properties should dovetail with low computational complexity [37]. To this end, several constraints are typically imposed in order to ensure the a priori identifiability of the mathematical model, whereas a posteriori identifiability is greatly considered during model selection. A model of plasma-insulin kinetics complements the s.c. insulin absorption model, which, except for Hovorka et al. [38], is represented by a single compartment with a nonsaturable elimination of insulin. In this section, before proceeding to the description of specific mechanistic or compartmental insulin pharmacokinetic models, we first delineate, according to Mosekilde et al. [20,23,34], the mechanisms per se that govern the absorption kinetics of s.c. administered regular insulin and the key modeling assumptions made.

4.2.1 Mechanisms of Subcutaneous Insulin Absorption

Oligomers of regular insulin reside in a dynamic equilibrium, with higher insulin concentrations in the s.c. tissue favoring oligomers of higher molecular weight [23]. Typically, only monomers (M), dimers (D), and hexamers (H) are considered such that

$$H \rightleftarrows 3D$$
$$D \rightleftarrows 2M,$$

$$(4.21)$$

which, by denoting the concentrations of $H, D,$ and M in the s.c. tissue by c_H, c_D and c_M (IU/mL), respectively, and applying the law of mass action to (4.21), is tantamount to:

$$\frac{dc_H}{dt} = P_{DH}\big(Q_{DH}c_D^3 - c_H\big),$$

$$(4.22)$$

$$\frac{dc_D}{dt} = P_{MD}\big(Q_{MD}c_M^2 - c_D\big).$$

$$(4.23)$$

Q_{DH} and Q_{MD} (mL^2/IU^2) are the equilibrium constants between H and D and between D and M, respectively, and P_{DH} and P_{MD} (min^{-1}) are the corresponding rate constants.

Following s.c. injection of regular insulin, insulin oligomers diffuse through the s.c. tissue assuming a time varying concentration gradient according to Fick's second law of diffusion:

$$\frac{\partial c_x}{\partial t} = D_x \nabla^2 c_x,$$

(4.24)

where x stands for $H, D,$ or M, D_x (cm^2/min) is the diffusion constant corresponding to x, and ∇^2 is the Laplace operator. D and M of insulin can penetrate the capillary membrane and be absorbed into plasma, whereas there is evidence of direct absorption of H into plasma, presumably, via the lymphatic system [23,39]. A first-order nonsaturable rate of absorption of insulin oligomers into plasma is considered:

$$\frac{\partial c_x}{\partial t} = - B_x c_x,$$

(4.25)

where B_x (min^{-1}) is the absorption rate constant corresponding to x (i.e., H, D, or M). Considering a 100% bioavailability of injected insulin, the elimination of insulin from plasma is typically modeled as a first-order nonsaturable process:

$$\dot{I}_p(t) = - k_e I(t) + \frac{1}{V_d} \int_{V_{SC}} (B_M c_M + B_D c_D + B_H c_H) dV_{s.c.},$$

(4.26)

where I_p (IU/mL) is the plasma-insulin concentration, k_e (min^{-1}) is the rate constant of plasma-insulin elimination, $V_{s.c.}$ is the s.c. volume, and V_d is the distribution volume of insulin.

4.2.2 Model 1: Mosekilde et al. [20]

A model of the absorption kinetics of s.c. injected regular insulin, formulated in terms of well-established physicochemical and pharmacokinetical principles (i.e., equilibration between different oligomeric forms of insulin, diffusion, reversible binding of insulin molecules in the s.c. tissue, and absorption), was proposed by Mosekilde et al. [20,40]. Three different forms of regular insulin are assumed to be present in the s.c. tissue: (1) free insulin in the hexameric form, (2) free insulin in the dimeric form, and (3) bound insulin denoting the temporary binding of insulin molecules in the s.c. tissue. Accordingly, the fraction of insulin dimers dissociating in monomers (i.e., the reaction $D \rightleftarrows 2M$) is considered as negligible. A quasi-stationary equilibrium is considered between hexameric and dimeric insulin during the entire absorption process. Bound insulin becomes considerable as insulin concentration reduces accounting for the tail of the absorption rate curve observed at very low concentrations [21]. It is further assumed that only the dimeric form of insulin can penetrate the capillary membrane and be absorbed into the plasma with a rate proportional to its concentration. Considering that insulin hexamers are the predominant form of insulin at higher concentrations and the insulin concentration lowering effect of diffusion is less significant at higher injection volumes, the latter hypotheses can explain the initial slow absorption phase observed for higher insulin concentrations and injection volumes [21], as well as, the inverse relationship between concentration of injected insulin and its rate of absorption.

A set of three coupled partial differential equations describes the pharmacokinetic processes as follows:

$$\frac{\partial c_H}{\partial t} = \underbrace{P_{DH}\left(Q_{DH}c_D^3 - c_H\right)}_{H \rightleftharpoons D \text{ transition}} + \underbrace{D_H \nabla^2 c_H}_{\text{diffussion}}, \tag{4.27}$$

$$\frac{\partial c_D}{\partial t} = -\underbrace{P_{DH}\left(Q_{DH}c_D^3 - c_H\right)}_{H \rightleftharpoons D \text{ transition}} + \underbrace{D_D \nabla^2 c_D}_{\text{diffusion}} - \underbrace{B_D c_D}_{\text{absorption}} - \underbrace{Sc_D(C - c_D) + \frac{c_B}{T}}_{\text{s.c. binding}}, \tag{4.28}$$

$$\frac{\partial c_B}{\partial t} = \underbrace{Sc_D v(C - c_B) - \frac{c_B}{T}}_{\text{s.c. binding}}. \tag{4.29}$$

where c_H, c_D, and c_B (IU/mL) denote the hexameric, dimeric, and bound insulin concentrations in the s.c. tissue, respectively. Only hexameric and dimeric insulin are supposed to diffuse in the s.c. tissue, where the diffusion constants are supposed to be the same for both insulin forms and equal to the diffusion constant of insulin in the water at 37°C, i.e., $D_H = D_D = 0.9 \times 10^{-4}$ cm^2/min. Provided that binding is significant only at low concentrations at which insulin dimers prevail, the binding rate is controlled by the concentration of dimeric insulin, c_D, with S (min^{-1}) being the binding rate constant, C (IU/cm^3) the binding capacity in the s.c. tissue and T (min) the lifetime of insulin in the bound state. Note that the local degradation of insulin in the s.c. insulin is considered relatively insignificant. The values of parameters $Q_{DH}, B_D, C,$ and T for a bolus injection in people with type 1 diabetes were determined based on specific features of insulin absorption curves provided by Binder et al. [21] and their values are given in Table 4.2. The values of rate constants P_{DH} and S need not be specified a priori as long as they are taken sufficiently high compared to B_D, such that a quasi-equilibrium is maintained between the three forms of insulin in the s.c. depot. Mosekilde et al. have chosen $P_{DH} = 0.5$ min^{-1}.

4.2.3 Model 2: Trajansoki et al. [32]

Trajanoski et al. [32] reduced the complexity of the model proposed by Mosekilde et al. [20] considering that the insulin binding in the s.c. tissue is clinically not relevant in the range of therapeutic concentrations (40 and 100 IU/mL) and injection volumes. In addition, the diffusion of insulin in the s.c. tissue is considered to be isotropic, i.e., homogeneous and with spherical symmetry with respect to the injection site, with r being the radial distance from

Table 4.2   Parameters of Insulin Absorption Models

Model #	Parameter	Unit	Value				
Mosekilde et al. [20]	D_H, D_D	cm²/min	0.9×10^{-4}				
	Q_{DH}	mL²/IU²	0.13				
	B_D	min⁻¹	1.3×10^{-2}				
	C	IU/cm³	0.05				
	T	min	800				
Trajansoki et al. [31,32]	D_H, D_D	cm²/min	0.9×10^{-4}				
	Q_{DH}	mL²/IU²	0.13				
	B_D	min⁻¹	1.3×10^{-2}				
	k_e	min⁻¹	0.09				
	V_d	L	12				
Tarin et al. [33]			Lispro Humalog Novorapid	Actrapid	Semilente	NPH (Protaphane)	Glargine (Lantus)
	D_H, D_H, D_B	cm²/min	3.36×10^{-4}	8.4×10^{-5}	8.4×10^{-5}	8.4×10^{-5}	8.4×10^{-5}
	Q_{DH}	mL²/IU²	4.75×10^{-4}	1.9×10^{-3}	7.6×10^{-2}	3.04	3.04
	B_D	min⁻¹	2.36×10^{-2}	1.18×10^{-2}	1.18×10^{-2}	1.18×10^{-2}	1.18×10^{-2}
	κ	mL/IU/min					0.01
	$c_{H,max}$	IU/mL					15
	d_b						0.1
Li et al. [35,36]	k	min⁻¹	2.35×10^{-5}				
	$C_{H,max}$	IU/mL	15				
	Q_{DH}	mL²/IU²	3.04				
	B_D	min⁻¹	0.02				
	r		0.2143				
	k_e	min⁻¹	0.0215				
Wilinska et al. [28]	k_{a1}	min⁻¹	1.12×10^{-2}				
	k_{a2}	min⁻¹	2.10×10^{-2}				
	k_e	min⁻¹	1.89×10^{-2}				
	k		0.67				
	V	L/kg	56.45×10^{-2}				
	MCR	L/kg/min	10.7×10^{-3}				
	$V_{max,LD}$	mU⁻¹/min	1.93				
	$k_{M,LD}$	mU	62.6				

the injection site. The modified model of s.c. insulin absorption, after neglecting (4.29) and eliminating the term $-Sc_D(C - c_B) + \frac{c_B}{T}$ in (4.28), becomes

$$\frac{\partial c_H(t,r)}{\partial t} = \underbrace{P_{DH}\left(Q_{DH}c_D^3(t,r) - c_H(t,r)\right)}_{H \rightleftarrows D \text{ transition}} + \underbrace{D_H \nabla^2 c_H(t,r)}_{\text{diffusion}}, \tag{4.30}$$

$$\frac{\partial c_D(t,r)}{\partial t} = -\underbrace{P_{DH}\left(Q_{DH}c_D^3(t,r) - c_H(t,r)\right)}_{H \rightleftarrows D \text{ transition}} + \underbrace{D_D \nabla^2 c_D(t,r)}_{\text{diffusion}} - \underbrace{B_D c_D(t,r)}_{\text{absorption}}. \tag{4.31}$$

The system of nonlinear partial differential equations has no closed solution and, therefore, a time and space discretization of the diffusion equation is implemented for the numerical calculation of c_D. First, the s.c. depot is divided into $i = 0, \ldots, n_c$ $(n_c = 15)$ spherical concentric shells, with V_0 being the volume of the injected insulin and $R_0 = \sqrt[3]{\frac{3V_0}{4\pi}}$ the radius of the innermost sphere. The diffusion equation corresponding to Fick's second law of diffusion is approximated by the following discretized equation:

$$\frac{\Delta c_{i+1}}{\Delta t} = \frac{c_{i+1}(k+1) - c_{i+1}(k)}{\Delta t} = \frac{1}{V_{i+1}}(f_i(k) - f_{i+1}(k)), \tag{4.32}$$

where $\Delta c_{i+1}/\Delta t$ stands for the time variation of the concentration of a generic substance inside the shell $i + 1$, the difference $(f_i(k) - f_{i+1}(k))$ describes the net difference between the incoming substance flow f_i and the outgoing substance flow f_{i+1} diffusing through the shell $i + 1$ at discrete time instant k, and $V_{i+1} = 4\pi/3(R_{i+1}^3 - R_i^3)$ is the volume of the considered shell. By employing Fick's first law of diffusion, the insulin flow f_i from the shell with radius $\overline{R}_i$ to the shell with radius $\overline{R}_{i+1}$ at any discrete time instant k is calculated by

$$f_i(k) = -\frac{4\pi d\overline{R}_i\overline{R}_{i+1}}{\overline{R}_{i+1} - \overline{R}_i}(c_{i+1}(k) - c_i(k)), \tag{4.33}$$

where c and d stand for a generic substance concentration inside the considered shell and diffusion constant, respectively, and $\overline{R}_{i+1} = \frac{1}{\sqrt[3]{2}\sqrt[3]{R_{i+1}^3 + R_i^3}}$ is defined as the radius that halves the volume of the shell $i + 1$.

After substitution of f_i, f_{i+1} in (4.32) according to (4.33), the corresponding discrete in space and time pharmacokinetic equations of (4.30) and (4.31) are given by

$$\begin{aligned}
\frac{c_{H,i+1}(k+1) - c_{H,i+1}(k)}{\Delta t} = \frac{3D_H}{R_{i+1}^3 - R_i^3} & \left[\frac{\overline{R}_{i+1}\overline{R}_{i+2}}{\overline{R}_{i+2} - \overline{R}_{i+1}}\left(c_{H,i+2}(k) - c_{H,i+1}(k)\right) \right. \\
& \left. - \frac{\overline{R}_i\overline{R}_{i+1}}{\overline{R}_{i+1} - \overline{R}_i}\left(c_{H,i+1}(k) - c_{H,i}(k)\right) \right] \\
& + P_{DH}\left(Q_{DH}c_{D,i+1}^3(k) - c_{H,i+1}(k)\right)
\end{aligned} \tag{4.34}$$

$$\begin{aligned}
\frac{c_{D,i+1}(k+1) - c_{D,i+1}(k)}{\Delta t} = \frac{3D_H}{R_{i+1}^3 - R_i^3} & \left[\frac{\overline{R}_{i+1}\overline{R}_{i+2}}{\overline{R}_{i+2} - \overline{R}_{i+1}}\left(c_{D,i+2}(k) - c_{D,i+1}(k)\right) \right. \\
& \left. - \frac{\overline{R}_i\overline{R}_{i+1}}{\overline{R}_{i+1} - \overline{R}_i}\left(c_{D,i+1}(k) - c_{D,i}(k)\right) \right] \\
& - P_{DH}\left(Q_{DH}c_{D,i+1}^3(k) - c_{H,i+1}(k)\right) - B_D c_{D,i+1}(k)
\end{aligned} \tag{4.35}$$

The boundary conditions of the model are (1) zero concentration is assigned to a shell with $i > n_c$, and (2) zero insulin flux from the hypothetical shell $i = -1$ to the shell $i = 0$ is considered. The initial conditions of the model are

$$c_{H,i}(0) = \begin{cases} \bar{c}_H, & 0 < i \le n_c \\ 0, & i > n_c \end{cases}$$

$$c_{D,i}(0) = \begin{cases} \bar{c}_D, & 0 < i \le n_c \\ 0, & i > n_c \end{cases},$$ (4.36)

with $\bar{c}_H$ and $\bar{c}_D$ being the initial concentration of hexameric and dimeric insulin, respectively, $\bar{I}$ the average insulin concentration of the depot, $Q_{DH}\bar{c}_D^3 = \bar{c}_H$, and $\bar{I} = \bar{c}_D + \bar{c}_H$.

Models (4.30) and (4.31) are also extended to include monomeric (rapid-acting) insulin analogues which feature a reduced tendency to self-association at pharmaceutical concentration and which s.c. absorption can be modeled by:

$$\frac{\partial c_M}{\partial t} = D_M \nabla^2 c_M - B_M c_M,$$ (4.37)

where c_M (IU/mL) denotes the concentration of monomeric insulin in the s.c. tissue, and D_M (cm^2/min) and B_M (min^{-1}) are the corresponding diffusion and absorption rate constants of monomeric insulin, respectively. The discretized form of (4.37) is obtained in a similar way to those of (4.30) and (4.31):

$$\frac{c_{M,i+1}(k+1) - c_{M,i+1}(k)}{\Delta t} = \frac{3D_M}{R_{i+1}^3 - R_i^3} \left[\begin{array}{l} \frac{\bar{R}_{i+1}\bar{R}_{i+2}}{\bar{R}_{i+2} - \bar{R}_{i+1}} \left(c_{M,i+2}(k) - c_{M,i+1}(k) \right) \\ - \frac{\bar{R}_i\bar{R}_{i+1}}{\bar{R}_{i+1} - \bar{R}_i} \left(c_{M,i+1}(k) - c_{M,i}(k) \right) \end{array} \right] - B_M c_{M,i+1}(k).$$ (4.38)

Wach et al. [31] further modified (4.37) to

$$\frac{\partial c_M(r,t)}{\partial t} = D_M \frac{1}{r^2} \frac{\partial}{\partial r} \left(r^2 \frac{\partial c_M}{\partial r} \right) - B_M c_M,$$ (4.39)

which, however, can be solved analytically by employing the Fourier transform method.

By assuming a single compartment for plasma-insulin kinetics, the plasma-insulin concentration following injection of regular insulin is given by:

$$\dot{I}_p(t) = -k_e I(t) + \frac{1}{V_d} \int_{V_{s.c.}} B_D c_D(r,t) dV_{s.c.},$$ (4.40)

where I_p is the plasma-insulin concentration, $V_{s.c.}$ is the complete s.c. volume, k_e (min^{-1}) is the rate constant of plasma-insulin elimination, and V_d is the plasma-insulin distribution volume [25].

The discretized form of (4.40) is given by

$$\frac{I_p(k+1) - I_p(k)}{\Delta t} = -k_e I_p(k) + \frac{1}{V_d} B_D \sum_{i=0}^{n_c} c_{D,i}(k) V_i.$$ (4.41)

The parameter values are derived from the literature [25,41,42] and are presented in Table 4.2 (according to [31]).

4.2.4 Model 3: Tarin et al. [33]

Tarin et al. extended the model originally presented in [20] and, subsequently, simplified and refined in [31,32] to describe the absorption kinetics of different s.c. administered insulin formulations including rapid-acting (Lispro, Aspart), short-acting (Regular), intermediate-acting (NPH), and long-acting (Glargine) analogues of insulin [33]. In addition to the chemical relationship between insulin dimers and hexamers, a virtual insulin association state is introduced, i.e., the bound state, to explain the kinetics of long-acting insulin analogues. Assuming homogeneity of the s.c. tissue and spherical symmetry with respect to the injection site, the diffusion of insulin, the molecular dissociation of insulin and the absorption of insulin into plasma are described by the following nonlinear partial differential equations:

$$\frac{\partial c_D(t,r)}{\partial t} = \underbrace{P_{\mathrm{DH}}\big(c_H(t,r) - Q_{\mathrm{DH}}c_D(t,r)^3\big)}_{H \rightleftarrows D \text{ transition}} - \underbrace{B_D c_D(t,r)}_{\text{absorption}} + \underbrace{D_D \nabla^2 c_D(t,r)}_{\text{diffusion}}, \tag{4.42}$$

$$\frac{\partial c_H(t,r)}{\partial t} = -\underbrace{P_{\mathrm{DH}}\big(c_H(t,r) - Q_{\mathrm{DH}}c_D(t,r)^3\big)}_{H \rightleftarrows D \text{ transition}} + \underbrace{\kappa c_B(t,r)\big(c_{H,\max} - c_H(t,r)\big)}_{B \rightarrow H \text{ transition}} + \underbrace{D_H \nabla^2 c_H(t,r)}_{\text{diffusion}}, \tag{4.43}$$

$$\frac{\partial c_B(t,r)}{\partial t} = -\underbrace{\kappa c_B(t,r)\big(c_{H,\max} - c_H(t,r)\big)}_{B \rightarrow H \text{ transition}} + \underbrace{d_B D_B \nabla^2 c_B(t,r)}_{\text{diffusion}}. \tag{4.44}$$

It holds that $D_H = D_D = D_B$, whereas a nondimensional factor $d_B \in [0, \ 1]$ is introduced to reduce the diffusion rate of the bound form given the limited solubility of Glargine insulin at the neutral PH of the injection site. Glargine insulin of hexameric form progressively disengages from the bound state, in which it is supposed to be initially residing, with a rate proportional to c_B and with a proportionality factor κ (mL/IU/min). The saturable solubility of the bound form is further modeled by introducing the parameter $c_{H,\max}$ (IU/mL), denoting the maximum concentration of hexameric insulin, and making the disengagement rate proportional to the difference $(c_{H,\max} - c_H(t,r))$. By assuming that only the dimeric form of insulin can be absorbed into the plasma, the exogenous insulin flow into the bloodstream at time t, $I_{\mathrm{ex}}(t)$ (IU/min), is given by

$$I_{\mathrm{ex}}(t) = B_D \int_{V_{\mathrm{s.c.}}} c_D(t,r)dV. \tag{4.45}$$

This model allows the description of all insulin formulations through the adequate selection of the parameters $Q_{\mathrm{DH}}, D_D, D_H, D_B, B_D, \kappa, c_{H,\max}$, and d_B. The parameters concerning insulin Glargine were estimated, through an iterative identification process, using the experimental data provided by Lepore et al. [43], whereas the parameters concerning the remaining insulin preparations were taken from the literature [32] (Table 4.2). As suggested in [25], the rate constant P_{DH} is considered equal to $P_{DH} = 0.5$ min^{-1} for all insulin preparations.

A three-compartment model is used to simulate the distribution and elimination of insulin in plasma [44]:

$$\dot{x}_p(t) = I_{ex}(t) - (m_{01} + m_{21} + m_{31})x_p(t) + m_{12}x_h(t) + m_{13}x_i(t), \tag{4.46}$$

$$\dot{x}_h(t) = -(m_{02} + m_{12})x_h(t) + m_{21}x_p(t), \tag{4.47}$$

$$\dot{x}_i(t) = -m_{13}x_i(t) + m_{31}x_p(t), \tag{4.48}$$

where x_p, x_h, and x_i (U) denote the insulin masses in the plasma, the liver and the interstitial tissue, respectively. The pair of m_{12} and m_{21} (min^{-1}) parameters accounts for the insulin transfer between plasma and liver. Similarly, the pair of m_{13} and m_{31} (min^{-1}) parameters accounts for the insulin transfer between plasma and interstitial tissue. Parameters m_{01} and m_{02} (min^{-1}) are the rate constants of plasma and hepatic insulin elimination, respectively. Given the lack of insulin secretion in people with type 1 diabetes, the only input to this physiological model is the exogenous insulin flow, $I_{ex}(t)$, obtained by (4.45).

Similarly to [31,32], the complete insulin absorption model in discretized form is expressed as

$$\frac{c_{H,i+1}(k+1) - c_{H,i+1}(k)}{\Delta t} = \frac{3D_H}{R_{i+1}^3 - R_i^3} \left[\begin{array}{l} \dfrac{\overline{R}_{i+1}\overline{R}_{i+2}}{\overline{R}_{i+2} - \overline{R}_{i+1}} \left(c_{H,i+2}(k) - c_{H,i+1}(k)\right) \\[2ex] - \dfrac{\overline{R}_i\overline{R}_{i+1}}{\overline{R}_{i+1} - \overline{R}_i} \left(c_{H,i+1}(k) - c_{H,i}(k)\right) \end{array} \right] \\ + P_{DH}\left(Q_{DH}c_{D,i+1}^3(k) - c_{H,i+1}(k)\right) + \kappa c_{B,i+1}(k)\left(c_{H,\max} - c_{H,i+1}(k)\right) \tag{4.49}$$

$$\frac{c_{D,i+1}(k+1) - c_{D,i+1}(k)}{\Delta t} = \frac{3D_D}{R_{i+1}^3 - R_i^3} \left[\begin{array}{l} \dfrac{\overline{R}_{i+1}\overline{R}_{i+2}}{\overline{R}_{i+2} - \overline{R}_{i+1}} \left(c_{D,i+2}(k) - c_{D,i+1}(k)\right) \\[2ex] - \dfrac{\overline{R}_i\overline{R}_{i+1}}{\overline{R}_{i+1} - \overline{R}_i} \left(c_{D,i+1}(k) - c_{D,i}(k)\right) \end{array} \right], \\ + P_{DH}\left(Q_{DH}c_{D,i+1}^3(k) - c_{H,i+1}(k)\right) - B_D c_{D,i+1}(k) \tag{4.50}$$

$$\frac{c_{B,i+1}(k+1) - c_{B,i+1}(k)}{\Delta t} = \frac{3d_B D_B}{R_{i+1}^3 - R_i^3} \left[\begin{array}{l} \dfrac{\overline{R}_{i+1}\overline{R}_{i+2}}{\overline{R}_{i+2} - \overline{R}_{i+1}} \left(c_{B,i+2}(k) - c_{B,i+1}(k)\right) \\[2ex] - \dfrac{\overline{R}_i\overline{R}_{i+1}}{\overline{R}_{i+1} - \overline{R}_i} \left(c_{B,i+1}(k) - c_{B,i}(k)\right) \end{array} \right]. \\ - \kappa c_{B,i+1}(k)\left(c_{H,\max} - c_{H,i+1}(k)\right) \tag{4.51}$$

The resulting exogenous insulin flow at time $k\Delta t$, $I_{ex}(k)$, is given by

$$I_{ex}(k) = B_D \sum_{i=0}^{n_c} c_{D,i}(k) V_i. \tag{4.52}$$

The boundary conditions, as well as, the initial conditions for all insulin formulations except insulin Glargine are the same with those specified in [31,32]. Regarding insulin Glargine, the initial concentration of the bound state in the innermost sphere is equal to the concentration of the injected insulin, whereas the initial concentrations of the hexameric and dimeric states are zero. For all other insulin formulations, the initial concentration of the bound state is equal to zero.

Using a state-space representation, the resulting discretized form of the system (4.46)–(4.48) is

$$x(k+1) = e^{A\Delta t} x(k) + \left(\int_0^{\Delta t} e^{A\tau} B_D dt \right) I_{ex}(k). \tag{4.53}$$

$$I_p(k) = Cx(k), \tag{4.54}$$

where $x = (x_p, x_h, x_i)^T$ is the state vector. The corresponding state, input and output matrices A, B, and C are

$$A = \begin{bmatrix} -(m_{01} + m_{21} + m_{31}) & m_{12} & m_{13} \\ m_{21} & -(m_{02} + m_{12}) & 0 \\ m_{31} & 0 & -m_{13} \end{bmatrix}, \quad B = \begin{bmatrix} 1 \\ 0 \\ 0 \end{bmatrix}, \quad C = \begin{bmatrix} \dfrac{1}{\text{plasma } b_w} \\ 0 \\ 0 \end{bmatrix}, \tag{4.55}$$

where plasma (mL/kg) is the plasma volume and b_w (kg) is a subject's body weight.

Fig. 4.3A shows the exogenous insulin flow profile of Aspart and Glargine insulin analogues resulting from the insulin therapy of a typical patient with type 1 diabetes for a time horizon of one day (Aspart insulin: 9:17 hour—2 U, 13:10 hour—8 U, 20:05 hour—10 U; Glargine: 0:00 hour—28 U). It can be seen that the profile varies substantially depending on the injected insulin doses and formulations, i.e., insulin Glargine has a slower onset of action and a longer duration of action than Aspart insulin, whose activity peaks rapidly. The plasma-insulin concentration of the combined effect of both insulin types is depicted in Fig. 4.3B. The long action of Glargine insulin, which resembles the basal insulin secretion of nondiabetic individuals, as well as the effect of Aspart insulin, which is used for controlling the postprandial hyperglycemia, can be observed.

4.2.5 Model 4: Li et al. [35,36]

Li and Kuang [35,36], based on the existing models [20,31–33,37], proposed the following model:

$$\dot{c}_B(t) = -k c_B(t) \frac{C_{H,\max}}{1 + c_H(t)}, \tag{4.56}$$

$$\dot{c}_H(t) = -P_{DH} \left(c_H(t) - Q_{DH} c_D^3(t) \right) + k c_B(t) \frac{C_{H,\max}}{1 + c_H(t)}, \tag{4.57}$$

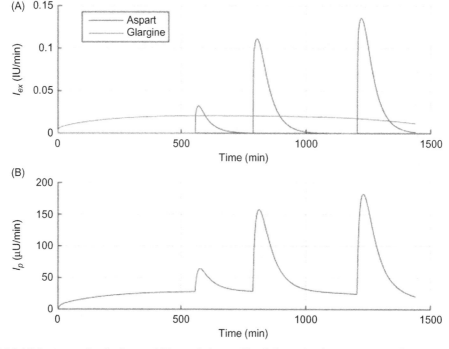

FIGURE 4.3 (A) Exogenous insulin flow and (B) cumulative profile of plasma-insulin concentration for a typical subject with type 1 diabetes (Aspart insulin: 9:17 hour—2 U, 13:10 hour—8 U, 20:05 hour—10 U; Glargine: 0:00 hour—28 U) as computed by the insulin model 3 [33].

$$\dot{c}_D(t) = P_{DH}\left(c_H(t) - Q_{DH}c_D^3(t)\right) - \frac{B_D c_D(t)}{1 + I_p(t)}, \tag{4.58}$$

$$\dot{I}_p(t) = \frac{rB_D c_D(t)}{1 + I_p(t)} - k_e I_p(t), \tag{4.59}$$

with initial conditions: (1) $c_H(0) > 0$, $c_D(0) = 0$, and $I_p(0) \geq 0$ in the case of regular insulin and insulin analogues except long-acting ones or (2) $c_B(0) > 0$, $c_H(0) = 0$, $c_D(0) = 0$, and $I_p(0) \geq 0$ in the case of long-acting insulin analogues. It has been presumed that the rate of dimers penetrating the capillary membrane is inversely proportional to the plasma-insulin concentration, as depicted by the term $-\left(B_D c_D(t)/(1 + I_p(t))\right)$ in (4.58) as well as the term $rB_D c_D(t)/\left(1 + I_p(t)\right)$ in (4.59) with $r \leq 1$. The gradual dissociation of hexameric insulin from the bound state, modeling the delay in absorption of long-acting insulin analogues, is represented by the term $-kc_B(t)(C_{H,max}/(1 + c_H(t)))$. The rate of transformation of bound insulin into hexameric insulin is assumed inversely proportional to c_H with maximum transformation capacity C_{max}, where k is the corresponding rate constant (min^{-1}).

4.2.6 Model 5: Wilinska et al. [28]

Wilinska et al. performed a comprehensive comparison study of 10 compartmental models of insulin Lispro kinetics after s.c. administration, which differed in the description of s.c.

insulin absorption and insulin clearance from plasma [28]. All models were a priori identifiable [45] and were estimated employing an iterative two-stage Bayesian method on 12-hour plasma-insulin concentration profiles of seven patients with type 1 diabetes under continuous s.c. insulin infusion therapy (continuous insulin infusion rate: 0.86 ± 0.27 U/h, bolus insulin delivery: 5.95 ± 2.37 U) [46,47]. The models were validated through assessing the physiological feasibility and the posterior identifiability of parameter estimates, and the distribution of residuals [48]. The dominant model, according to the Bayesian information criterion [49], considering two, slow and fast, channels of insulin absorption kinetics in the s.c. tissue and including a saturable local degradation of insulin at the injection site, is described as

$$\frac{dQ_{1a}}{dt} = ku - k_{a1}Q_{1a} - \text{LD}_a, \tag{4.60}$$

$$\frac{dQ_{1b}}{dt} = (1-k)u - k_{a2}Q_{1b} - \text{LD}_b, \tag{4.61}$$

$$\frac{dQ_2}{dt} = k_{a1}Q_{1a} - k_{a1}Q_2, \tag{4.62}$$

$$\frac{dQ_3}{dt} = k_{a1}Q_2 + k_{a2}Q_{1b} - k_eQ_3, \tag{4.63}$$

where u (mU/min) is the insulin input, Q_{1a} and Q_{1b} (mU) represent the mass of insulin in the slow absorption channel comprising of two compartments, Q_2 (mU) is the mass of insulin in the fast absorption channel, V (L/kg) is the insulin distribution volume, k (dimensionless) is the proportion of total input flux passing through the slow absorption channel, k_{a1}, k_{a2}, and k_e (min^{-1}) are transfer rates, and LD$_a$ and LD$_b$ (mU/min) represent local insulin degradation rates at the injection site. The Michaelis−Menten kinetics is assumed for LD$_a$ and LD$_b$:

$$\text{LD}_a = V_{\text{max,LD}}Q_{1a}/(k_{M,LD} + Q_{1a}), \tag{4.64}$$

$$\text{LD}_b = V_{\text{max,LD}}Q_{1b}/(k_{M,LD} + Q_{1b}), \tag{4.65}$$

where $V_{\text{max,LD}}$ (mU/min) is the saturation level and $K_{M,LD}$ (mU) is the value of insulin mass at which insulin degradation is equal to half of its maximal value. The parameter estimates of the model are shown in Table 4.2, with Wilinska et al. remarking on considerable inter-subject variability across all individual parameter estimates. The mean value of k indicates that 67% (interquartile range: 53%−82%) of delivered insulin passes through the slow absorption channel with a mean absorption rate k_{a1} of 0.011 (interquartile range: 0.004−0.029) min^{-1} and the remaining 33% passes through the fast channel with a mean absorption rate k_{a2} of 0.021 (interquartile range: 0.011−0.040) min^{-1}. In addition, the mean values of $V_{\text{max,LD}} = 1.93$ (interquartile range: 0.62−6.03) mU/min and $K_{M,LD} = 62.6$ mU (interquartile range: 62.6−62.6) indicate that the effect of local degradation is not insignificant in the range of therapeutic insulin concentrations. It should be noted that although parameters k_e and V were not physiologically feasible, their product, the metabolic clearance rate, attained physiological feasibility and, actually, was almost identical with that obtained by Kraegen et al. [25] and Shimoda et al. [27].

The widespread suggestion that insulin clearance from plasma follows linear kinetics was corroborated by Wilinska et al. with models imposing nonlinear Michaelis−Menten dynamics on insulin clearance not being *a posteriori* identifiable. On the contrary, the remote effect of insulin on its volume of distribution, which was modeled in a Michaelis−Menten form, was not confirmed. Models assuming nonlinear dynamics and saturability of insulin absorption rate with increasing insulin dose proved borderline identifiable, with the estimates of some parameters exhibiting high degree of uncertainty. In addition, the effect of insulin delivery mode i.e., s.c. bolus injection or continuous s.c. infusion, as well as, of insulin association state i.e., monomeric and dimeric on insulin absorption rate was not observed.

4.3 Glucose Absorption After Oral Ingestion

The time course of the rate of appearance (Ra) of ingested glucose into plasma is mainly regulated by the rate of gastric emptying of ingested glucose, the rate of intestinal glucose absorption into plasma and the hepatic uptake. Mathematical modeling of the Ra focuses on the description of gastric emptying function and the intestinal absorption of luminal glucose [50−52]. The oral glucose minimal model [12−14] has been proven a significant tool for the identification of Ra models, obviating the need for the direct measurement of glucose Ra using tracer-based methodologies [53,54].

4.3.1 Model 1: Hovorka et al. [50]

A simple two-compartment model of intestinal glucose absorption was incorporated into a nonlinear model predictive controller of glucose concentration in subjects with type 1 diabetes during fasting conditions [50]. Assuming identical transfer rate constants between the two compartments equal to $1/t_{max,G}$, the rate of appearance of ingested glucose in plasma, Ra (mg/min), is described as

$$Ra(t) = \frac{DA_G t e^{-t/t_{max,G}}}{t_{max,G}^2},$$

(4.66)

where $t_{max,G}$ (min) is the time to peak Ra, D (mg) is the amount of carbohydrates digested and A_G is the carbohydrate bioavailability. Both $t_{max,G}$ and A_G were considered constants and were derived from the literature (Table 4.3).

4.3.2 Model 2: Lehmann and Deutsch [51]

The time course of appearance in plasma of glucose after oral ingestion is determined by assuming a trapezoidal gastric emptying function, a single compartment for the intestine and first-order kinetics of intestinal glucose absorption [51]. The amount of glucose in the

Table 4.3 Parameters of Glucose Absorption Models

Model	Parameter	Unit	Value	
Hovorka et al. [50]	$t_{max,G}$	min	40	
	A_G		0.80	
Lehmann and Deutsch [51]	k_{abs}	min^{-1}	1/60	
	V_{max}	mg/min	360	
Dalla Man et al. [8,52]			*Normal*	*Type 2 diabetes*
	k_{max}	min^{-1}	0.0558	0.0465
	k_{min}	min^{-1}	0.0080	0.0076
	k_{abs}	min^{-1}	0.057	0.023
	k_{21}	min^{-1}	0.0558	0.0465
	f		0.90	0.90
	α	mg^{-1}	0.00013	0.00006
	b		0.82	0.68
	β	mg^{-1}	0.00236	0.00023
	c		0.01	0.09
Wong et al. [57]	$G_{empt,max}$	g/min	1.1	
	V_d	L/kg	0.22	
Salinari et al. [53]			*Normal*	*Type 2 diabetes*
	k	min^{-1}	2.13×10^2	3.21×10^2
	Γ^a	min^{-1}	1.83×10^2	5.09×10^2
	z_1	cm	0	
	σ_1	cm	20	
	z_2	cm	350	
	σ_2	cm	120	
	β		1.1	
	f		0.87	
	L	cm	600	
	u	cm/min	3	

[a]Instead of c, the z-averaged absorption rate coefficient Γ is reported, computed as the integral of $\gamma(z)$ divided by L.

intestine, i.e., q_{gut} (mg), following the ingestion of a meal containing D mg of glucose equivalent carbohydrates, is defined as

$$\dot{q}_{gut}(t) = - \underbrace{k_{abs}q_{gut}(t)}_{Ra} + \underbrace{G_{empt}(t)}_{\text{gastric emptying}} , \qquad (4.67)$$

where G_{empt} (mg/min) is the rate of gastric emptying and k_{abs} (min^{-1}) is the rate constant of intestinal absorption. The function G_{empt} is described by:

$$G_{empt}(t) = \begin{cases} (V_{max}/T_{asc})t, & t < T_{asc} \\ V_{max}, & T_{asc} \le t < T_{asc} + T_{max} \\ V_{max} - (V_{max}/T_{desc})(t - T_{asc} - T_{max}), & T_{asc} + T_{max} \le t < T_{asc} + T_{desc} \\ 0, & \text{otherwise} \end{cases}, \qquad (4.68)$$

where the time interval T_{max} for which the rate of gastric emptying is constant and maximum, i.e., V_{max} (mg/min), is a function of the carbohydrate content of the meal:

$$T_{max}(D) = \frac{2D - V_{max}(T_{asc} + T_{des})}{2V_{max}}, \tag{4.69}$$

whereas the time intervals T_{asc} and T_{desc} corresponding to the rising up and dropping periods, respectively, of the trapezoidal function have a default value 30 minutes. Nevertheless, in the case where D is less than the critical value of $D_{crit} = (T_{asc} + T_{desc})V_{max}/2$ (≈ 10.8g), G_{empt} is reduced to a triangular function (i.e., $T_{max} = 0$) and T_{asc} and T_{desc} are defined as

$$T_{asc}(D) = T_{desc}(D) = \frac{2D}{V_{max}}. \tag{4.70}$$

The rate of appearance of ingested glucose in plasma, i.e., Ra (mg/min), is described by the first term of (4.67):

$$Ra(t) = k_{abs}q_{gut}(t). \tag{4.71}$$

The values of the model parameters k_{abs} and V_{max} have been derived from Berger and Rodbard [55] and Guyton et al. [56] and are assumed to be patient independent (Table 4.3).

4.3.3 Model 3: Dalla Man et al. [8,52]

Dalla Man et al. [8,52] proposed a three-compartment model of Ra incorporating nonlinear dynamics of gastric emptying process and, similarly to Lehmann et al. [51], assuming a constant rate of intestinal glucose absorption.

The stomach is represented by two compartments:

$$\dot{q}_{sto1}(t) = -k_{21}q_{sto1}(t) + D\delta(t), \tag{4.72}$$

$$\dot{q}_{sto2}(t) = -k_{empt}q_{sto2}(t) + k_{21}q_{sto1}(t), \tag{4.73}$$

where q_{sto1} (mg) and q_{sto2} (mg) are the amounts of glucose in the stomach corresponding to the solid and liquid state of glucose, $\delta(t)$ is the impulse function, D (mg) is the amount of ingested glucose, k_{21} (min^{-1}) is the rate constant of grinding and k_{empt} (min^{-1}) is the rate of gastric emptying. k_{empt} is modeled as a nonlinear function of the total amount of glucose in the stomach $q_{sto} = q_{sto1} + q_{sto2}$:

$$k_{empt}(q_{sto}) = k_{min} + \frac{k_{max} - k_{min}}{2}\left\{\tanh\left[\alpha(q_{sto} - bD)\right] - \tanh\left[\beta(q_{sto} - cD)\right] + 2\right\}. \tag{4.74}$$

As is shown in Fig. 4.4, k_{empt} is initially (i.e., $q_{sto} = D$) maximum and equal to k_{max}, then it decreases to its minimum value k_{min} with rate $\alpha = 5/(2D(1 - b))$ (mg^{-1}) and returns to k_{max} with rate $\beta = 5/(2Dc)$ (mg^{-1}) at $q_{sto} = 0$, where $k_{empt} = (k_{max} - k_{min})/2$ at points bD and cD.

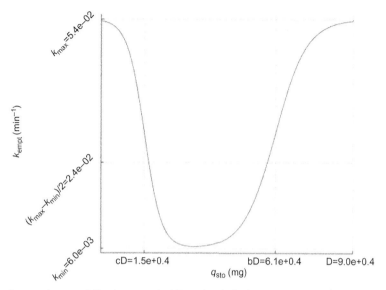

FIGURE 4.4 Gastric emptying rate following a meal of 90 g of carbohydrates as computed by the meal model 3 [52].

The intestine is represented by a single compartment and q_{gut} (mg), the glucose mass in the intestine, is given as

$$\dot{q}_{gut}(t) = -k_{abs}q_{gut}(t) + k_{empt}q_{sto2}(t) \tag{4.75}$$

Subsequently, the appearance rate of glucose in plasma Ra (mg/min/kg) is computed as

$$Ra(t) = fk_{abs}q_{gut}(t) \tag{4.76}$$

where k_{abs} (min^{-1}) is the rate constant of intestinal absorption and f is the fraction of the intestinal absorption which actually appears in plasma.

The model is a priori uniquely identifiable. It was identified and validated on Ra data, which were measured with the tracer-to-tracee ratio clamp technique during a mixed meal in normal subjects and subjects with type 2 diabetes. All parameters were estimated with good precision by constrained nonlinear least squares, after imposing $k_{21} = k_{max}$, and their values are reported in Table 4.3.

4.3.4 Model 4: Wong et al. [57]

A single compartment representing the stomach, a linear gastric emptying rate and a linear intestinal absorption rate with a maximum value $G_{empt,max}$ are the main assumptions made in [57] in order to describe Ra:

$$\dot{q}_{sto}(t) = -k_{empt}q_{sto}(t) + u_{CHO}(t), \tag{4.77}$$

$$\dot{q}_{gut}(t) = -\min(k_{abs}q_{gut}(t), k_{abs,max}) + k_{empt}q_{sto}(t), \tag{4.78}$$

$$Ra(t) = \frac{\min(k_{abs}q_{gut}(t), G_{empt,max})}{0.18(V_d bw)}, \tag{4.79}$$

where $q_{sto}(t)$ (g) and $q_{gut}(t)$ represent the mass of glucose in the stomach and the intestine, respectively, u_{CHO} is the glucose input (g/min) (i.e., meal carbohydrate content), V_d is the glucose plasma distribution volume (L/kg), and bw (kg) is the subject's body weight. The rate constants k_{empt} and k_{abs} were identified on Ra data [13], whereas $G_{empt,max}$ and V_d are considered constant and equal to 1.1 g/min and 0.22 L/kg, respectively.

4.3.5 Model 5: Salinari et al. [53]

Salinari et al. postulated a rather mechanistic model of the Ra of exogenous glucose in plasma which is mainly differentiated in the description of the transit of glucose along the intestinal lumen and the transporter-mediated absorption of luminal glucose by the enterocytes (intestinal absorptive cells) [53]. As discussed in Chapter 2, Pathophysiology and Management of Type 1 Diabetes, the release of the gastrointestinal inhibitory polypeptide (GIP) and glucagon-like peptide-1 (GLP-1) incretin hormones is associated with glucose ingestion. On this basis, Salinari et al. expressed GIP and GLP-1 kinetics in terms of the rate of intestinal glucose absorption, which was proven useful in the parameter estimation of the Ra model. In particular, their model is identified on OGTT and GLP-1 concentration data.

The small intestine is associated with a longitudinal coordinate z, measuring the distance from the pylorus ($z = 0$), and the amount of glucose in the intestinal lumen per unit length at time t is denoted by $q(z,t)$ (mmol/cm) with $q(z,0) = 0$. Assuming that glucose moves through the lumen at a constant velocity u and that glucose absorption by the enterocytes follows a first-order linear kinetics with a rate coefficient $\gamma = \gamma(z)$, a mass conservation equation for q is given by

$$\frac{\partial q}{\partial t} + u\frac{\partial q}{\partial z} = -\gamma q, \quad z \geq 0, \ t \geq 0. \tag{4.80}$$

At $z = 0$, glucose influx is taken equal to the rate of gastric emptying, i.e., $G_{empt}(t)$ (mmol/L), thus the following boundary condition is defined:

$$q(0,t) = \begin{cases} (1/u)G_{empt}(t), & 0 \leq t \leq \theta \\ 0, & t \geq \theta \end{cases}, \tag{4.81}$$

where θ is the total time required for the gastric emptying of a glucose bolus. $G_{empt}(t)$ of a glucose bolus of D mmol is computed by representing the fraction of glucose retained in the stomach at time t by a power exponential function $h(t) = \exp[-(kt)^\beta]$ [58,59]:

$$G_{empt}(t) = -D \times \frac{dh}{dt} = D\beta k^\beta t^\beta \exp\left[-(kt)^\beta\right]. \tag{4.82}$$

Finally, the solution of (4.80) is given by

$$q(z,t) = \begin{cases} q(0, t - z/u)\exp\left[-(1/u)\int_0^z \gamma(z')dz'\right], & 0 \leq t - z/u \leq \theta, z \geq 0 \\ 0, & \text{elsewhere} \end{cases}. \tag{4.83}$$

Experimental evidence suggests glucose transporters are nonuniformly distributed along the small intestine, with proximal intestine, i.e., duodenum and jejunum, accumulating higher percentages of glucose transporters compared with the distant one, i.e., ileum. To this end, two glucose transporters, a proximal and a distant one, are assumed to be present. The rate per unit length of intestinal glucose absorption and delivery to portal blood associated with the first transporter, ρ_1 (mmol/cm/min), is expressed as follows:

$$\rho_1(z, t) = F_1(z)\frac{c(z, t)}{K_{M,1} + c(z, t)} \overset{c(z,t) \ll K_{M,1}}{\cong} \frac{F_1(z)}{K_{M,1}}c(z, t) = \gamma_1(z)q(z, t), \tag{4.84}$$

where $c(z, t) = q(z, t)/A(z)$, with $A(z)$ the intestine cross-sectional area at z, the maximal rate $F_1(z)$ is nonzero for those z values where the specified transported is expressed, $K_{M,1}$ is the Michaelis–Menten constant and $\gamma_1(z) = F_1(z)/(K_{M,1}A(z))$. Similarly, $\rho_2(z, t) = \gamma_2(z)q(z, t)$ and the total transport rate, ρ, equals to

$$\rho(z, t) = \left[\gamma_1(z) + \gamma_2(z)\right]q(z, t). \tag{4.85}$$

The absorption coefficients $\gamma_1(z)$ and $\gamma_2(z)$ are modeled as piecewise constant functions or Gaussian functions. Integrating $\rho(z, t)$ over the length L of the small intestine and denoting by f the fraction of total glucose absorbed at time t that reaches the plasma, the *Ra* of exogenous glucose is given as

$$Ra(t) = f \int_0^L \gamma(z)q(z, t)dz, t \geq 0. \tag{4.86}$$

A closed form of (4.86) is obtained under the assumption of an exponential $G_{empt} = Dk\exp(-kt)$ (by setting $\beta = 1$ in (4.82)) and a constant, with respect to z, rate coefficient γ. Thus, the luminal glucose density $q(z, t)$ for $z \in [0, L]$ is simplified to

$$q(z, t) = \begin{cases} \dfrac{Dk}{u}\exp\left[-k(t - z/u)\right]\exp(-\gamma z/u), & 0 \leq t - z/u \\ 0, & \text{elsewhere} \end{cases}, \tag{4.87}$$

and, subsequently, *Ra* becomes

$$Ra(t) = \begin{cases} fD\dfrac{k\gamma}{k - \gamma}[\exp(-\gamma t) - \exp(-kt)], & 0 \leq t \leq L/u \\ fD\dfrac{k\gamma}{k - \gamma}\left[\exp\left[-k(t - L/u) - \gamma L/u\right] - \exp(-kt)\right], & t > L/u \end{cases}. \tag{4.88}$$

The OGTT minimal model [13,14], complemented with the equation of GLP-1 kinetics (described by Equation 7 in the original paper [53]), was fitted on OGGT and GLP-1 concentration data from healthy controls and patients with type 2 diabetes. Note that the absorption coefficients $\gamma_1(z)$ and $\gamma_2(z)$ were assumed normally distributed with means z_1 and z_2, standard deviations σ_1 and σ_2, and proportionality coefficients c_1 and c_2 with $c_1 = c_2/2$ and $c = c_2$. The parameters k and c were estimated from data, whereas the remaining ones (i.e., z_1, σ_1, z_2, σ_2, β, f, L, and u) were considered constants (Table 4.3). Salinari et al. reported a strong correlation between the estimated insulin sensitivity and the measured one by the euglycemic hyperinsulinemic clamp in both controls ($r = 0.929$) and patients with type 2 diabetes ($r = 0.886$).

4.4 Effect of Physical Exercise on Glucose–Insulin Dynamics

4.4.1 Model 1: Lenart and Parker [60]

The pioneer study by Lenart and Parker [60] points out the key physiological changes in glucose–insulin metabolism during exercise and further develops Sorensen's physiological model of glucose metabolism [61] to incorporate the effects of short-term moderate-intensity exercise. Starting from the quantification of exercise intensity and proceeding to a comprehensive modeling of blood flow distribution, glucose and insulin uptake and hepatic glucose production during exercise, the study by Lenart and Parker serves as a springboard to gain an understanding of the most essential aspects in exercise modeling, through the prism of an existing and well-established compartmental modeling approach.

The exercise intensity is quantified using the oxygen uptake, which is denoted by VO_2 (mL O_2/kg/min) and is expressed as a percentage of an individual's maximum rate of oxygen uptake (VO_2^{max}):

$$PVO_2^{max} = \frac{VO_2}{VO_2^{max}} \times 100\%, \tag{4.89}$$

with the average PVO_2^{max} at the basal state being equal to 8%. PVO_2^{max} during an exercise bout is estimated by the following differential equation considering that it reaches its ultimate level within 4–5 minutes after the onset of the exercise and it remains constant afterwards:

$$\frac{dPVO_2^{max}}{dt} = -\frac{5}{3}PVO_2^{max} + \frac{5}{3}ePVO_2^{max}, \tag{4.90}$$

where $ePVO_2^{max}$ is the ultimate (target) exercise intensity level. The increased oxygen and glucose requirements by the exercising muscle induce a redistribution of the blood flow through the circulatory system, with peripheral blood flow increasing with exercise intensity. Therefore, the dynamics of blood flow in individual tissues during exercise are modeled as linear functions of PVO_2^{max} using the percentage changes derived by Chapman and Mitchell [62].

The effect of exercise on peripheral glucose uptake (PGU) rate is represented by a dimensionless multiplier, M_{PGU}^E:

$$M_{PGU}^E = 1 + \frac{PGU_A \times PAMM \times 28}{35}. \tag{4.91}$$

PGU_A (mg/min/kg_{muscle}) is the active muscle peripheral glucose uptake rate and PAMM is the percentage of active muscle mass, taking the basal PGU equal to 35 mg/min and the skeletal muscle mass approximately equal to 28 kg in an average 70 kg weighted human. The glucose uptake by the adipose tissue is considered negligible. PGU_A has been shown to progressively increase with the duration of exercise and reach a steady-state plateau value (i.e., $ePGU_A$) at $t = 90$ minutes, before decreasing due to the depletion of hepatic glycogen. PGU_A dynamics for $t \leq 90$ minutes are consistently reproduced by:

$$\frac{d\text{PGU}_A}{dt} = -\frac{1}{30}\text{PGU}_A + \frac{1}{30}e\text{PGU}_A, \tag{4.92}$$

where the $ePGU_A$ value depends on the exercise intensity level ($ePGU_A = 32$ mg ($min^{-1}kg^{-1}$muscle) for 30% PVO_2^{max}; $ePGU_A = 85$ mg/min/kg_{muscle} for 60% PVO_2^{max}).

Similarly to PGU, the effect of exercise on the hepatic glucose production (HGP) rate is represented by a dimensionless multiplier, M_{HGP}^E:

$$M_{HGP}^E = 1 + \frac{\text{HGP}_A \times \text{PAMM}}{155}, \tag{4.93}$$

where HGP_A is the augmented rate of HGP, mainly by glycogenolysis, compensating for the increased glucose uptake in the exercising tissue; HGP_A is assumed to be approximately equal to PGU_A. The value of 155 mg/min corresponds to the basal HGP.

During exercise, the increased blood flow to the exercising muscle results in increased insulin uptake (PIU) by 3.4 times the basal level. Accordingly, this increase in PIU is described as a function of PAMM:

$$M_{PIU}^E = 1 + 2.4 \times \text{PAMM}. \tag{4.94}$$

As is shown in Fig. 4.5, model predictions of arterial glucose concentration are consistent with published data in the literature for exercise durations up to 90 minutes

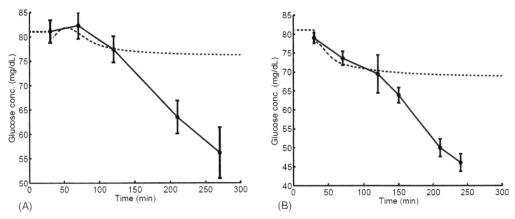

FIGURE 4.5 Published and predicted arterial glucose profiles to 2-legged exercise with a step to (A) 30% VO_2^{max} and (B) 60% VO_2^{max}, at $t = 30$ min, and a constant insulin infusion rate 24.0 mU/min [60].

($t \leq 90$ minutes). The deviation of the modified Sorensen's model output from the measured arterial glucose concentration profile for $t \leq 90$ minutes is attributed to the fact that glycogen dynamics are not included in it ($\text{HGP}_A \approx \text{PGA}_A$) [60,63].

4.4.2 Model 2: Derouich and Boutayeb [64]

The effect of physical activity on glucose–insulin dynamics was primarily introduced in Bergman's minimal model [7,10] by Derouich and Boutayeb, showing its role in improving insulin sensitivity and regulating blood glucose concentration in normal people and patients with diabetes [64]. The following model is considered:

$$\frac{dG(t)}{dt} = -(1 + q_2)X(t)G(t) + (p_1 + q_1)(G_b - G(t)) + g_{\text{inf}}(t), \tag{4.95}$$

$$\frac{dX(t)}{dt} = (p_3 + q_3)(I(t) - I_b) - p_2X(t), \tag{4.96}$$

where $G(t)$ and $I(t)$ represent the glucose and insulin concentrations in plasma, respectively, with G_b and I_b denoting their corresponding basal values and $G(0) = G_0, X(0) = X_0$, and $I(0) = I_0$, and $X(t)$ is the insulin concentration in the interstitial space. The parameters p_1, p_2, and p_3 originate from Bergman's minimal model, whereas the parameters q_1, q_2, and q_3 incorporate the effect of physical activity and increase with the intensity of exercise; in particular, q_1 and q_3 express the increment in glucose and insulin utilization, respectively, and q_2 the increment in insulin sensitivity. The perturbation term $g_{\text{inf}}(t)$, denoting the glucose infusion rate at time t, is hereon introduced to study the effect of exercise on glucose disappearance.

The behavior of the system (4.95) and (4.96) is studied at equilibrium, where we obtain

$$X^* = \frac{p_3 + q_3}{p_2}(I_e - I_b), \tag{4.97}$$

$$\begin{aligned} g_{\text{inf}}^* &= (1 + q_2)X^*G^* - (p_1 + q_1)(G_b - G^*) \\ &= \frac{(1 + q_2)(p_3 + q_3)}{p_2}(I_e - I_b)G^* - (p_1 + q_1)(G_b - G^*). \end{aligned} \tag{4.98}$$

G^* and I_e are plasma-glucose and plasma-insulin concentrations at equilibrium, respectively, and g_{inf}^* is the amount of glucose ingested such that equilibrium is maintained. Insulin sensitivity, S_{1I}, is then defined as

$$\begin{aligned} S_{1I} = \frac{\partial^2 g_{\text{inf}}^*}{\partial I_e \partial G^*} &= \frac{\partial \left(\frac{\partial g_{\text{inf}}^*}{\partial G^*} \right)}{\partial I_e} = \frac{\partial \left(\frac{(p_3 + q_3)(1 + q_2)}{p_2}(I_e - I_b) + (p_1 + q_1) \right)}{\partial I_e} \\ &= \frac{(p_3 + q_3)(1 + q_2)}{p_2}, \end{aligned} \tag{4.99}$$

which, when $q_2 = 0$ and $q_3 = 0$ (at rest), becomes:

$$S_{0I} = \frac{p_3}{p_2}.$$ (4.100)

Comparing (4.99) with (4.100), it can be observed that $S_{0I} < S_{1I}$, which corroborates the beneficial effect of physical activity on insulin sensitivity. Note that, as it is expected, the variation of g_{inf}^* with respect to G^* (i.e., $\partial g_{inf}^* / \partial G^*$) is resolved as a linear function of the increase of insulin $(I_e - I_b)$ where the constant term involves the q_1 parameter. Hence, G^* is a decreasing function of $I = I_e - I_b$:

$$G^*(I) = \frac{(p_1 + q_1)G_b + g_{inf}^*}{\dfrac{(1 + q_2)(p_3 + q_3)I}{p_2} + (p_1 + q_1)}.$$ (4.101)

The two extreme cases

$$\lim_{I \to 0} G^*(I) = G_b + \frac{g_{inf}^*}{(p_1 + q_1)},$$ (4.102)

$$\lim_{I \to \infty} G^*(I) = 0,$$ (4.103)

indicate that paucity of insulin, even when physical activity is performed, can lead to hyperglycemia and, on the contrary, excess of insulin can lead to severe hypoglycemia. Indeed, the first extreme case approximates the glycemic state of type 1 diabetes prior to the initiation of insulin therapy by considering $I_e \approx 0$ and $I_b \approx 0$ in (4.101). Similarly, the case of non-insulin dependent type 2 diabetes is approximated by considering $I_e \approx 0$ in (4.101):

$$G^*(I) = \frac{(p_1 + q_1)G_b + g_{inf}^*}{(p_1 + q_1) - \dfrac{(1 + q_2)(p_3 + q_3)I_b}{p_2}}.$$ (4.104)

Fig. 4.6 illustrates the time course of plasma-glucose concentration, and interstitial and plasma-insulin concentrations in type 1 diabetes with and without physical activity, which confirm the proper adjustment of insulin therapy and carbohydrates intake to physical activity intensity has the potential to reduce the risk of hypoglycemia during exercise.

4.4.3 Model 3: Breton [65]

Breton et al. [65] postulated a modified version of Bergman's minimal model [7,10] accounting for the effect of physical activity and in which, in contrast to [64] where only model's parameterization was augmented, the intensity of physical activity is quantified by means of an individual's heart rate (HR). Bergman's minimal model is complemented with

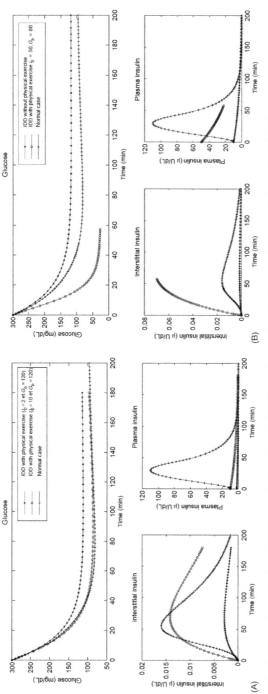

FIGURE 4.6 Effect of exercise ($q_1 = 0.0028$, $q_2 = 0.75$, and $q_3 = 0.00005$) on glucose–insulin dynamics in type 1 diabetes for (A) different initial plasma-insulin concentrations and (B) a large amount of injected insulin. *Reprinted from Derouich, M. and A. Boutayeb, The effect of physical exercise on the dynamics of glucose and insulin. J Biomech, 2002. 35(7): p. 911–917, Copyright © 2002 Elsevier Science Ltd. All rights reserved, with permission from Elsevier.*

variables Y and Z describing the increments in glucose utilization and insulin sensitivity, respectively:

$$\frac{dG(t)}{dt} = -p_1(G(t) - G_b) - (1 + \alpha Z(t))X(t)G(t) - \beta Y(t)G(t) + \frac{D}{V_G}, \tag{4.105}$$

$$\frac{dX(t)}{dt} = p_3(I(t) - I_b) - p_2 X(t), \tag{4.106}$$

$$\frac{dY(t)}{dt} = -\frac{1}{\tau_{HR}} Y(t) + \frac{1}{\tau_{HR}} (HR - HR_b), \tag{4.107}$$

$$\frac{dZ(t)}{dt} = -\left(f(Y(t)) + \frac{1}{\tau} \right) Z(t) + f(Y(t)), \tag{4.108}$$

$$f(Y(t)) = \frac{\left(\dfrac{Y(t)}{aHR_b} \right)^n}{1 + \left(\dfrac{Y(t)}{aHR_b} \right)^n}, \tag{4.109}$$

where the notation for the compartments G, X, and I is identical to that by Derouich and Boutayeb [64] and HR_b denotes the basal heart rate. Equation (4.107), with $\tau_{HR} = 5$ minutes, aims at capturing the energy expenditure variation during exercise. Equation (4.108) captures a rapid increase in Z during exercise (with a rate constant $f(Y(t)) + 1/\tau$) and a slow decrease in Z following exercise (with a rate constant $1/\tau$), where both τ and n are set such that they allow the detection of HR spikes greater or equal to 1.1 HR_b (i.e., $a = 1.1$). The model parameters reported in Table 4.4 were estimated from experimental data, by recursively minimizing a weighted least-squares function with Bayesian constraints assuring physiological validity of the estimated values; 21 patients with type 1 diabetes underwent a hyperinsulinemic−euglycemic clamp protocol including an initial euglycemic period, followed by a 15-minute exercise period at $50\%\mathrm{PVO}_2^{max}$ (maximum rate of oxygen uptake) and a 30-minute recovery period. Population values were used for the parameters of Bergman's minimal model related to plasma-insulin concentration due to the lack of such measurements during the protocol. The resulting model improved the original model's (with p_2 constrained such that $p_2 > 0.01$) weighted mean square error in predicting glucose dynamics during and after exercise from 17.7 to 7.7 mg/dL. Authors underline that hepatic glucose production (glycogenolysis or gluconeogenesis) was suppressed during the protocol precluding any modeling effort of these processes.

4.4.4 Model 4: Dalla Man et al. [66]

Dalla Man et al. [66], paralleling Breton [65], enhanced the modeling capabilities of the University of Virginia/Padova type 1 diabetes simulator [19,52]. The physical activity effect is incorporated into insulin-dependent glucose utilization, U_{id}, assuming that insulin action increases proportionally to the intensity and duration of exercise:

$$U_{id}(t) = \frac{V_{m0}(1 + \beta Y(t)) + V_{mx}(1 + \alpha Z(t)W(t))(X(t) + I_b) - V_{mx}I_b}{K_m[1 - \gamma Z(t)W(t)(X(t) + I_b)] + G_t(t)} G_t(t). \tag{4.110}$$

Table 4.4 Parameters of Exercise Models

Model	Parameter	Unit	Value
Breton [65]	G_b	mg/dL	172
	p_1	min^{-1}	4.10×10^{-3}
	p_2	min^{-1}	1.55×10^{-2}
	α		0.974
	β		3.39×10^{-4}
	V_G	dL/kg	2.028
Dalla Man et al. [66]	A		3×10^{-4}
	β	bpm^{-1}	0.01
	γ		1×10^{-7}
	α		0.1
	τ_{HR}	min	5
	τ_{in}	min	1
	τ_{ex}	min	600
	n		4
Roy and Parker [67]	a_1	mL/kg min^2	0.00158
	a_2	min^{-1}	0.056
	a_3	mL/kg min^2	0.00195
	a_4	min^{-1}	0.0485
	a_5	μU mL/min	0.00125
	a_6	min^{-1}	0.075
	k	mL/kg min^2	0.0108
	T_1	min	6

Y and f follow (4.107) and (4.109), respectively, whereas Z is modified to:

$$\frac{dZ(t)}{dt} = -\left(\frac{f(Y(t))}{\tau_{in}} + \frac{1}{\tau_{ex}}\right)Z(t) + f(Y(t)), \qquad (4.111)$$

such that the decreasing rate of Z following exercise is driven by a separate time constant $\tau_{ex} \gg \tau_{in}$ capturing the slow decay of insulin sensitivity after exercise. The intensity and duration of exercise is quantified by the area under the curve ($HR(t) - HR_b$), denoted by W:

$$W(t) = \begin{cases} \int_0^t (HR(t) - HR_b)dt, & t < t_z \\ 0, & \text{otherwise} \end{cases}, \qquad (4.112)$$

where $t_z = 3\tau_{ex}$ is the time at which $Z(t)$ returns to zero. We recall that X (pmol/L) and G_t (mg/kg) are described by (4.12) and (4.8), respectively. In summary, $V_{m0}\beta Y(t)$ represents the transient increase in insulin-independent glucose clearance, and $V_{mx}(1 + \alpha Z(t)W(t))(X(t) + I_b)$ in tandem with $K_m[1 - \gamma Z(t)W(t)(X(t) + I_b)]$ represent the so-called rapid-on/slow-off increase in insulin sensitivity.

Model predictions, using literature-derived parameters (Table 4.4), were assessed on 100 in silico subjects with type 1 diabetes under several experimental conditions combining different levels of exercise intensity (1.5 HR$_b$ and 2.0 HR$_b$) and duration (15 and 30 minutes). The model produces a reasonable glucose infusion rate under steady state conditions (during a hyperinsulinemic−euglycemic clamp protocol). Reasonable plasma-glucose concentration profiles are also obtained for the case where exercise is performed at fasting or after meal intake and insulin administration (with a carbohydrate to insulin ratio equal to 15 g/U). Nevertheless, the validity of the model needs to be in vivo demonstrated.

4.4.5 Model 5: Roy and Parker [67]

The model proposed by Roy and Parker [67] constitutes an extension of Bergmans's minimal model [7,10] including changes in glucose−insulin dynamics due to short- or long-term mild-to-moderate intensity exercise. The exercise intensity is quantified using PVO_2^{max}; however, an estimated, instead of a measured PVO_2^{max} value, is used according to:

$$\dot{PVO}_2^{max}(t) = -0.8 PVO_2^{max}(t) + 0.8 u_3(t), \tag{4.113}$$

with $PVO_2^{max}(0) = 0$ and $u_3(t)$ is the ultimate exercise intensity level above the basal level; assuming the basal level of PVO_2^{max} of an individual at rest equal to 8%, $u_3(t)$ ranges from 0% to 92%. In addition, the integrated exercise intensity, $A(t)$, is used as a measure of energy expenditure:

$$\dot{A}(t) = \begin{cases} u_3(t), & u_3(t) > 0 \\ -\dfrac{A(t)}{0.001}, & u_3(t) = 0, \end{cases} \tag{4.114}$$

where $u_3(t) = 0$ signals the end of the physical activity and the fast return of $A(t)$ to the basal level.

The effect of exercise on the rates of hepatic glycogenolysis G_{prod} (mg/min), glucose uptake G_{up} (mg/min) and insulin elimination I_e (μU/mL/min) is modeled by the following equations:

$$\dot{G}_{prod}(t) = a_1 PVO_2^{max}(t) - a_2 G_{prod}(t), \tag{4.115}$$

$$\dot{G}_{up}(t) = a_3 PVO_2^{max}(t) - a_4 G_{up}(t), \tag{4.116}$$

$$\dot{I}_e(t) = a_5 PVO_2^{max}(t) - a_6 I_e(t), \tag{4.117}$$

$$\dot{G}_{gly}(t) = \begin{cases} 0, & A(t) < A_{TH} \\ k, & A(t) \geq A_{TH} \\ -\dfrac{G_{gly}}{T_1}, & u_3(t) = 0 \end{cases}, \tag{4.118}$$

where G_{gly} accounts for the decrease in G_{prod} by a factor of k (min^{-1}) when $A(t)$ exceeds the critical threshold of A_{TH} during prolonged exercise. A_{TH} is represented as a function of $u_3(t)$ and t_{gly}, the duration of exercise at intensity $u_3(t)$ before G_{prod} starts to decrease, as follows:

$$A_{TH} = u_3(t)t_{gly}(u_3(t)) = u_3(t)(-1.1521u_3(t) + 87.481), \tag{4.119}$$

with the linear fit $t_{gly}(u_3(t)) = -1.1521u_3(t) + 87.481$ being estimated from experimental data ($R^2 = 0.991$). In (4.118), when $u_3(t) = 0$, G_{prod} increases by a factor of $\frac{G_{gly}}{T_1}$ (min^{-1}) as a result of the enhanced postexercise gluconeogenesis from lactate and the, subsequent, replenishment of hepatic glycogen. Finally, Bergman's minimal model is modified by the addition of the terms $-I_e(t)$ and $BW/V_G(G_{prod}(t) - G_{gly}(t)) - BW/V_G G_{up}(t)$ in the equations describing the plasma-glucose and insulin concentrations, respectively, where BW (kg) is the body weight of the subject and V_G ($V_G = 117.0$ dL) is the glucose distribution volume. The parameters of the exercise model were estimated from experimental data of healthy individuals using nonlinear least squares (Table 4.4); however, it was validated on data from both healthy people and people with type 1 diabetes.

The intensity of the exercise (intense walking) as recorded by the activity device over time for a typical patient is shown in Fig. 4.7A along with the simulated metabolic response of the patient (Fig. 4.7B and C). We mention that PVO$_2^{max}$ is calculated according to

$$PVO_2^{max} = \frac{VO_2}{VO_2^{max}} = \frac{3.5MET}{VO_2^{max}}, \tag{4.120}$$

where MET (kcal/kg/min) is the metabolic equivalent defined as the ratio of metabolic rate during a specific physical activity to a reference metabolic rate, set by convention to 3.5 mL O$_2$/kg/min. MET is provided by the SenseWear Armband (BodyMedia Inc.) physical activity monitor which estimates MET every 1 minute collecting physiological data at 32 Hz from the following sensors: (1) a 3-axis accelerometer, (2) a galvanic skin response sensor, (3) a heat flux sensor, and (4) an electronic thermometer. In addition, VO$_2^{max}$ is derived from reference tables. Fig. 4.7B illustrates the glucose uptake rate (G_{up}) and the hepatic glucose production rate ($G_{prod} - G_{gly}$) during and after exercise, where it can be observed that the effects of exercise progressively attenuate during the recovery period. The rate of insulin removal from plasma (I_e), as shown in Fig. 4.7C, exhibits a similar behavior.

This chapter covered the most representative paradigms of physiologically-based mathematical models regarding: (1) subcutaneously administered insulin kinetics, (2) gastric emptying and intestinal absorption kinetics of ingested glucose, and (3) the effect of exercise on endogenous glucose production and utilization. Our aim was to provide the reader with the information necessary to understand the relevant input modeling approaches which we will refer to in the following chapters. Chapter 5, Linear Time Series Models of Glucose Concentration, deals with linear dynamical models of glucose dynamics in type 1 diabetes focusing on the identification and validation of autoregressive and moving average approaches, with or without exogenous inputs.

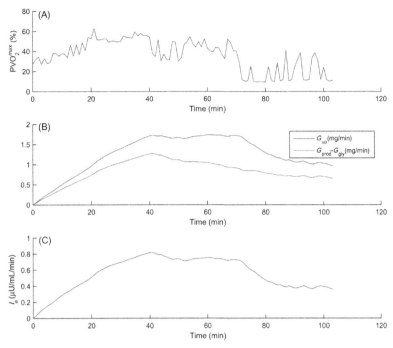

FIGURE 4.7 The effects of an exercise event on metabolism of a typical subject with type 1 diabetes. (A) Data from sensors, (B) glucose uptake and production rate as computed by the exercise model 5, (C) insulin removal rate as computed by the exercise model 5 [67].

References

[1] Cobelli C, Carson E. 5—Modeling the system. Introduction to modeling in physiology and medicine. Burlington: Academic Press; 2008. p. 75—157.

[2] Cobelli C, Carson E. 6—Model identification. Introduction to modeling in physiology and medicine. Burlington: Academic Press; 2008. p. 159—68.

[3] Cobelli C, Carson E. 7—Parametric modeling—the identifiability problem. Introduction to modeling in physiology and medicine. Burlington: Academic Press; 2008. p. 169—94.

[4] Cobelli C, Carson E. 8—Parametric models—the estimation problem. Introduction to modeling in physiology and medicine. Burlington: Academic Press; 2008. p. 195—234.

[5] Cobelli C, Carson E. 10—Model validation. Introduction to modeling in physiology and medicine. Burlington: Academic Press; 2008. p. 257—67.

[6] Cobelli C, et al. Diabetes: models, signals, and control. IEEE Rev Biomed Eng 2009;2:54—96.

[7] Bergman RN, et al. Quantitative estimation of insulin sensitivity. Am J Physiol 1979;236(6):E667—77.

[8] Dalla Man C, Rizza RA, Cobelli C. Meal simulation model of the glucose—insulin system. IEEE Trans Biomed Eng 2007;54(10):1740—9.

[9] Wilinska ME, Hovorka R. Simulation models for in-silico evaluation of closed-loop insulin delivery systems in type 1 diabetes. In: Marmarelis V, Mitsis G, editors. Data-driven modeling for diabetes: diagnosis and treatment. Berlin, Heidelberg: Springer Berlin Heidelberg; 2014. p. 131—49.

[10] Bergman RN, Phillips LS, Cobelli C. Physiologic evaluation of factors controlling glucose tolerance in man: measurement of insulin sensitivity and beta-cell glucose sensitivity from the response to intravenous glucose. J Clin Invest 1981;68(6):1456−67.

[11] Cobelli C, Caumo A, Omenetto M. Minimal model SG overestimation and SI underestimation: improved accuracy by a Bayesian two-compartment model. Am J Physiol 1999;277(3 Pt 1):E481−8.

[12] Cobelli C, et al. The oral minimal model method. Diabetes 2014;63(4):1203−13.

[13] Dalla Man C, et al. Minimal model estimation of glucose absorption and insulin sensitivity from oral test: validation with a tracer method. Am J Physiol Endocrinol Metab 2004;287(4):E637−43.

[14] Dalla Man C, et al. Insulin sensitivity by oral glucose minimal models: validation against clamp. Am J Physiol Endocrinol Metab 2005;289(6):E954−9.

[15] Vicini P, Caumo A, Cobelli C. The hot IVGTT two-compartment minimal model: indexes of glucose effectiveness and insulin sensitivity. Am J Physiol 1997;273(5 Pt 1):E1024−32.

[16] Toffolo G, Cobelli C. The hot IVGTT two-compartment minimal model: an improved version. Am J Physiol Endocrinol Metab 2003;284(2):E317−21.

[17] Ferrannini E, Cobelli C. The kinetics of insulin in man. I. General aspects. Diabetes Metab Rev 1987;3(2):335−63.

[18] Dalla Man C, et al. GIM, simulation software of meal glucose−insulin model. J Diabetes Sci Technol 2007;1(3):323−30.

[19] Kovatchev BP, et al. In silico preclinical trials: a proof of concept in closed-loop control of type 1 diabetes. J Diabetes Sci Technol 2009;3(1):44−55.

[20] Mosekilde E, et al. Modeling absorption kinetics of subcutaneous injected soluble insulin. J Pharmacokinet Biopharm 1989;17(1):67−87.

[21] Binder C, et al. Insulin pharmacokinetics. Diabetes Care 1984;7(2):188−99.

[22] Heinemann L. Variability of insulin absorption and insulin action. Diabetes Technol Ther 2002;4(5):673−82.

[23] Rasmussen CH, et al. Absorption kinetics of insulin mixtures after subcutaneous administration. In: Mosekilde E, Sosnovtseva O, Rostami-Hodjegan A, editors. Biosimulation in biomedical research, health care and drug development. Vienna: Springer Vienna; 2012. p. 329−59.

[24] Kobayashi T, et al. The pharmacokinetics of insulin after continuous subcutaneous infusion or bolus subcutaneous injection in diabetic patients. Diabetes 1983;32(4):331−6.

[25] Kraegen EW, Chisholm DJ. Insulin responses to varying profiles of subcutaneous insulin infusion: kinetic modelling studies. Diabetologia 1984;26(3):208−13.

[26] Puckett WR, Lightfoot EN. A model for multiple subcutaneous insulin injections developed from individual diabetic patient data. Am J Physiol 1995;269(6 Pt 1):E1115−24.

[27] Shimoda S, et al. Closed-loop subcutaneous insulin infusion algorithm with a short-acting insulin analog for long-term clinical application of a wearable artificial endocrine pancreas. Front Med Biol Eng 1997;8(3):197−211.

[28] Wilinska ME, et al. Insulin kinetics in type-1 diabetes: continuous and bolus delivery of rapid acting insulin. IEEE Trans Biomed Eng 2005;52(1):3−12.

[29] Wong J, et al. A subcutaneous insulin pharmacokinetic model for computer simulation in a diabetes decision support role: validation and simulation. J Diabetes Sci Technol 2008;2(4):672−80.

[30] Lv D, et al. Pharmacokinetic model of the transport of fast-acting insulin from the subcutaneous and intradermal spaces to blood. J Diabetes Sci Technol 2015;9(4):831−40.

[31] Wach P, et al. Numerical approximation of mathematical model for absorption of subcutaneously injected insulin. Med Biol Eng Comput 1995;33(1):18−23.

[32] Trajanoski Z, et al. Pharmacokinetic model for the absorption of subcutaneously injected soluble insulin and monomeric insulin analogues. Biomed Tech (Berl) 1993;38(9):224−31.

[33] Tarin C, et al. Comprehensive pharmacokinetic model of insulin Glargine and other insulin formulations. IEEE Trans Biomed Eng 2005;52(12):1994–2005.

[34] Soeborg T, et al. Absorption kinetics of insulin after subcutaneous administration. Eur J Pharm Sci 2009;36(1):78–90.

[35] Li J, Johnson JD. Mathematical models of subcutaneous injection of insulin analogues: a mini-review. Discrete Continuous Dyn Syst Ser B 2009;12(2):401–14.

[36] Li J, Kuang Y. Systemically modeling the dynamics of plasma insulin in subcutaneous injection of insulin analogues for type 1 diabetes. Math Biosci Eng 2009;6(1):41–58.

[37] Nucci G, Cobelli C. Models of subcutaneous insulin kinetics. A critical review. Comput Methods Progr Biomed 2000;62(3):249–57.

[38] Hovorka R, et al. Five-compartment model of insulin kinetics and its use to investigate action of chloroquine in NIDDM. Am J Physiol 1993;265(1 Pt 1):E162–75.

[39] Kurtzhals P, Ribel U. Action profile of cobalt(III)-insulin. A novel principle of protraction of potential use for basal insulin delivery. Diabetes 1995;44(12):1381–5.

[40] Mosekilde E, Sosnovtseva OV, Holstein-Rathlou NH. Mechanism-based modeling of complex biomedical systems. Basic Clin Pharmacol Toxicol 2005;96(3):212–24.

[41] Kang S, et al. Subcutaneous insulin absorption explained by insulin's physicochemical properties. Evidence from absorption studies of soluble human insulin and insulin analogues in humans. Diabetes Care 1991;14(11):942–8.

[42] Robertson DA, et al. Metabolic effects of monomeric insulin analogues of different receptor affinity. Diabet Med 1992;9(3):240–6.

[43] Lepore M, et al. Pharmacokinetics and pharmacodynamics of subcutaneous injection of long-acting human insulin analog glargine, NPH insulin, and ultralente human insulin and continuous subcutaneous infusion of insulin lispro. Diabetes 2000;49(12):2142–8.

[44] Cobelli C, et al. An integrated mathematical-model of the dynamics of blood-glucose and its hormonal-control. Math Biosci 1982;58(1):27–60.

[45] Saccomani MP, et al. Chapter 4—A priori identifiability of physiological parametric models. Modeling methodology for physiology and medicine. San Diego: Academic Press; 2001. p. 77–105.

[46] Steimer JL, et al. Alternative approaches to estimation of population pharmacokinetic parameters: comparison with the nonlinear mixed-effect model. Drug Metab Rev 1984;15(1–2):265–92.

[47] Hovorka R, Hovorka R, Vicini P. Chapter 5—Parameter estimation A2—Carson, Ewart. In: Cobelli C, editor. Modeling methodology for physiology and medicine. San Diego: Academic Press; 2001. p. 107–51.

[48] Carson ER, Cobelli C, Finkelstein L. The mathematical modeling of metabolic and endocrine systems: model formulation, identification, and validation. New York: J. Wiley; 1983.

[49] Schwarz G. Estimating the dimension of a model. Ann. Statist. 1978;6(2):461–4.

[50] Hovorka R, et al. Nonlinear model predictive control of glucose concentration in subjects with type 1 diabetes. Physiol Meas 2004;25(4):905–20.

[51] Lehmann ED, Deutsch T. A physiological model of glucose–insulin interaction in type 1 diabetes mellitus. J Biomed Eng 1992;14(3):235–42.

[52] Dalla Man C, Camilleri M, Cobelli C. A system model of oral glucose absorption: validation on gold standard data. IEEE Trans Biomed Eng 2006;53(12 Pt 1):2472–8.

[53] Salinari S, Bertuzzi A, Mingrone G. Intestinal transit of a glucose bolus and incretin kinetics: a mathematical model with application to the oral glucose tolerance test. Am J Physiol Endocrinol Metab 2011;300(6):E955–65.

[54] Herrero P, et al. A simple robust method for estimating the glucose rate of appearance from mixed meals. J Diabetes Sci Technol 2012;6(1):153–62.

[55] Berger M, Rodbard D. Computer simulation of plasma insulin and glucose dynamics after subcutaneous insulin injection. Diabetes Care 1989;12(10):725−36.

[56] Guyton JR, et al. A model of glucose−insulin homeostasis in man that incorporates the heterogeneous fast pool theory of pancreatic insulin release. Diabetes 1978;27(10):1027−42.

[57] Wong XW, et al. Development of a clinical type 1 diabetes metabolic system model and in silico simulation tool. J Diabetes Sci Technol 2008;2(3):424−35.

[58] Elashoff JD, Reedy TJ, Meyer JH. Analysis of gastric emptying data. Gastroenterology 1982;83 (6):1306−12.

[59] Schirra J, et al. Gastric emptying and release of incretin hormones after glucose ingestion in humans. J Clin Invest 1996;97(1):92−103.

[60] Lenart PJ, Parker RS. Modeling exercise effects in type I diabetic patients. IFAC Proc Vol 2002;35 (1):247−52.

[61] Parker RS, et al. Robust $H\infty$ glucose control in diabetes using a physiological model. AIChE J 2000;46 (12):2537−49.

[62] Chapman CB, Mitchell JH. The physiology of exercise. Sci Am 1965;212:88−96.

[63] Hernandez-Ordonez M, Campos-Delgado DU. An extension to the compartmental model of type 1 diabetic patients to reproduce exercise periods with glycogen depletion and replenishment. J Biomech 2008;41(4):744−52.

[64] Derouich M, Boutayeb A. The effect of physical exercise on the dynamics of glucose and insulin. J Biomech 2002;35(7):911−17.

[65] Breton MD. Physical activity—the major unaccounted impediment to closed loop control. J Diab Sci Technol (Online) 2008;2(1):169−74.

[66] Man CD, Breton MD, Cobelli C. Physical activity into the meal glucose−insulin model of type 1 diabetes: in silico studies. J Diabetes Sci Technol 2009;3(1):56−67.

[67] Roy A, Parker RS. Dynamic modeling of exercise effects on plasma glucose and insulin levels. J Diabetes Sci Technol 2007;1(3):338−47.

Linear Time Series Models of Glucose Concentration

5.1 Generalized Model Structure of a Linear Time-Invariant System

A time-invariant linear causal single-input–single-output (SISO) system subject to an additive random disturbance v, as we have seen in Chapter 3, Methodology for Developing a Glucose Prediction Model, is represented by the parameterized, with respect to $\theta \in R^m$, transfer functions $G(q, \theta)$, and $H(q, \theta)$ such that:

$$y(t) = G(q, \theta)u(t) + H(q, \theta)\varepsilon(t), \tag{5.1}$$

$$G(q, \theta) = \sum_{n=1}^{\infty} g_n(\theta)q^{-n}, \tag{5.2}$$

$$H(q, \theta) = 1 + \sum_{n=1}^{\infty} h_n(\theta)q^{-n}, \tag{5.3}$$

where u is the system's input, y is the system's output, and $\{\varepsilon(t)\}$ is a sequence of independent random variables with zero mean and finite variance λ (white noise process) [1]. Provided that transfer functions $G(q)$ and $H(q)$ are stable (i.e., $\sum_{n=1}^{\infty} |g_n(\theta)| < \infty$ and $\sum_{n=0}^{\infty} |h_n(\theta)| < \infty$) and $u(t)$ is a quasistationary signal with spectrum $\Phi_u(t)$, the characteristics of (5.1) in the frequency domain are described by (1) the complex-valued function $G(e^{i\omega})$, with $-\pi \leq \omega \leq \pi$, denoting the frequency response of the system $G(q)u(t)$ and (2) the function $\lambda|H(e^{i\omega})|^2$, with $-\pi \leq \omega \leq \pi$, denoting the spectrum $\Phi_v(\omega)$ of the stochastic process $v(t) = H(q)\varepsilon(t)$ [1]. Frequency-domain expressions pertaining to (5.1) are widely covered in [1].

Given $y(s)$, $u(s)$, and $v(s)$ for $s \leq t - 1$, the one-step-ahead prediction $\hat{y}(t|\theta)$ of $y(t)$ is computed as follows:

$$\hat{y}(t|\theta) = H^{-1}(q, \theta)G(q, \theta)u(t) + \left(1 - H^{-1}(q, \theta)\right)y(t), \tag{5.4}$$

where the filter $H^{-1}(q, \theta) = 1/H(q, \theta) = \sum_{n=1}^{\infty} \tilde{h}_n(\theta)q^{-n}$ is assumed to be stable (i.e., $\sum_{n=0}^{\infty} |\tilde{h}_n(\theta)| < \infty$). The corresponding prediction error is

$$e(t) = y(t) - \hat{y}(t|\theta) = -H^{-1}(q, \theta)G(q, \theta)u(t) + H^{-1}(q, \theta)y(t). \tag{5.5}$$

Personalized Predictive Modeling in Type 1 Diabetes. DOI: http://dx.doi.org/10.1016/B978-0-12-804831-3.00005-4

Similarly, should $y(s)$ and $u(s')$ are known for $s \leq t - k$ and $s' \leq t - 1$, respectively, the k-step-ahead prediction of $y(t)$ is

$$\hat{y}(t|\theta) = \overline{H}_k(q, \theta)H^{-1}(q, \theta)G(q, \theta)u(t) + \left(1 - \overline{H}_k(q, \theta)H^{-1}(q, \theta)\right)y(t), \qquad (5.6)$$

where $\overline{H}_k(q, \theta)$ is a polynomial of q^{-1} of order $k - 1$ defined as $\overline{H}_k(q, \theta) = \sum_{n=0}^{k-1} h_n(\theta)q^{-n}$, whereas the prediction error is a moving average (MA) process of $e(t)$:

$$e_k(t) = y(t) - \hat{y}(t|\theta) = \overline{H}_k(q, \theta)e(t). \qquad (5.7)$$

Eq. (5.1) resolves into (5.8) when G and H are considered rational functions of q^{-1}:

$$A(q)y(t) = \frac{B(q)}{F(q)}u(t) + \frac{C(q)}{D(q)}\varepsilon(t), \qquad (5.8)$$

where $A(q)$, $B(q)$, $C(q)$, $D(q)$, and $F(q)$ are polynomials of the backward shift operator q^{-1} (i.e., $q^{-1}y(t) = y(t - 1)$) of order n_a, n_b, n_c, n_d, and n_f, respectively, and their coefficients form the model parameters $\theta \in R^m$ (Fig. 5.1A). Accordingly, the one-step-ahead prediction rule becomes

$$\hat{y}(t|\theta) = \frac{D(q)B(q)}{C(q)F(q)}u(t) + \left(1 - \frac{D(q)A(q)}{C(q)}\right)y(t). \qquad (5.9)$$

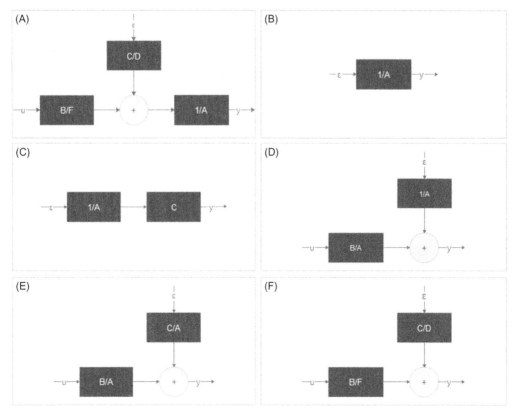

FIGURE 5.1 (A) General transfer function model, (B) AR model, (C) ARMA model, (D) ARX model, (E) ARMAX model, (F) BJ model.

An innate delay of n_u samples, before the effect of u on y is observed, can be incorporated in the numerator of G in (5.8) which, given that $\overline{B}(q)$ is a polynomial of q^{-1} of order $n_b - 1$, becomes $q^{-n_u}\overline{B}(q)$.

5.1.1 Training and Evaluation

Linear model selection, estimation, and validation follow the principles provided in Chapter 3, Methodology for Developing a Glucose Prediction Model. A sequence of steps for the identification of a general transfer function model (GTFM), as it is defined by (5.8), is suggested in Table 5.1. The identification of models in (5.8) form consists in learning the coefficients of the polynomials $A(q)$, $B(q)$, $C(q)$, $D(q)$, and $F(q)$ by least squares, according to which, as it has been described in Chapter 3, Methodology for Developing a Glucose Prediction Model, the error function $E(\theta)$ is defined in terms of the residual sum of squares $\sum_{i=1}^{N_{Z_{train}}} e_i^2 = \sum_{i=1}^{N_{Z_{train}}} (y(t_i) - \hat{y}(t_i|\theta))^2$ associated with a training set Z_{train} of size $N_{Z_{train}}$. Regularized least squares is typically employed as a means of controlling the values of the parameters and, in turn, balancing the bias and the variance of the model. The order of polynomials is typically determined via K-fold cross-validation on Z_{train} or based on the Akaike information criterion (AIC) [2], the corrected AIC (AICc) [3,4] or the Bayesian information criterion (BIC) [or minimum description length (MDL)] [5,6]. The hyperparameter set can be expanded by adding input delays; however, input delays can be determined prior to model identification by exploiting *a priori* knowledge or by exploring the dataset (e.g., nonparametric estimation of the impulse responses). It should be noted that regularization avoids specifying model hyperparameters (i.e., n_a, n_b, n_c, n_d, and n_f). In addition, an external cross-validation may be applied to reduce the bias in error estimation.

Table 5.1 Training and Evaluation Procedure of a General Transfer Function Model

Input: Z_{train}, Z_{test}

Model selection:

(1) Optimize hyperparameters n_a, n_b, n_c, n_d, and n_f by:

   (a) K-fold cross-validation on Z_{train}, or

   (b) information criteria evaluation (i.e., AIC, AICc, BIC, or MDL) on a validation set Z_{val}.

Linear system identification:

(2) Compute $A(q)$, $B(q)$, $C(q)$, $D(q)$, and $F(q)$ by least squares or regularized least squares on Z_{train}:

$$E(\theta) = \sum_{i=1}^{N_{Z_{train}}} e_i^2 = \sum_{i=1}^{N_{Z_{train}}} (y(t_i) - \hat{y}(t_i|\theta))^2$$

$$\theta = \left[a_1, \ldots, a_{n_a}, b_1, \ldots, b_{n_b}, c_1, \ldots, c_{n_c}, d_1, \ldots, d_{n_d}, f_1, \ldots, f_{n_f},\right]^T$$

(3) Compute 1-step-ahead (5.4) and k-step-ahead (5.6) prediction models.

Model evaluation:

(4) Evaluate goodness-of-fit on Z_{test} by:

   (a) Error measures (e.g., RMSE, FIT%, J)

   (b) Whiteness of residuals

   (c) Comparison of $G(e^{j\omega})$ and $\lambda|H(e^{j\omega})|^2$ with their nonparametric estimates.

Output: $A(q)$, $B(q)$, $C(q)$, $D(q)$, and $F(q)$

All statistical measures and procedures reported in Section 3.4 can be employed to assess the performance of linear models on the test set Z_{test}. In this chapter, we provide two additional measures which are utilized in the related literature, namely the percentage of FIT and the percentage of the variance accounted for:

$$\text{FIT} = \left(1 - \frac{\|y - \hat{y}\|_2}{\|y - \bar{y}\|_2}\right) \times 100\%, \tag{5.10}$$

$$\text{VAF} = \left(1 - \frac{Var(y - \hat{y})}{Var(y)}\right) \times 100\%, \tag{5.11}$$

where $\bar{y}$ is the average value of y. The realization of the output's disturbance as a stationary stochastic process, which is independent of the system's input, further imposes that the autocorrelation of residuals and the covariance between the residuals and past inputs should not be significant. In addition, the comparison of the Bode diagram of the linear model's frequency response ($G(e^{i\omega})$) and its noise spectrum ($\lambda |H(e^{i\omega})|^2$) with their nonparametric estimates (i.e., Blackman–Tuckey approach [1]), in tandem with the evaluation of the physiological validity of the estimated parameters and their variances, can reveal the consistency of model behavior.

5.2 Autoregressive and Moving Average Models

5.2.1 Basic Concepts of Autoregressive and Moving Average Models

Autoregressive (AR) and ARMA models have provided a linear framework to the approximation of the dynamics of the glucose system in both type 1 and type 2 diabetes. The subcutaneous (s.c.) glucose concentration time series $y(t)$ is considered a stationary process subject to an additive random disturbance $v(t)$. In the absence of the system's input u, the generalized model structure of a time-invariant linear causal SISO system is reduced to

$$A(q)y(t) = \frac{C(q)}{D(q)}\varepsilon(t), \tag{5.12}$$

where $A(q)$, $C(q)$, and $D(q)$ are polynomials of q^{-1}, and $\varepsilon(t)$ is a white noise process.

As it is illustrated in Fig. 5.1B, AR models consider $C(q) = D(q) = 1$ and system's output $y(t)$ is modeled as

$$A(q)y(t) = \varepsilon(t) \Rightarrow y(t) = \frac{1}{A(q)}\varepsilon(t), \tag{5.13}$$

where $A(q) = 1 + a_1 q^{-1} + \cdots + a_{n_a} q^{-n_a}$, and n_a is the AR model order. In accordance with (5.1), the transfer function of $v(t)$ equals

$$H(q, \theta) = \frac{1}{A(q)}, \tag{5.14}$$

and the parameter vector $\theta \in R^m$ equals $\theta = [a_1, \ldots, a_{n_a}]^T$. Therefore, based on (5.9), the one-step-ahead prediction of $y(t)$ constitutes a linear combination of previous glucose samples:

$$\hat{y}(t|\theta) = (1 - A(q))y(t) = -\sum_{l=1}^{n_a} a_l q^{-l} y(t). \tag{5.15}$$

In the case where $D(q) = 1$, $y(t)$ is modeled as an ARMA process:

$$A(q)y(t) = C(q)\varepsilon(t) \Rightarrow y(t) = \frac{C(q)}{A(q)}\varepsilon(t), \tag{5.16}$$

with $A(q) = 1 + a_1 q^{-1} + \cdots + a_{n_a} q^{-n_a}$, $C(q) = 1 + c_1 q^{-1} + \cdots + c_{n_c} q^{-n_c}$, n_a representing the AR model order, and n_c representing the MA model order. The transfer function of the ARMA process, $H(q, \theta)$, is given in terms of the transfer function $1/A(q)$ of the AR model and the transfer function $C(q)$ of the MA model:

$$H(q, \theta) = \frac{C(q)}{A(q)}, \tag{5.17}$$

where $\theta = [a_1, \ldots, a_{n_a}, c_1, \ldots, c_{n_c}]^T$ (Fig. 5.1C). The corresponding, one-step-ahead prediction of $y(t)$ is given by

$$\hat{y}(t|\theta) = \left(1 - \frac{A(q)}{C(q)}\right)y(t). \tag{5.18}$$

In both AR and ARMA models, the k-step-ahead prediction of $y(t)$ is computed by

$$\hat{y}(t|\theta) = \left(1 - \overline{H}_k(q, \theta)H^{-1}(q, \theta)\right)y(t), \tag{5.19}$$

supposing that we have observed $y(s)$ for $s \leq t - k$.

5.2.2 Glucose Prediction Applications

Table 5.2 presents the main studies proposing AR models of the s.c. glucose concentration in people with diabetes, which were identified by prediction error methods (PEM) and were evaluated by different statistical measures and for different values of prediction horizon [7−9].

Gani et al. [7] proposed an AR model of order 30, AR(30), which parameters were obtained through regularized least squares on smoothed continuous glucose monitoring (CGM) data. The Tikhonov approach was applied both for smoothing the raw CGM data as well as for regularizing the parameter estimates, whereas the order of the model was selected through crossvalidation. The quality of predictions was assessed through: (1) the root mean squared error (RMSE) between the predicted and the smoothed glucose signal and (2) the time lag corresponding to the maximum of the crosscorrelation function between the

Table 5.2 Studies Employing AR Models to Short-Term Prediction of Subcutaneous Glucose Concentration in Diabetes

Study	Model	Prediction Horizon	Evaluation Measures	Dataset	Prediction Performance
Gani et al. [7]	Ordinary least squares or regularized AR(30)	30, 60, 90 min	RMSE Time lag	Nine people with type 1 diabetes [10] CGM Device: iSense, iSense Corp. Sampling Interval: 1 min Monitoring Period: 5 days	*RMSE* 30 min: 0.1 ± 0.02 mmol/L 60 min: 0.7 ± 0.1 mmol/L 90 min: 1.6 ± 0.2 mmol/L	*Time lag* 30 min: 0.2 ± 0.4 min 60 min: 12.3 ± 2.8 min 90 min: 38.4 ± 5.2 min
Gani et al. [8]	Regularized AR(30)	30 min	RMSEClarke error grid analysis	Study 1 Nine people with type 1 diabetes [10] CGM device: iSense, iSense Corp. Monitoring period: 5 days Sampling interval: 1 min	Same-subject *RMSE* 30 min: 0.17 ± 0.02 mmol/L *Time lag* 30 min: 0.6 ± 1.7 min *Clarke EGA—Zone A:* 30 min: 99.0%	Cross-subject *RMSE* 30 min: 0.18 ± 0.03 mmol/L *Time lag* 30 min: 0.3 ± 1.2 min	Cross-study *RMSE* 30 min: 0.17 ± 0.03 mmol/L *Time lag* 30 min: 0.4 ± 1.4 min
				Study 2 Study 2: 18 children with type 1 diabetes CGM device: Guardian RT, Medronic Inc. Sampling interval: 5 min Monitoring period: 6 days	Same-subject *RMSE* 30 min: 0.21 ± 0.06 mmol/L *Time lag* 30 min: 0.0 ± 0.0 min *Clarke EGA—Zone A:* 30 min: 99.3%	Cross-subject *RMSE* 30 min: 0.21 ± 0.07 mmol/L *Time lag* 30 min: 0.1 ± 0.8 min	Cross-study *RMSE* 30 min: 0.22 ± 0.08 mmol/L *Time lag* 30 min: 0.2 ± 1.0 min
				Study 3 Study 3: 7 people with type 2 diabetes CGM device: Dexcom, Dexcom Inc. Sampling interval: 5 min Monitoring period: 56 days	Same-subject *RMSE* 30 min: 0.16 ± 0.03 mmol/L *Time lag* 30 min: 0.0 ± 0.0 min *Clarke EGA—Zone A:* 30 min: 99.5%	Cross-subject *RMSE* 30 min: 0.16 ± 0.03 mmol/L *Time lag* 30 min: 0.0 ± 0.0 min	Cross-study *RMSE* 30 min: 0.17 ± 0.03 mmol/L *Time lag* 30 min: 0.0 ± 0.0 min
Lu et al. [9]	Regularized AR(30)	0:5:50 min	RMSE	Nine people with type 1 diabetes [8] CGM device: iSense, iSense Corp Sampling interval: 1 min Monitoring period: 5 days			

predicted and the smoothed glucose signal. The dataset comprised nine subjects with type 1 diabetes which were monitored over 5 days. The training and test set were each comprised of 2000 samples, where the sampling interval of CGM measurements was $T = 1$ min. Moreover, the stationarity of the glucose time series was verified before the analysis. The estimated AR coefficients of the derived AR model reflected the temporal behavior of the autocorrelation function of the glucose signal, leading to stable accurate 30-minutes predictions with negligible RMSE (0.1 ± 0.02 mmol/L) and time lags (0.2 ± 0.4 minutes). The prediction accuracy decreased with increasing prediction horizon, with prediction horizons of 60 and 90 minutes being associated with higher errors (0.7 ± 0.1 mmol/L and 1.6 ± 0.2 mmol/L, respectively) and clinically acceptable time lags (12.3 ± 2.8 and 38.4 ± 5.2 minutes, respectively). Gani et al. demonstrated, additionally, that deriving AR models directly from raw CGM data yields unphysiologic AR parameters and stable predictions which time lags, however, equal to the prediction horizon, presumably, due to the high-frequency noise not allowing the identification of any but the first AR parameter. Smoothing of raw CGM data without regularizing AR parameters resulted also in parameters exhibiting an inconsistent, oscillatory behavior (with their values not gradually decreasing as the parameter index increases), and accurate, though, highly unstable predictions when white noise was added.

In a subsequent study [8], Gani et al. proved that a regularized AR(30) model trained on smoothed CGM glucose data can serve as a universal, individual-independent predictive model of short-term (30 minutes or less) dynamics of s.c. glucose concentration regardless of diabetes type, CGM device, and interindividual differences. The same-subject, cross-subject, and cross-study predictions were identical in terms of the RMSE, with Clarke error grid analysis (EGA) results corroborating their high accuracy. The analysis of the power spectrum density (PSD) of the glucose concentration signals of people with type 1 or type 2 diabetes, coming from three different studies, showed the four frequency bands, as characterized by Rahaghi et al. [11], are retained across different individuals. In addition to this, the invariance of the AR parameters on a periodic signal's (as s.c. glucose concentration) amplitude and phase, and their sole dependency on its frequency contributes to the similarity of the AR models. Nevertheless, the need for filtering out the high-frequency dynamics (with periods <60 minutes) in the glucose signal and regularizing the AR fitting method was stressed for obtaining physiologically plausible AR parameters and robust models.

Lu et al. [9] investigated the predictive capacity of the frequency bands of the s.c. glucose signal, which resemble those of the blood glucose signal [11], in AR modeling of the short-term glucose dynamics in type 1 diabetes. Four bandpass filters were developed, where each band is characterized by the periodicity of glucose signal's oscillations (Band I: 5−15 minutes, Band II: 60−120 minutes, Band III: 150−500 minutes, Band IV: ≥700 minutes). Of note, the high-frequency band, i.e., Band I, which is associated with rapid pulsatile insulin secretion by pancreatic β-cells in healthy individuals, is devoid of any significant physiological information in the case of type 1 diabetes and, should be treated as noise [12,13]. In addition, multibandpass filters were developed for each of the three pairwise combinations of the Bands II−IV. The same training and testing AR configuration as in [7] was applied in each of the bands, whereas, for comparison purposes, a reference AR model was developed using the overall spectrum of the glucose signal except Band I. First, Lu et al. showed that Bands III and IV account for the majority of the s.c. glucose signal's PSD, whereas $\sim 1.5\%$ and $\sim 0.6\%$ of PSD fall into Band II and Band I, respectively. As expected, the PSDs estimated by the sub band AR models were less resolved than those obtained from the raw glucose signal. Comparing the predictive capacity of the developed sub band AR models, the authors showed that: (1) the reference AR model yielded the smallest RMSE across the 0−50 minutes prediction horizons, capturing the entire frequency information of the s.c. glucose concentration signal, (2) the AR models concerning the medium-frequency dynamics (Band II or Band III) resulted in negligible RMSEs (<3 mg/dL) and exhibited comparable performance to the reference model for prediction horizons <25 minutes, (3) Band III models outperformed Band II models for longer prediction horizons (25−50 minutes), (4) Band IV model, which had systematically inferior performance for horizons <40 minutes, outperformed Band II and III models for prediction horizons >45 minutes, and (5) models combining Band II, with either Band III or Band IV, were compared well with the reference model over the 0−50 prediction horizon range and outperformed each of the models based on a single band; the latter is rational considering that Band II represents the glucose dynamics in response to meal intake and insulin injections. The utmost conclusion of Lu et al. study was that the need to explicitly represent and model exogenous inputs for short-term (0−50 minutes) glucose concentration predictions is obviated as long as Bands II, III, and IV are captured by an AR model.

5.3 Autoregressive and Moving Average Models with Extra Inputs

5.3.1 Basic Concepts of Autoregressive and Moving Average Models with Extra Inputs

The AR with extra inputs (ARX) models, the ARMA with extra inputs (ARMAX) models, and the Box−Jenkins (BJ) models, which has been extensively applied in glucose predictive modeling, derive from (5.8) by properly setting some of the polynomials $A(q)$, $B(q)$, $C(q)$, $D(q)$, or $F(q)$ equal to one.

5.3.1.1 ARX Models
An ARX model is defined as

$$A(q)y(t) = B(q)u(t) + \varepsilon(t) \Rightarrow y(t) = \frac{B(q)}{A(q)}u(t) + \frac{1}{A(q)}\varepsilon(t), \tag{5.20}$$

having set $C(q) = D(q) = F(q) = 1$, with $A(q) = 1 + a_1 q^{-1} + \cdots + a_{n_a}q^{-n_a}$, $B(q) = b_1 q^{-1} + \cdots + b_{n_b}q^{-n_b}$. As it is shown in Fig. 5.1D, the transfer functions of the system are

$$G(q, \theta) = \frac{B(q)}{A(q)}$$

$$H(q, \theta) = \frac{1}{A(q)},$$

(5.21)

and $\theta = [a_1, \ldots, a_{n_a}, b_1, \ldots, b_{n_b}]^T$. In line with (5.9), we can obtain

$$\begin{aligned}\hat{y}(t|\theta) &= B(q)u(t) + (1 - A(q))y(t) \\ &= b_1 u(t-1) + \cdots + b_{n_b} u(t-n_b) - a_1 y(t-1) - \cdots - a_{n_a} y(t-n_a) = \theta^T \phi(t)\end{aligned}$$

(5.22)

where $\phi(t) = [u(t-1), \ldots, u(t-n_b), -y(t-1), \ldots, -y(t-n_a)]^T$. It is obvious that an ARX model is equivalent to a linear regression model of the form (3.13), which means that ordinary or regularized least squares methods can be applied to the estimation of model parameters θ.

5.3.1.2 ARMAX Models
ARMAX models derive from (5.8) by setting $D(q) = F(q) = 1$:

$$A(q)y(t) = B(q)u(t) + C(q)\varepsilon(t) \Rightarrow y(t) = \frac{B(q)}{A(q)}u(t) + \frac{C(q)}{A(q)}\varepsilon(t),$$

(5.23)

with $A(q) = 1 + a_1 q^{-1} + \cdots + a_{n_a} q^{-n_a}$, $B(q) = b_1 q^{-1} + \cdots + b_{n_b} q^{-n_b}$, and $C(q) = 1 + c_1 q^{-1} + \cdots + c_{n_c} q^{-n_c}$. We can see that system disturbances are modeled as an MA process of white noise, with the transfer functions of the system being

$$G(q, \theta) = \frac{B(q)}{A(q)}$$

$$H(q, \theta) = \frac{C(q)}{A(q)},$$

(5.24)

and $\theta = [a_1, \ldots, a_{n_a}, b_1, \ldots, b_{n_b}, c_1, \ldots, c_{n_c}]^T$ (Fig. 5.1E). Correspondingly, the one-step-ahead prediction rule is given by

$$\hat{y}(t|\theta) = \frac{B(q)}{C(q)}u(t) + \left(1 - \frac{A(q)}{C(q)}\right)y(t).$$

(5.25)

5.3.1.3 Box–Jenkins Models
The BJ model is derived from (5.8) by setting $A(q) = 1$:

$$y(t) = \frac{B(q)}{F(q)}u(t) + \frac{C(q)}{D(q)}\varepsilon(t),$$

(5.26)

with $B(q) = b_1 q^{-1} + \cdots + b_{n_b} q^{-n_b}$, $C(q) = 1 + c_1 q^{-1} + \cdots + c_{n_c} q^{-n_c}$, $D(q) = 1 + d_1 q^{-1} + \cdots + d_{n_d} q^{-n_d}$, and $F(q) = 1 + f_1 q^{-1} + \cdots + f_{n_f} q^{-n_f}$. Unlike ARX and ARMAX models, the transfer functions G and H are expressed independently of the polynomial $A(q)$:

$$G(q, \theta) = \frac{B(q)}{F(q)}$$
$$H(q, \theta) = \frac{C(q)}{D(q)}, \tag{5.27}$$

with $\theta = [b_1, \ldots, b_{n_b}, c_1, \ldots, c_{n_c}, d_1, \ldots, d_{n_d}, f_1, \ldots, f_{n_f},]^T$ (Fig. 5.1F), and, following (5.9) the one-step-ahead prediction rule becomes

$$\hat{y}(t|\theta) = \frac{D(q)B(q)}{C(q)F(q)} u(t) + \left(1 - \frac{D(q)}{C(q)}\right) y(t). \tag{5.28}$$

5.3.2 Glucose Prediction Applications

Table 5.3 presents the state-of-the-art studies which employ linear time-invariant models with extra inputs to predict short-term s.c. glucose dynamics. In Stahl et al. [14], a number of linear system identification models, i.e., ARMA, ARMAX, and GTFM, were evaluated on interpolated blood glucose concentration values aiming at providing reasonably accurate 2-h-ahead predictions. Data were collected from one subject with type 1 diabetes during ambulatory conditions, with the first week of data comprising the training set and the second week of data comprising the test set. Compartmental modeling of the insulin (Input 1) and glucose (Input 2) fluxes formed the main exogenous inputs to the system. Though an ARMA model of order $n_a = 6$ and $n_c = 1$ [ARMA(6,1)], as specified by both the AIC and the MDL criteria, resulted in uncorrelated residuals and an almost perfect FIT% of 99.7% for one-step-ahead predictions (corresponding to 15 minutes), its performance worsened to 56.15% for eight-step-ahead predictions (corresponding to 2 hours). An ARMAX model of order $n_a = 6$, $n_{b1} = 2$, $n_{b2} = 1$, and $n_c = 1$ [ARMAX(6,2,1,1)] induced correlated residuals and a slight improvement of the FIT% to 59.11%, as compared with the ARMA(6,1) model. The separation of system dynamics by a GTFM model of order $n_a = 5$, $n_{b1} = 2$, $n_{b2} = 3$, $n_{f1} = 1$, $n_{f2} = 1$, $n_c = 3$, and $n_d = 2$ [GTFM (5,2,3,1,1,3,2)] did reduce the autocorrelation of the residuals and increased the predictive capacity of 2-h-ahead predictions to 60.83%. However, the spectral coherence between the input and output variables indicated the presence of nonlinear system dynamics and, potentially, unrepresented inputs and unmeasured disturbances.

Proper input excitation, as captured by the insulin-to-carbohydrate ratio (ICR), was linked with the generalization capability of ARX, ARMAX, and BJ models in a simulation study by Finan et al. [15]. The physiological model of Hovorka et al. [16], describing the s.c.-to-intravenous insulin absorption as well as the glucose rate of appearance following a meal, was employed for generating different scenarios of input excitation over a 24-hour period. Quantifying the degree of linear dependence between the two input vectors by the condition

Table 5.3 Studies Employing Linear System Models with Extra Inputs to Short-Term Prediction of Subcutaneous Glucose Concentration in Diabetes

Study	Model	Input	Prediction Horizon	Evaluation Measures	Dataset	Prediction Performance		
Stahl et al. [14]	Ordinary least squares GTFM (5,2,3,1,1,3,2)	Blood glucose concentration Insulin and carbohydrate compartmental modeling	15:15:120 min	Residual autocorrelation analysis FIT%	1 person with type 1 diabetes Monitoring period: 2 weeks	*FIT%* 60 min: 60.83%		
Finan et al. [15]	Ordinary least square ARX, ARMAX, BJ	Blood glucose concentration Insulin and carbohydrate compartmental modeling [16]	1-h, 2-h, Infinite-step-ahead	FIT% RAD Clarke error grid analysis	In silico type 1 diabetes data	*ARMAX* *FIT%* 1-h: 77% 2-h: 65% *RAD%:* 1-h: 4.7% 2-h: 6.3% *Clarke EGA—* *Zone A:* 1-h: 99% 2-h: 94%	*BJ* *FIT%* 1-h: 73% 2-h: 59% *RAD%:* 1-h: 5.2% 2-h: 7.4% *Clarke EGA—* *Zone A:* 1-h: 97% 2-h: 92%	*ARX* *FIT%* 1-h: 51% 2-h: 25% *RAD%:* 1-h: 7.6% 2-h: 12.9% *Clarke EGA—* *Zone A:* 1-h: 89% 2-h: 70%
Cescon & Johansson [17]	Ordinary least square ARMAX models	Linearly interpolated blood glucose and insulin concentration Insulin and carbohydrate compartmental modeling [18]	30, 60, 90, 120 min	FIT% VAF%	Nine people with type 1 diabetes [19] Monitoring period: 3 days Sampling interval: 1 min	*FIT%* 30 min: 68.19 ± 8.83 60 min: 41.15 ± 15.81 90 min: 23.42 ± 20.71 120 min: 12.67 ± 25.02 *VAF%* 30 min: 89.27 ± 5.82 60 min: 63.75 ± 20.85 90 min: 39.15 ± 37.54 120 min: 21.12 ± 53.47		
Cescon et al. [20]	Subspace-based multistep models	CGM Insulin and carbohydrate compartmental modeling	Case A: 10, 20, 30 min Case B: 30, 60, 90, 120 min	Prediction error standard deviation Absolute error Relative error CG-pEGA CG-rEGA ISO (%)	Nine people with type 1 diabetes [19] CGM device: Abbot Freestyle Navigator Sampling interval: 10 min Monitoring period: 3 days Sampling interval: 10 min	*Prediction error standard deviation* *Case A* 10 min: 3.66 ± 0.99 mg/dL 20 min: 9.44 ± 2.63 mg/dL 30 min: 15.58 ± 4.87 mg/dL *Case B* 30 min: 19.77 ± 7.46 mg/dL 60 min: 39.44 ± 16.11 mg/dL 90 min: 52.28 ± 21.04 mg/dL 120 min: 59.56 ± 24.44 mg/dL		

(Continued)

Table 5.3 (Continued)

Study	Model	Input	Prediction Horizon	Evaluation Measures	Dataset	Prediction Performance	
Zhao et al [21]	Latent variable-based model without or with extra inputs (i.e., LV, LVX)	CGM data Second-order transfer function models of insulin and meal intake [22]	0–60 min	RMSE Clarke error grid analysis	In-silico data/University of Virginia/ University of Padova simulator	LV—Case 1 *RMSE* 30 min: 11.2 ± 1.1 mg/dL 60 min: 18.8 ± 3.1 mg/dL *Clarke EGA—Zone A:* 30 min: 96.4% ± 1.5% 60 min: 83.5% ± 5.3%	LVX—Case 1 *RMSE* 30 min: 8.9 ± 0.7 mg/dL 60 min: 14.6 ± 1.2 mg/dL *Clarke EGA—Zone A:* 30 min: 97.9% ± 0.7% 60 min: 89.7% ± 2.3%
					Seven people with type 1 diabetesCGM device: DexCom 7 Plus, DexComMonitoring Period: -Sampling interval: 5 min	LV *RMSE* 15 min: 11.3 ± 2.4 mg/dL 30 min: 19.7 ± 3.3 mg/dL 45 min: 26.0 ± 3.8 mg/dL 60 min: 31.2 ± 4.0 mg/dL *Clarke EGA—Zone A:* 15 min: 96.4% ± 2.0% 30 min: 84.9% ± 7.6% 45 min: 76.3% ± 10.2% 60 min: 68.4% ± 9.6%	LVX *RMSE* 15 min: 11.1 ± 2.4 mg/dL 30 min: 18.7 ± 3.7 mg/dL 45 min: 24.4 ± 4.7 mg/dL 60 min: 29.2 ± 5.5 mg/dL *Clarke EGA—Zone A:* 15 min: 96.8% ± 1.8% 30 min: 86.1% ± 7.5% 45 min: 78.8% ± 9.9% 60 min: 72.1% ± 10.6%
Zhao et al [23,24]	ARX, Model migration	CGM data Second-order transfer function models of insulin and meal intake [22]	30 min	RMSE CG-rEGA	In silico data/University of Virginia/ University of Padova simulator	*RMSE* Adolescents:14.85 ± 4.94 mg/dL Adults: 10.98 ± 2.10 mg/dL Children: 18.56 ± 10.29 mg/dL *CG-rEGA—Zone A* Adolescents: 70.76% ± 1.31% Adults: 70.50% ± 0.57% Children: 66.87% ± 5.71%	

number of the input matrix $[u_1(t), u_2(t)]$, where $u_1(t)$ and $u_2(t)$ represent the amount of insulin bolus and meal carbohydrate content, respectively; they demonstrated that the median FIT% of ARMAX and BJ models in the case of 1-hour ahead predictions is negatively correlated with the condition number ($r = -0.86$ and $r = -0.88$, respectively), whereas these correlations are weaker for 2-hour ahead predictions ($r = -0.64$ and $r = -0.82$, respectively). On the other hand, the median FIT% of ARX models, which is inferior compared with the other two models, is correlated with the condition number to a significantly lesser extent, with $r = -0.43$ and $r = -0.39$ for 1 and 2-hour ahead predictions, respectively. In addition, the impulse response characteristics (i.e., the maximum change in glucose concentration and the time to maximum change in response to an insulin bolus, the maximum change in glucose concentration and the time to maximum change in response to a meal intake) of the identified models indicate that datasets with higher level of excitation tend to estimate better the dynamics of the system, which is more apparent for ARMAX and BJ models. Overall, (1) ARMAX models outperformed BJ and ARX models predicting glycemic excursions accurately and with small delays, (2) BJ models were found susceptible to erratic predictions, and (3) ARX models produced a significantly delayed output.

An attempt to address input collinearity in glucose prediction models was also made by Zhao et al. by using latent variable models [21]. The proposed scheme combined partial least squares regression and canonical correlation analysis and, as a result, the inferred uncorrelated input variables, which comprise linear combinations of the input, shared the maximum covariance and correlation with the output variable. In particular, the input concerning the estimated carbohydrate content of meals, and the s.c. administered insulin doses was described by their corresponding finite impulse response functions [22]. The method was evaluated on 10 in silico subjects from the University of Virginia/Padova type 1 diabetes simulator [25] as well as on 7 subjects with type 1 diabetes monitored in ambulatory conditions. In particular, three simulation scenarios were implemented with different ICR values (Case I: ideal ICR, Case II: 30% increase in ICR, and Case III: 30% decrease in ICR) so as to excite different modes of the system. Both univariate and multivariate latent variable models (LV and LVX, respectively) were compared and contrasted with the respective AR and ARX models in terms of the RMSE and the Clarke EGA from 1- to 12-step-ahead predictions with a sampling interval of 5 minutes. Regarding the in silico subjects, (1) LV and AR models had a similar performance in all three simulation scenarios and for all prediction horizons, (2) LVX and ARX models performed equally well in Case 1 clearly outperforming AR and LV models for prediction horizons ≥ 30 minutes, and (3) LVX maintained their high accuracy in Cases II and III unlike ARX models, which RMSE, as prediction horizon increased (≥ 30 minutes), became comparable to the RMSE that would be incurred by assigning the current glucose concentration value as the estimate of future measurements. Retrospective evaluation on clinical data revealed, though to a lesser extent, the predominance of LVX models for prediction horizons ≥ 30 minutes, with the ARX model performing better than the univariate models (i.e., AR and LV models).

Cescon et al. [17] carried out a detailed comparison of ARMAX and state-space models of the glucose system in terms of stability, uncorrelated (white noise) residuals, and physiologically sensible responses to 1 IU of insulin and 10 g of carbohydrates. The data, which were collected in a clinical trial carried out in the framework of the DIAdvisor project [19], were equally divided into training and test sets. The input of the models encompassed past values of the interpolated plasma insulin concentration and the rate of appearance of glucose into plasma following carbohydrate intestinal absorption [18], and the output was interpolated blood glucose concentration. Individual-specific ARMAX models of order in the range $1 \leq n_a \leq 10$, $1 \leq n_{bi} \leq 10$, $1 \leq n_c \leq 10$, and $1 \leq n_{u_i} \leq 3$, with $i = 1, 2$, which were identified by PEM, satisfied the above criteria and achieved a value of VAF $\geq 50\%$ on 60 minutes-ahead predictions in the majority of patients; nevertheless, the requirement of FIT $\geq 50\%$ on 60 minutes-ahead predictions was not achieved. The coherence spectra between the inputs and the output variables supported the low excitation the input signals providing the system with because of the concurrent and, more importantly, in a specified ratio intake of insulin and carbohydrates.

The problem of multistep-ahead prediction of s.c. glucose concentration in type 1 diabetes was, subsequently, treated by Cescon et al. in the context of a subspace-based multiple-input–multiple-output model with $u \in R^m$ the input, $y \in R^l$ the output, $x \in R^n$ the state, and $\varepsilon \in R^l$ the zero-mean white noise process uncorrelated with u [20]. The future values of the s.c. glucose concentration from the current time t up to the time $t + f - 1$ were assembled into an f-dimensional column vector $\hat{y}^f$ which was expressed as a linear combination of the past joint input–output data $z^p = \begin{bmatrix} u^p & y^p \end{bmatrix}^T \in R^{(l+m)p}$ and the future input $u^f \in R^{mf}$ within the time intervals $[t - p, t - 1]$ and $[t, t + f - 1]$, respectively:

$$\hat{y}^f = \hat{\Gamma} z^p + \hat{\Lambda} u^f, \tag{5.29}$$

Physiological models were employed to reconstruct the rate of appearance of ingested glucose into plasma from the meal carbohydrate content and the plasma insulin concentration from the administered insulin [18], which form the input $u \in R^2$ of the model. The optimization of the $\hat{\Gamma} \in R^{lp \times (l+m)p}$ and $\hat{\Lambda} \in R^{lp \times mf}$ matrices was formulated as a least squares problem [26], which solution requires that: (1) the input signals are persistently exciting of order at least mf, (2) the intersection of the spans of the Hankel matrices Z^p, and U^f should be zero. In addition, it is suggested that $p \geq \max\{n, \tau\}$, with n being the model order and $\tau \leq f$ the number of steps ahead that one wishes to investigate. Note that the model output is, finally, not dependent on the state x and, thus, the model order n needs not to be directly specified. The same dataset as in [17] was utilized, where the first half of the data was used in the estimation of $\hat{\Gamma}$ and $\hat{\Lambda}$ matrices and the second one in the model testing. Cescon et al. compared the predictive performance of two different model configurations, i.e., Case A with $\tau_{\max} = 30$ minutes and Case B with $\tau_{\max} = 120$ minutes (i.e., $f = \tau_{\max}/T$ where $T = 10$ minutes is the sampling interval), and results suggested that p should not be given $\gg \tau$. Moreover, the assessment of the predicted s.c. glucose signal taking as reference the blood glucose signal (Table 5.3), and, in parallel, the comparison with a Kalman-based ARMAX model of third order demonstrated the competitiveness of their approach.

The feasibility of an individual-independent AR short-term (<60 minutes) glucose prediction model in different frequency ranges of the s.c. glucose signal has been demonstrated

[8,24]. Nevertheless, the existent interpatient variability in response to exogenous inputs indicates training and testing of multivariate glucose models need to be applied individually, as is the case in the aforementioned studies. Zhao et al. proposed a methodology for rapid identification of ARX models of s.c. glucose concentration in type 1 diabetes by utilizing the concept of model migration [23]. In particular, (1) a base ARX model, with the same input configuration as in [21] is first estimated by least squares using data from one subject and (2) for each new subject, the parameters concerning the exogenous inputs (i.e., $B_1(q)$ and $B_2(q)$ with input 1 and input 2 describing insulin and carbohydrate responses, respectively) are properly customized using a small amount of data capturing the properties of the glucose system. Base model refinement constitutes an iterative procedure, where parameter update (increment or decrement by a predefined step) is determined according to the sign of the difference $\text{mean}(\hat{y}) - \text{mean}(y)$ such that (1) if $\text{mean}(\hat{y}) - \text{mean}(y) > 0$ then $B_1(q)$ is increased or $B_2(q)$ is decreased and (2) if $\text{mean}(\hat{y}) - \text{mean}(y) < 0$ then $B_1(q)$ is decreased or $B_2(q)$ is increased. In a proof-of-concept study including 30 in silico subjects from the University of Virginia/Padova type 1 diabetes simulator [25], Zhao et al. experimented with different simulation scenarios (Case I: ideal ICR, Case II: 30% increase in ICR, Case III: 30% decrease in ICR, and Case IV: Case I with bolus insulin being injected 30 minutes later after the respective meal) and demonstrated no statistically significant differences in prediction accuracy between ARX models based on model migration method and individualized ones for a prediction horizon of ≤ 30 minutes. For longer prediction horizons, the individualized ARX models produced a considerably lower RMSE as long as training and test data concern the same Case; otherwise, ARX models relying on model migration performed slightly better. The latter behavior was attributed to the propensity of individualized models to data overfitting. Nevertheless, global ARX modeling was found inferior to both individualized and model migration identification methods.

5.4 Computational Experiments

Both the time- and frequency-domain behavior of linear time-invariant models of the s.c. glucose concentration in type 1 diabetes, and more specifically of AR and ARX models, is demonstrated in this section. The experiments were conducted using the MATLAB System Identification Toolbox.

5.4.1 Identification of AR Models of Glucose Concentration

The first part of the analysis is based on data from one subject with type 1 diabetes (i.e., Subject 1) following multiple-dose insulin therapy and without significant micro- and macrovascular complications. During the observation period, the subject was obliged to abstain from any structured exercise program and was counseled to follow a 1400-calorie daily diet. The glycemic profile of the patient was recorded using the Medtronic IPro2 CGM system (Medtronic Minimed Inc.) in ambulatory conditions over a 7-day period (Mean $\pm$ SD: 118.03 $\pm$ 33.03 mg/dL, 10th percentile: 73.00 mg/dL, 90th percentile: 169.90 mg/dL, interquartile range: 47.00 mg/dL), with a sampling interval T of glucose measurements equal to 5 minutes. The corresponding ambulatory glucose profile (AGP) report [27] is presented in Fig. 5.2. The CGM dataset, as it is shown in Fig. 5.3, is split into two parts, with the first half of the CGM data (i.e., from Day 2 to Day 4) constituting the training set and the second half of the CGM data (i.e., from Day 5 to Day 7) constituting the test set. The spectrum plot of the CGM time series of Subject 1, as it is estimated by the Blackman–Tukey procedure, is illustrated in Fig. 5.4, where we can observe both the low- and high-frequency dynamics of the full dataset are well represented by the training and test sets.

An AR model of order $n_a = 7$ is identified via least squares on the training set. The order of the polynomial A, i.e., $n_a = 7$, has been selected according to the MDL criterion, with the value of n_a varying from 1 to 10. As it is shown in Fig. 5.5, the normalized sum of the squared error regarding the one-step-ahead predictions remains approximately constant for $n_a = 7, \ldots, 10$, whereas the improvement is marginal for $n_a = 4, \ldots, 10$. For comparison purposes, regularized least squares is also utilized having set $n_a = 25$. In particular, regularized least squares is implemented by using a tune/correlated (TC) kernel matrix, which hyperparameters are obtained via marginal likelihood maximization [28]. The estimated polynomial A of the AR model is

$$A(q) = 1 - 1.8981q^{-1} + 0.4106q^{-2} + 0.7061q^{-3} + 0.2379q^{-4} \\ - 0.4662q^{-5} - 0.1636q^{-6} + 0.1736q^{-7}, \tag{5.30}$$

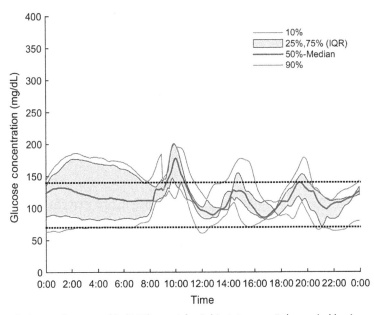

FIGURE 5.2 The ambulatory glucose profile (AGP) report for Subject 1 over a 7-day period having excluded the first day of CGM.

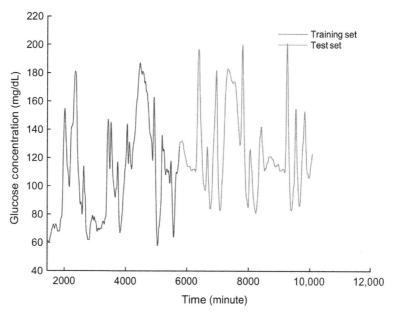

FIGURE 5.3 The CGM time series of Subject 1 having been split into training and test sets.

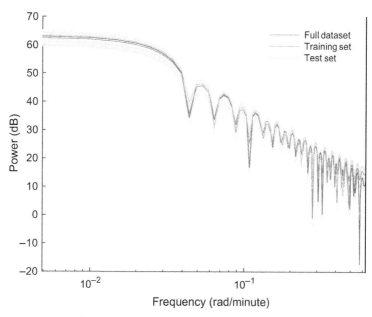

FIGURE 5.4 Estimated spectrum of the CGM time series of Subject 1 with confidence bounds corresponding to 3 standard deviations.

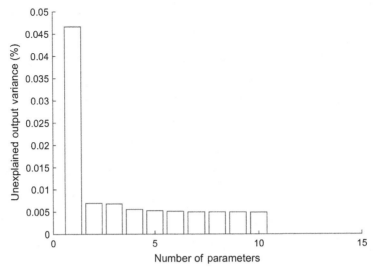

FIGURE 5.5 AR model one-step-ahead prediction error vs number of parameters (n_a). The unexplained output variance (in %) is quantified by the normalized sum of the squared prediction error.

and the corresponding pole-zero configuration of the transfer function $H(q, \theta) = 1/A(q)$ is portrayed in Fig. 5.6. The regularized coefficient estimates reflect a similar glucose autocorrelation dependency for $i \leq 6$, whereas they are close to zero for $i \geq 7$:

$$
\begin{aligned}
A(q) = 1 & - 1.8739q^{-1} + 0.3586q^{-2} + 0.6851q^{-3} + 0.2829q^{-4} - 0.3411q^{-5} - 0.2249q^{-6} - 0.0286q^{-7} \\
& + 0.0530q^{-8} + 0.1035q^{-9} + 0.0862q^{-10} - 0.0128q^{-11} - 0.1168q^{-12} - 0.0464q^{-13} + 0.0404q^{-14} \\
& + 0.0522q^{-15} + 0.0302q^{-16} - 0.0206q^{-17} - 0.0223q^{-18} - 0.0228q^{-19} - 0.0091q^{-20} + 0.0125q^{-21} \, , \\
& + 0.0185q^{-22} + 0.0121q^{-23} - 0.0029q^{-24} - 0.0130q^{-25}
\end{aligned}
$$

(5.31)

and, accordingly, the poles and zeros of the regularized AR model are close to those of the AR model for $i = 1, \ldots, 6$ (Fig. 5.6). The rational function $H(q, \theta)$ of both models has one pole approximately equal to 0.99, and the remainder of poles and zeros lie inside the unit circle. In addition, the impulse response of $H(q)$ is estimated with a high variance (Fig. 5.7).

The validation of the model, by using the test set, commences with the comparison between the power spectrum of the additive disturbance $v = H(q)\varepsilon(t)$ of the AR and regularized AR models and the spectrum of the true system (depending on the test data). As it is shown in Fig. 5.8, there exists a low agreement between the estimated parametric and the nonparametric noise spectra. We can observe in Fig. 5.9 that residuals of one-step-ahead predictions of the AR model are correlated for $\tau = 3$ and $\tau = 4$, likewise the whiteness test of the residuals of the regularized AR model (Fig. 5.10) supports that their autocorrelation does not lie in the confidence region for $\tau = 4$. Thus, the error term $\varepsilon(t)$ in (5.13) cannot be regarded as white noise. The predictive performance of both models is evaluated for multiple prediction horizons of 5, 15, 30, 45, 60, 90, and 120 minutes, which correspond to 1, 3, 6, 9,

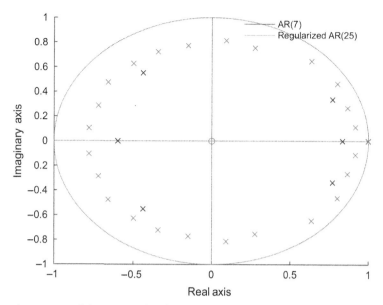

FIGURE 5.6 The pole-zero map of the estimated AR(7) and regularized AR(25) models for Subject 1.

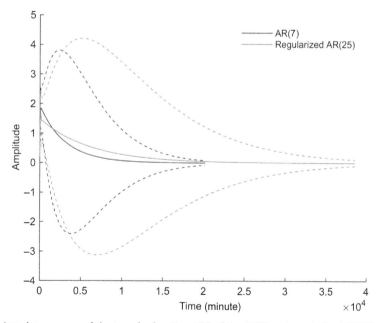

FIGURE 5.7 The impulse response of the transfer function $H(q)$ of the AR(7) and regularized AR(25) models for Subject 1 with confidence intervals corresponding to 3 standard deviations.

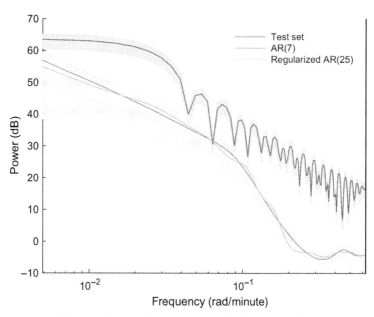

FIGURE 5.8 Power spectrum of the stochastic stationary process $H(q)\varepsilon(t)$ of the AR(7) and regularized AR(25) models for Subject 1 with confidence intervals corresponding to three standard deviations.

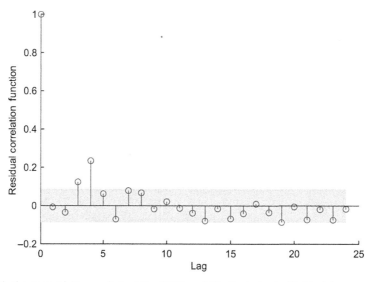

FIGURE 5.9 Residual autocorrelation analysis of the AR(7) model in the test set of Subject 1.

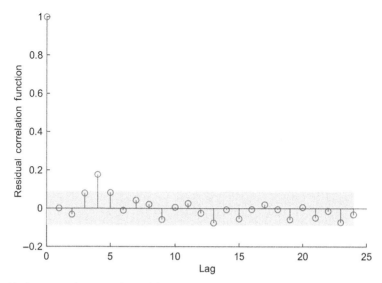

FIGURE 5.10 Residual autocorrelation analysis of the AR(7) model in the test set of Subject 1.

Table 5.4   Validation of AR(7) Model of Subject 1

Prediction Horizon	Model	Evaluation Measures				
		RMSE (mg/dL)	FIT(%)	ESOD$_{norm}$	Time Gain (min)	*J*
5 min	AR(7)	0.77	0.97	3.15	5.00	3.15
	ARr(7)	0.75	0.97	2.90	5.00	2.90
15 min	AR(7)	2.93	0.90	24.52	10.00	12.26
	ARr(7)	2.82	0.90	22.42	10.00	11.21
30 min	AR(7)	8.78	0.69	84.77	15.00	28.26
	ARr(7)	8.44	0.70	80.49	15.00	26.83
45 min	AR(7)	15.72	0.44	118.63	20.00	29.66
	ARr(7)	14.93	0.47	110.28	20.00	27.57
60 min	AR(7)	22.00	0.22	119.82	20.00	29.95
	ARr(7)	20.71	0.27	114.32	20.00	28.58
90 min	AR(7)	31.27	− 0.10	121.31	20.00	30.33
	ARr(7)	29.02	− 0.03	105.71	20.00	26.43
120 min	AR(7)	37.27	− 0.32	127.68	20.00	31.92
	ARr(7)	33.98	− 0.20	85.50	15.00	28.50

12, 18, and 24 samples ahead. The goodness-of-fit as well as the continuous glucose error grid analysis (CG-EGA) concerning the estimated models are presented in Tables 5.4 and 5.5, respectively. Predictions up to 15 minutes ahead are associated with a high FIT%, and the corresponding time gain is comparable to the prediction horizon. The increase of the prediction horizon induces a substantial deterioration both in the FIT% and the ESOD$_{norm}$,

Table 5.5 CG-EGA of Predictions of AR(7) Model of Subject 1

Prediction Horizon	Model	Hypoglycemia			Euglycemia			Hyperglycemia		
		AR	BE	ER	AR	BE	ER	AR	BE	ER
5 min	AR(7)	NaN	NaN	NaN	100.00	0.00	0.00	100.00	0.00	0.00
	ARr(7)	NaN	NaN	NaN	100.00	0.00	0.00	100.00	0.00	0.00
15 min	AR(7)	NaN	NaN	NaN	99.75	0.25	0.00	95.92	0.00	4.08
	ARr(7)	NaN	NaN	NaN	99.75	0.25	0.00	95.92	0.00	4.08
30 min	AR(7)	NaN	NaN	NaN	93.00	6.88	0.12	77.55	20.41	2.04
	ARr(7)	NaN	NaN	NaN	93.73	6.02	0.25	79.59	18.37	2.04
45 min	AR(7)	NaN	NaN	NaN	86.98	12.53	0.49	69.39	26.53	4.08
	ARr(7)	NaN	NaN	NaN	87.10	12.41	0.49	67.35	26.53	6.12
60 min	AR(7)	NaN	NaN	NaN	85.26	14.00	0.74	61.22	26.53	12.24
	ARr(7)	NaN	NaN	NaN	85.63	13.64	0.74	59.18	30.61	10.20
90 min	AR(7)	NaN	NaN	NaN	81.33	18.43	0.25	65.31	22.45	12.24
	ARr(7)	NaN	NaN	NaN	84.15	15.60	0.25	65.31	22.45	12.24
120 min	AR(7)	NaN	NaN	NaN	78.87	20.02	1.11	71.43	14.29	14.29
	ARr(7)	NaN	NaN	NaN	85.50	14.13	0.37	77.55	8.16	14.29

with the time gain being reduced to 20 minutes for a prediction horizon ≥ 45 minutes. The CG-EGA corroborates the increase of erroneous readings in the hyperglycemic region as prediction horizon increases, whereas a considerable percentage of predictions concerning euglycemic and hyperglycemic reference values are classified as benign errors. Regularization yields slightly more precise and smoother predictions; though, both AR solutions are comparable with respect to the CG-EGA for prediction horizons ≤ 90 minutes. The six-step-ahead (i.e., 30 minutes) predictions of the AR and the regularized AR models are shown in Fig. 5.11.

5.4.2 Identification of ARX Models of Glucose Concentration

The second part of computational experiments approximates the glucose system through a multiple-input single-output linear time-invariant model having two observable input variables (i.e., food and insulin intake). One subject with type 1 diabetes (i.e., Subject 2), following multiple-dose insulin therapy and without significant micro- and macrovascular complications, was observed under free-living conditions for 13 consecutive days [29]. The patient was equipped with the Guardian Real-Time CGM system (Medtronic Minimed Inc.), with $T = 5$ minutes, and, additionally, information on food intake and s.c. insulin injections was recorded on a daily basis using a specially designed paper diary. The nutritional content of each meal was postanalyzed by a certified dietician. The AGP profile of the glucose dataset over the observational period is depicted in Fig. 5.12 accompanied by the following statistics: Mean $\pm$ SD: 143.10 ± 43.05 mg/dL, 10th percentile: 90.00 mg/dL, 90th percentile: 204.00 mg/dL, interquartile range: 62.00 mg/dL. The physiological models of Tarin et al. [30] and Lehmann et al. [31] are employed to assess the absorption kinetics of subcutaneously administered insulin

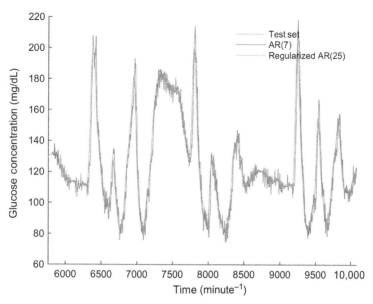

FIGURE 5.11 Six-step-ahead predictions (i.e., 30 minutes) of s.c. glucose concentration based on the AR(7) and regularized AR(25) models for Subject 1.

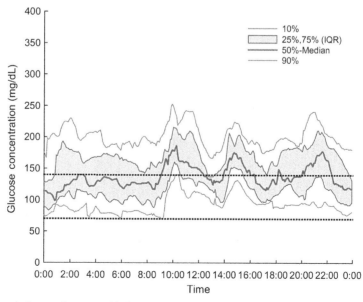

FIGURE 5.12 The ambulatory glucose profile (AGP) report for Subject 2 over a 12-day period having excluded the first day of CGM.

and, subsequently, compute the time course of plasma insulin concentration I_p(IU/mL), and the time course of the rate of appearance of ingested glucose into plasma, Ra (mg/min), respectively. As we can observe in Fig. 5.13, the input–output dataset is split up into four separate segments because of missing output data. In particular, the first two data segments form the training set and the two last data segments form the test set. The impulse response of the system is shown in Fig. 5.14, where we can observe the low excitation I_p is injecting into the system. In addition, the nonparametric spectral analysis of the dataset is depicted in Figs. 5.15 and 5.16.

A regularized ARX model, consisting of a TC kernel, is estimated and compared with the univariate regularized AR model. Following [1], a single regularized least squares optimization problem is considered such that

$$E(\theta) = \left(\sum_{t \in T^1} (y(t) - \hat{y}(t|\theta))^2 + \lambda \theta^T P \theta \right) + \cdots + \left(\sum_{t \in T^4} (y(t) - \hat{y}(t|\theta))^2 + \lambda \theta^T P \theta \right), \qquad (5.32)$$

where T^i is the index set of the ith segment, and each of the models $\hat{y}(t|\theta)$ is assigned zero initial conditions. The orders of the impulse responses, which correspond to the orders of

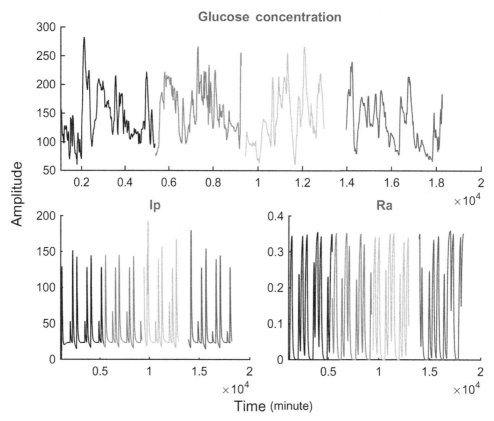

FIGURE 5.13 The input–output data of Subject 2 having been split up into four data segments.

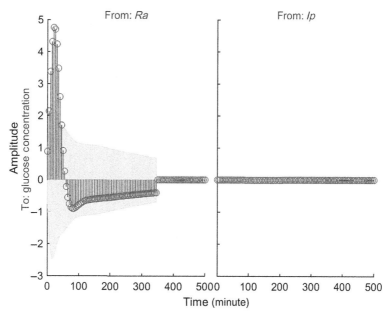

FIGURE 5.14 Transient response analysis of *Ra* and I_p time series of Subject 2.

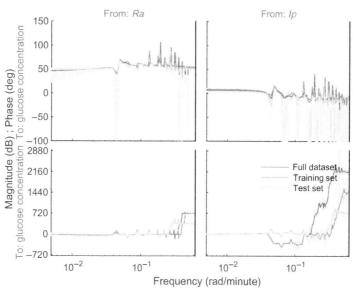

FIGURE 5.15 Bode plots of the frequency response of the output with respect to the system's inputs with confidence bounds corresponding to three standard deviations.

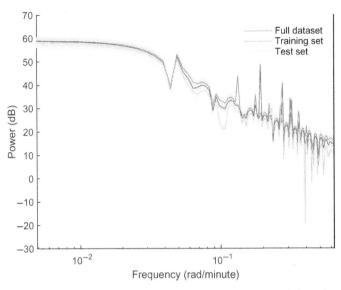

FIGURE 5.16 Estimated noise spectrum of the CGM time series of Subject 2 with confidence bounds corresponding to three standard deviations.

the polynomials A, B_1, and B_2, and the corresponding delays are set equal to $n_a = 25$, $n_{b_1} = 50$, $n_{b_2} = 50$, $n_{u_1} = 10$, $n_{u_2} = 10$, whereas the regularization hyperparameters are determined via marginal likelihood optimization [28]. Both models are stable provided that the poles and zeros of the transfer functions $G(q, \theta)$ and $H(q, \theta)$ are all located inside the unit circle (Fig. 5.17). Nevertheless, the inclusion of the extra inputs reduces the variance of the estimated coefficients as it is translated into the confidence intervals of the impulse response of $H(q)$ (Fig. 5.18). In addition, the noise spectra of both solutions are almost identical (Fig. 5.19).

The six-step-ahead (i.e., 30 minutes) predictions of the regularized AR and the ARX models are illustrated in Figs. 5.20 and 5.21. Tables 5.6 and 5.7 present the evaluation of both models, with respect to basic statistics for the residuals and the CG-EGA, for a prediction horizon of 5, 15, 30, 45, 60, 90, and 120 minutes. The contribution of the extra inputs in the overall model performance (Table 5.6) is evident in both Segment 1 and Segment 2 for horizons ≥ 30 minutes; multivariate solution results in lower errors, higher regularity of predictions, and lower time lags between the predicted and the actual glucose trajectories. The CG-EGA renders ARX models more advantageous in the hyperglycemic region, which is getting more pronounced as prediction horizon increases. On the contrary, multivariate predictions are more erratic in the hypoglycemic region. On top of these, the bode plot of the cross-spectrum between the input and the output clearly shows that ARX models are incapable of representing the true impulse responses of the system (Fig. 5.22).

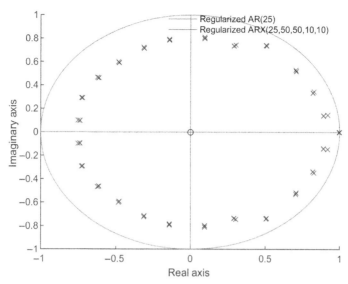

FIGURE 5.17 The pole-zero map of the estimated regularized AR(25) and regularized ARX(25,50,50,10,10) models for Subject 2.

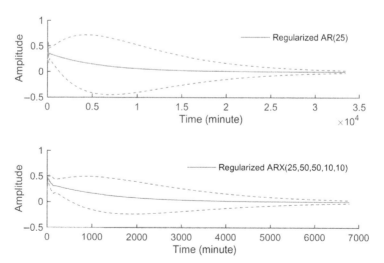

FIGURE 5.18 The impulse response of the transfer function $H(q)$ of the regularized AR(25) and regularized ARX (25,50,50,10,10) models for Subject 2 with confidence intervals corresponding to three standard deviations.

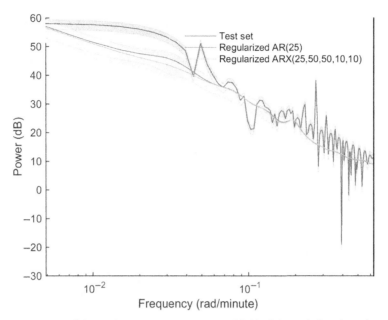

FIGURE 5.19 Power spectrum of the stochastic stationary process $H(q)\varepsilon(t)$ of the AR(25) and regularized ARX (25,50,50,10,10) models for Subject 2 with confidence intervals corresponding to three standard deviations.

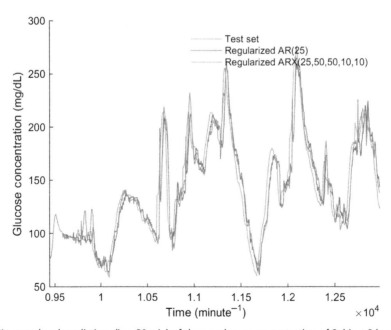

FIGURE 5.20 Six-step-ahead predictions (i.e., 30 min) of the s.c. glucose concentration of Subject 2 based on the regularized AR(25) and regularized ARX(25,50,50,10,10) models as applied in Segment 1.

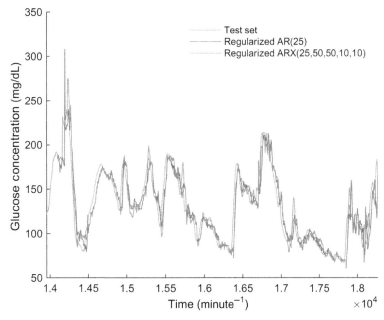

FIGURE 5.21 Six-step-ahead predictions (i.e., 30 min) of the s.c. glucose concentration of Subject 2 based on the regularized AR(25) and regularized ARX(25,50,50,10,10) models as applied in Segment 2.

Table 5.6   Validation of ARX Model of Subject 2

		Segment 1					Segment 2				
Prediction Horizon	Model	RMSE (mg/dL)	FIT (%)	ESOD$_{norm}$	Time Gain (min)	J	RMSE (mg/dL)	FIT (%)	ESOD$_{norm}$	Time Gain (min)	J
5 min	AR	3.38	0.93	3.72	0.00	Inf	3.38	0.91	3.58	0.00	Inf
	ARX	3.38	0.93	3.50	0.00	Inf	2.58	0.93	2.02	5.00	2.02
15 min	AR	8.81	0.81	9.22	5.00	9.22	8.49	0.78	8.83	5.00	8.83
	ARX	8.81	0.81	7.93	5.00	7.93	7.64	0.81	3.89	5.00	3.89
30 min	AR	17.00	0.64	11.03	5.00	11.03	15.00	0.62	10.57	5.00	10.57
	ARX	16.45	0.65	8.48	10.00	4.24	13.77	0.65	4.38	10.00	2.19
45 min	AR	24.60	0.48	11.71	5.00	11.71	20.68	0.47	11.10	5.00	11.10
	ARX	23.02	0.51	8.04	10.00	4.02	18.55	0.53	4.00	15.00	1.33
60 min	AR	30.97	0.34	9.79	5.00	9.79	25.79	0.34	9.30	5.00	9.30
	ARX	28.30	0.40	6.36	10.00	3.18	22.76	0.42	3.81	15.00	1.27
90 min	AR	40.33	0.14	7.54	0.00	Inf	33.73	0.14	7.17	0.00	Inf
	ARX	35.56	0.24	5.25	15.00	1.75	28.52	0.27	4.21	20.00	1.05
120 min	AR	45.87	0.02	5.59	0.00	Inf	38.77	0.01	6.25	0.00	Inf
	ARX	40.02	0.15	4.54	10.00	2.27	32.45	0.17	4.31	5.00	4.31

Table 5.7 CG-EGA of Predictions of ARX Model of Subject 2

| Prediction Horizon | Model | Segment 1 | | | | | | | | | Segment 2 | | | | | | | | |
| | | Hypoglycemia | | | Euglycemia | | | Hyperglycemia | | | Hypoglycemia | | | Euglycemia | | | Hyperglycemia | | |
		AR	BE	ER	AR	BE	ER	AR	BE	ER	AR	BE	ER	AR	BE	ER	AR	BE	ER
5 min	AR	100.00	0.00	0.00	97.83	2.17	0.00	95.27	3.55	1.18	100.00	0.00	0.00	98.26	1.61	0.13	96.91	2.06	1.03
	ARX	100.00	0.00	0.00	97.83	2.17	0.00	94.67	3.55	1.78	100.00	0.00	0.00	98.13	1.74	0.13	97.94	2.06	0.00
15 min	AR	100.00	0.00	0.00	95.28	4.53	0.20	84.02	8.88	7.10	100.00	0.00	0.00	93.17	6.29	0.54	82.47	13.40	4.12
	ARX	100.00	0.00	0.00	96.26	3.54	0.20	83.43	7.69	8.88	100.00	0.00	0.00	92.64	6.83	0.54	87.63	9.28	3.09
30 min	AR	82.76	0.00	17.24	91.34	8.46	0.20	76.33	13.61	10.06	100.00	0.00	0.00	89.83	8.84	1.34	79.38	16.49	4.12
	ARX	68.97	0.00	31.03	91.73	7.68	0.59	77.51	14.79	7.69	100.00	0.00	0.00	90.36	8.03	1.61	87.63	9.28	3.09
45 min	AR	58.62	0.00	41.38	90.16	9.25	0.59	69.23	18.93	11.83	100.00	0.00	0.00	88.62	10.44	0.94	78.35	16.49	5.15
	ARX	58.62	0.00	41.38	90.94	8.86	0.20	75.15	15.38	9.47	100.00	0.00	0.00	90.36	8.57	1.07	86.60	9.28	4.12
60 min	AR	48.28	3.45	48.28	90.35	9.06	0.59	69.82	18.93	11.24	100.00	0.00	0.00	87.28	11.51	1.20	81.44	14.43	4.12
	ARX	48.28	3.45	48.28	90.75	8.86	0.39	75.15	15.98	8.88	100.00	0.00	0.00	88.76	10.31	0.94	93.81	4.12	2.06
90 min	AR	31.03	0.00	68.97	90.16	8.46	1.38	68.05	13.02	18.93	100.00	0.00	0.00	87.55	10.98	1.47	83.51	11.34	5.15
	ARX	24.14	0.00	75.86	92.13	7.09	0.79	78.70	9.47	11.83	100.00	0.00	0.00	89.96	9.24	0.80	94.85	4.12	1.03
120 min	AR	10.34	0.00	89.66	89.76	9.65	0.59	69.82	10.65	19.53	100.00	0.00	0.00	88.89	9.37	1.74	84.54	11.34	4.12
	ARX	6.90	0.00	93.10	91.14	8.46	0.39	75.15	10.06	14.79	100.00	0.00	0.00	90.90	8.70	0.40	93.81	4.12	2.06

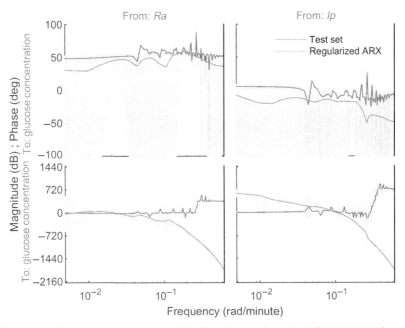

FIGURE 5.22 Bode plot of the deterministic process $G(q)u(t)$ in the regularized ARX(25,50,50,10,10) model of Subject 2 with confidence intervals corresponding to three standard deviations.

5.5 Discussion and Conclusions

Linear system identification is an asset for the exploration of the dynamics of the s.c. glucose in type 1 diabetes in the time and frequency domain. Literature suggests that AR models can effectively explain the variance of the s.c. glucose signal for very short-term prediction horizons (up to 15 minutes), whereas accurate predictions for higher horizons have been reported when the high frequencies of the glucose signal are not modeled. Moreover, should the frequency content of the glucose signal is adequately described, then AR model portability among patients is feasible. The incorporation of extra inputs in ARX, ARMAX, BJ, and state-space models does improve the performance of univariate linear models; however, this is more prominent for in silico data. Nevertheless, predictions for horizons ≥ 30 minutes cannot be totally characterized accurate irrespective of the selected model structure, which can be explained by the innate nonlinearity and nonstationarity of the glucose system, as well as, by the deficient input excitation. According to competitive learning, the modes of the glucose system which can actually be represented as a linear function of the inputs, presumably the low-frequency glycemic dynamics associated with circadian or ultradian rhythms, need to be learned.

In this chapter, we experimented with two type 1 diabetes subjects monitored under ambulatory conditions. We demonstrated that both ordinary as well as regularized least squares yield stable AR models featuring no white noise residuals, a rough approximation of the noise spectrum, and a fair predictive capacity up to ≤ 30-minute horizons. The extra inputs (i.e., Ra and I_p), provided for Subject 2, contributed to more precise and clinically acceptable predictions, which is getting more evident as horizon increases. In addition, the variance of the estimate noise spectrum is considerably reduced, whereas the frequency response of the system $G(q)u(t)$ resembles the behavior of a low-pass filter and, thus, deviates from the true system's behavior. We should mention that the analysis performed herein is purely for demonstration purposes, and these preliminary results should only be considered as indicative.

References

[1] Lennart L, editor. System identification (2nd ed.): Theory for the user. New Jersey: Prentice Hall PTR; 1999.

[2] Akaike H. A new look at the statistical model identification. IEEE Trans Autom Control 1974;19 (6):716−23.

[3] Zucchini W. An introduction to model selection. J Math Psychol 2000;44(1):41−61.

[4] Hurvich CM, Tsai CL. Regression and time-series model selection in small samples. Biometrika 1989;76 (2):297−307.

[5] Schwarz G. Estimating the dimension of a model. Ann Stat 1978;6(2):461−4.

[6] Rissanen J. Modeling by shortest data description. Automatica 1978;14(5):465−71.

[7] Gani A, et al. Predicting subcutaneous glucose concentration in humans: data-driven glucose modeling. IEEE Trans Biomed Eng 2009;56(2):246−54.

[8] Reifman J, et al. Predictive monitoring for improved management of glucose levels. J Diabetes Sci Technol 2007;1(4):478−86.

[9] Gani A, et al. Universal glucose models for predicting subcutaneous glucose concentration in humans. IEEE Trans Inf Technol Biomed 2010;14(1):157−65.

[10] Lu Y, et al. The importance of different frequency bands in predicting subcutaneous glucose concentration in type 1 diabetic patients. IEEE Trans Biomed Eng 2010;57(8):1839−46.

[11] Rahaghi FN, Gough DA. Blood glucose dynamics. Diabetes Technol Ther 2008;10(2):81−94.

[12] Lu Y, et al. The importance of different frequency bands in predicting subcutaneous glucose concentration in type 1 diabetic patients. IEEE Trans Biomed Eng 2010;57(8):1839−46.

[13] Gough DA, Kreutz-Delgado K, Bremer TM. Frequency characterization of blood glucose dynamics. Ann Biomed Eng 2003;31(1):91−7.

[14] Breton MD, Shields DP, Kovatchev BP. Optimum subcutaneous glucose sampling and Fourier analysis of continuous glucose monitors. J Diab Sci Technol (Online) 2008;2(3):495−500.

[15] Stahl F, Johansson R. Diabetes mellitus modeling and short-term prediction based on blood glucose measurements. Math Biosci 2009;217(2):101−17.

[16] Finan DA, et al. Effect of input excitation on the quality of empirical dynamic models for type 1 diabetes. AIChE J 2009;55(5):1135−46.

[17] Hovorka R, et al. Nonlinear model predictive control of glucose concentration in subjects with type 1 diabetes. Physiol Meas 2004;25(4):905−20.

[18] Cescon M, Johansson R. Linear modeling and prediction in diabetes physiology. In: Marmarelis V, Mitsis G, editors. Data-driven modeling for diabetes. Berlin Heidelberg: Springer; 2014. p. 187−222.

[19] Dalla Man C, Camilleri M, Cobelli C. A system model of oral glucose absorption: validation on gold standard data. IEEE Trans Biomed Eng 2006;53(12 Pt 1):2472–8.

[20] Poulsen JU, et al. A diabetes management system empowering patients to reach optimised glucose control: from monitor to advisor. Conf Proc IEEE Eng Med Biol Soc 2010;2010:5270–1.

[21] Cescon M, Johansson R, Renard E. Subspace-based linear multi-step predictors in type 1 diabetes mellitus. Biomed Signal Proc Control 2015;22:99–110.

[22] Kovatchev BP, et al. In silico preclinical trials: a proof of concept in closed-loop control of type 1 diabetes. J Diabetes Sci Technol 2009;3(1):44–55.

[23] Zhao C, et al. Predicting subcutaneous glucose concentration using a latent-variable-based statistical method for type 1 diabetes mellitus. J Diabetes Sci Technol 2012;6(3):617–33.

[24] Verhaegen M. Identification of the deterministic part of MIMO state space models given in innovations form from input-output data. Automatica 1994;30(1):61–74.

[25] Zhao C, Sun Y, Zhao L. Interindividual glucose dynamics in different frequency bands for online prediction of subcutaneous glucose concentration in type 1 diabetic subjects. AIChE J 2013;59(11):4228–40.

[26] Zhao C, Yu C. Rapid model identification for online subcutaneous glucose concentration prediction for new subjects with type I diabetes. IEEE Trans Biomed Eng 2015;62(5):1333–44.

[27] Grosman B, et al. Zone model predictive control: a strategy to minimize hyper- and hypoglycemic events. J Diabetes Sci Technol 2010;4(4):961–75.

[28] Bergenstal RM, et al. Recommendations for standardizing glucose reporting and analysis to optimize clinical decision making in diabetes: the Ambulatory Glucose Profile (AGP). Diabetes Technol Ther 2013;15(3):198–211.

[29] Pillonetto G, et al. Kernel methods in system identification, machine learning and function estimation: a survey. Automatica 2014;50(3):657–82.

[30] Georga E, et al. Data mining for blood glucose prediction and knowledge discovery in diabetic patients: the METABO diabetes modeling and management system. Conf Proc IEEE Eng Med Biol Soc 2009;2009:5633–6.

[31] Tarin C, et al. Comprehensive pharmacokinetic model of insulin Glargine and other insulin formulations. IEEE Trans Biomed Eng 2005;52(12):1994–2005.

[32] Lehmann ED, Deutsch T. A physiological model of glucose–insulin interaction in type 1 diabetes mellitus. J Biomed Eng 1992;14(3):235–42.

6

Nonlinear Models of Glucose Concentration

6.1 Problem Formulation

Consider a sequence of input–output pairs $Z = \{(x^i, y_i)\}_{i=1}^{N}$, where $(x^i, y_i) \in Z = X \times Y$, $X \subseteq R^d$ and $Y \subseteq R$. Each sample $(x^i, y_i) \equiv (x(t_i - kT), y(t_i))$ associates the input vector x^i corresponding to observations up to time $t_i - kT$ with the current observation of subcutaneous (s.c.) glucose concentration y_i at time t_i, where k is the prediction step and T is the glucose sampling interval. For ease of notation we will assume $t_{i+1} - t_i = T$. An approximation $f:R^d \rightarrow R$ of the true mapping is learnt in the context of linear, with respect to their parameters $\theta \in R^m$, models of the form:

$$f(x, \theta) = \theta^T \phi(x) + b, \tag{6.1}$$

in which $\phi \in R^m$ is a vector of nonlinear basis functions and b is the bias parameter. The function $f:R^d \rightarrow R$ maps the input vector $x \in R^d$, which describes input up to time $t - kT$, to the glucose concentration at time t, with t being the time for which the prediction is made and kT the prediction horizon. Table 6.1 outlines the model selection, identification, and evaluation process given a nonlinear model M, a training set Z_{train} and a test set Z_{test}. Similarly to linear model construction, an external crossvalidation may be applied in order to obtain a less biased estimation of model's performance. Table 6.2 presents the state-of-the-art studies treating the short-term prediction of s.c. glucose concentration as a linear regression problem.

Table 6.1 Training and Evaluation Procedure of Linear Regression Models

Input: Z_{train}, Z_{test}, Model M
Model Selection:
1. Optimize model M (6.1) hyperparameters by K-fold crossvalidation on Z_{train}
Nonlinear System Identification:
2. Compute $\theta \in R^m$ on Z_{train} by applying the training algorithm associated with model M (6.1)
3. Compute the k-step-ahead prediction model. For instance,
    a. Feed-forward neural network (6.4)
    b. Gaussian processes (6.10)
    c. Support vector regression (6.12)
Model Evaluation:
4. Evaluate goodness of fit on Z_{test} by error measures and procedures (e.g., root mean squared error (RMSE), FIT%, J)
Output: $\theta \in R^m$

Table 6.2 Studies Employing Linear Regression Models to Short-Term Prediction of Subcutaneous Glucose Concentration in Diabetes

Study	Model	Input	Prediction Horizon	Evaluation Measures	Dataset	Prediction Performance
Zecchin et al. [1]	FFNN & First-order recursive autoregressive model Nonpersonalized model	Continuous Glucose Monitoring (CGM) Carbohydrate compartmental modeling [2]	30 min	RMSE Time Gain $ESOD_{norm}$ J	In-silico data/University of Virginia/University of Padova Simulator Fifteen people with type 1 diabetes CGM device: Freestyle Navigator, Abbott Diabetes Care Sampling interval: 1 min Monitoring period: 7 days	RMSE 9.4 ± 1.5 mg/dL Time Gain 24.9 ± 4.4 min $ESOD_{norm}$ 1.9 ± 0.2 J 3.1 ± 1.2 RMSE 14.0 ± 4.1 mg/dL Time Gain 16.2 ± 3.7 min $ESOD_{norm}$ 2.7 ± 1.6 J 10.8 ± 7.4
Zecchin et al. [3,4]	Jump neural network Nonpersonalized model	CGM Carbohydrate compartmental modeling [2]	30 min	RMSE Time Gain $ESOD_{norm}$	Twenty people with type 1 diabetes CGM device: Dexcom Seven Plus, Dexcom Sampling interval: 5 min Monitoring period: 2–3 days	RMSE 16.6 ± 3.1 mg/dL Time Gain 18.5 ± 3.4 min $ESOD_{norm}$ 9.6 ± 1.6
Zarkogianni et al. [5]	SOM Physical activity: energy expenditure	CGM Physical activity: energy expenditure	30, 60, 120 min	RMSE Correlation coefficient (CC) (%) MARD Continuous Glucose Error Grid Analysis (CG-EGA)	Ten people with type 1 diabetes CGM device: Guardian RT, Medtronic Inc. Sampling interval: 5 min Monitoring period: 6 days	**Case 1** *RMSE* 30 min: 12.29 ± 2.27 mg/dL 60 min: 21.06 ± 3.20 mg/dL 120 min: 33.68 ± 5.26 mg/dL *CC%* 30 min: 97.92 ± 0.70 60 min: 94.00 ± 1.77 120 min: 84.22 ± 4.87 *MARD* 30 min: 5.34 ± 1.08 60 min: 9.36 ± 1.95 120 min: 15.99 ± 3.14 *CG-EGA (accurate readings)* 30 min: Hypo 91.11% Hyper 88.59% 60 min: Hypo 78.47% Hyper 86.96% 120 min: Hypo 56.40% Hyper 84.73% **Case 2** *RMSE* 30 min: 11.42 ± 2.33 mg/dL 60 min: 19.58 ± 3.80 mg/dL 120 min: 31.00 ± 6.07 mg/dL *CC%* 30 min: 98.14 ± 0.37 60 min: 94.26 ± 1.27 120 min: 84.28 ± 6.54 *MARD* 30 min: 5.19 ± 1.48 60 min: 8.95 ± 2.24 120 min: 14.56 ± 3.46 *CG-EGA (accurate readings)* 30 min: Hypo 89.10% Hyper 90.65% 60 min: Hypo 76.70% Hyper 89.06% 120 min: Hypo 58.77% Hyper 86.17%

Reference	Models	Features	Prediction horizon	Evaluation metrics	Dataset	Case 1	Case 6
Georga et al. [6]	SVR	CGM, Carbohydrate and insulin compartmental modeling [7, 8], Physical activity: energy expenditure, Time of the day	5, 15, 30, 60, 120 min	RMSE, Correlation coefficient, CG-EGA	Fifteen people with type 1 diabetes. CGM device: Guardian RT, Medtronic Inc. Sampling interval: 5 min. Monitoring period: 12.5 ± 4.6 days	RMSE 15 min: 9.05 ± 2.24 mg/dL 30 min: 15.29 ± 2.76 mg/dL 60 min: 24.19 ± 3.78 mg/dL 120 min: 33.04 ± 6.49 mg/dL *Correlation coefficient* 15 min: 0.98 ± 0.01 30 min: 0.95 ± 0.01 60 min: 0.87 ± 0.05 120 min: 0.72 ± 0.12 *CG-EGA (accurate readings)* 15 min: Hypo 95 32% Hyper 81.84% 30 min: Hypo 81.94% Hyper 76.05% 60 min: Hypo 42.56% Hyper 70.21% 120 min: Hypo 16.20% Hyper 66.34%	RMSE 15 min: 5.21 ± 1.58 mg/dL 30 min: 6.03 ± 1.67 mg/dL 60 min: 7.14 ± 1.84 mg/dL 120 min: 7.62 ± 1.81 mg/dL *Correlation coefficient* 15 min: 0.90 ± 0.00 30 min: 0.99 ± 0.00 60 min: 0.99 ± 0.01 120 min: 0.99 ± 0.01 *CG-EGA (accurate readings)* 15 min: Hypo 96.75% Hyper 90.00% 30 min: Hypo 94.05% Hyper 89.28% 60 min: Hypo 90.59% Hyper 87.45% 120 min: Hypo 90.05% Hyper 83.29%
Georga et al. [9]	SVR, Random forests, RRelief	CGM, Carbohydrate and insulin compartmental modeling [7,8], Physical activity: energy expenditure, Time of the day 1	30, 60 min	RMSE	Fifteen people with type 1 diabetes. CGM device: Guardian RT, Medtronic Inc. Sampling interval: 5 min. Monitoring period: 12.5 ± 4.6 days	SVR-RF *RMSE* 30 min: 5.7 ± 1.5 mg/dL 60 min: 6.4 ± 2.1 mg/dL	SVR-RRelief *RMSE* 30 min: 5.9 ± 1.4 mg/dL 60 min: 6.8 ± 2.0 mg/dL
Ståhl et al. [10]	Sliding window, Bayesian model averaging, Linear state-space models, Recursive ARX model, Kernel-based model	CGM, Carbohydrate and insulin compartmental modeling [2]	60 min 40 min	RMSE, Clarke Error Grid Analysis	In-silico data/University of Virginia/University of Padova Simulator Six people with type 1 diabetes. CGM device: Freestyle Navigator, Abbot Diabetes Care, Dexcom Seven Plus, Dexcom. Sampling interval: Monitoring period: 3 days	*RMSE* Mode A: 8.4 mg/dL Mode B: 7.6 mg/dL Mode A + B: 8.1 mg/dL Trial B Median RMSE/RMSE$_{best}$ [min−max] 1.03 [0.75−1.04] CG-EGA−Zones A + B 95.5%	Trial C Median RMSE/RMSE$_{best}$ [min−max] 1.03 [0.94−1.05] CG-EGA−Zones A + B 95.3%

6.2 Neural Networks

6.2.1 Basic Concepts of Neural Networks

Feed-forward neural networks (FFNNs) are universal function approximators of the class of linear regression models:

$$f(x, \theta) = \sum_{j=0}^{m} \theta_j \phi_j(x) = \theta^T \phi(x), \tag{6.2}$$

where $\theta = (\theta_0, \ldots, \theta_m)^T$ are model parameters and $\phi = (\phi_0, \ldots, \phi_m)^T$ is a vector of nonlinear parametric basis functions, with θ_0 being the bias parameter and $\phi_0(x) = 1$. Each basis function $\phi_j(x)$ constitutes itself a nonlinear function of a linear combination of the input $x \in R^d$ [11]:

$$\phi_j(x) = h\left(\sum_{i=0}^{d} w_{ji}^{(1)} x^i\right), \tag{6.3}$$

where the coefficients $w_{ji}^{(1)}$, with $i = 1, \ldots, d$, and $w_{j0}^{(1)}$ ($x^0 = 1$) are the weights and biases, respectively, corresponding to the links between the input and the jth node of the hidden layer of the FFNN, and h is a nonlinear differentiable activation function which is typically implemented as a sigmoidal function. According to (6.2), the output of a FFNN is formulated as follows:

$$y_l(x, w) = \sum_{j=0}^{m} w_{lj}^{(2)} \phi_j(x) = \sum_{j=0}^{m} w_{lj}^{(2)} h\left(\sum_{i=0}^{d} w_{ji}^{(1)} x^i\right), \tag{6.4}$$

where $\phi_0(x) = 1$, and similarly to (6.3), the coefficients $w_{lj}^{(2)}$, with $l = 1, \ldots, L$, and $w_{l0}^{(2)}$ are the weights and biases of the links between the hidden layer and the lth node of the output layer of the FFNN. The weights $w^{(1)} \in R^{d \times m}$ and $w^{(2)} \in R^{m \times L}$ are concatenated into the parameter vector $\theta = \left[w^{(1)}, w^{(2)}\right]^T$.

Given a training set Z_{train} of size $N_{Z_{train}}$, iterative nonlinear optimization methods are employed to locate the parameters θ which minimize the defined error function $E(\theta)$:

$$\theta^{(\tau+1)} = \theta^{(\tau)} + \Delta\theta^{(\tau)}, \tag{6.5}$$

where τ is the iteration step, also called an epoch. $\Delta\theta^{(\tau)}$ is typically specified with respect to the gradient of the error function $\nabla E(\theta)$ (e.g., gradient descent, conjugate gradients), which is efficiently computed by the error backpropagation method [12]. At each iteration step τ, the whole training set is processed in order to evaluate $\nabla E(\theta)$ at $\theta^{(\tau)}$ and, then, $\theta^{(\tau+1)}$ is updated based on (6.5). Note that the error function $E(\theta)$, irrespective of its form (it is typically defined as the sum of squared residuals), is a nonconvex function of θ and, therefore, multiple reruns of the optimization algorithm need to be performed in order to avoid a local minimum solution. As we have discussed in Chapter 3, Methodology for Developing a Glucose Prediction Model, regularization as well as early stopping can be used to balance the bias and the variance of an FFNN. The generalization performance of an FFNN is also highly affected by the value of the hyper-parameter m, which is determined by crossvalidation over the training set Z_{train}. Alternatively, a large value of m is selected and regularization is used to control model's complexity.

The extreme learning machine (ELM) method has been proposed for training single hidden layer FFNNs [13]. ELM is a universal learner featuring a high computational efficiency accompanied by a high accuracy, which makes ELM well-suited for large-scale real-time data processing. Given a new input $x \in R^d$, the output of ELM is expressed as follows:

$$f(x) = \sum_{j=1}^{m} \theta_j h_j(x) = \theta^T h(x), \tag{6.6}$$

where $\theta = (\theta_1, \ldots, \theta_m)^T$ is the weight vector between the hidden layer of m nodes and the output node, $h = [h_1, \ldots, h_m]^T$ is the ELM nonlinear feature mapping and each $h_i(x)$ can be a nonlinear piecewise continuous function which parameters are randomly generated from any continuous probability distribution [13]. By formulating ELM optimization as a regularized least squares problem, θ is written in closed form as follows:

$$\theta^* = H^T \left(HH^T + \frac{I}{C} \right)^{-1} Y, \tag{6.7}$$

where H is defined as $H = [h(x^1), \ldots, h(x^N)]^T$, the output vector $Y = [y_1, \ldots, y_N]^T$, I is the $N \times N$ identity matrix, and C is the regularization parameter. Note that the elements $\langle h(x^i), h(x^j) \rangle$ of the $N \times N$ matrix $K = HH^T$ can be expressed via a kernel function κ deriving a kernel-based representation of the ELM function [14]:

$$f(x) = \left[\kappa(x, x^1), \ldots, \kappa(x, x^N) \right] \left(K + \frac{I}{C} \right)^{-1} Y. \tag{6.8}$$

6.2.2 Glucose Prediction Applications

Zecchin et al. proposed a hybrid scheme combining a FFNN with a linear model to describe both nonlinear and linear s.c. glucose system dynamics 30 minutes ahead [1]. The glucose concentration at time t is predicted as the sum of the linear model's output $\hat{y}_l(t)$ and the error $\hat{e}(t)$ associated with $\hat{y}_l(t)$ as it is estimated by the FFNN, i.e., $\hat{y}(t) = \hat{y}_l(t) + \hat{e}(t)$. The linear model has been postulated as a first-order polynomial which parameters are learnt recursively by weighted least squares [15]. The FFNN is comprised of one hidden layer with $H = 8$ neurons having a tangent sigmoid activation function, and one output layer with one neuron having a linear function. The FFNN estimates the error $\hat{e}(t) = y(t) - \hat{y}_l(t)$ as a function of (1) the error $e(t - kT) = y(t - kT) - \hat{y}_l(t - kT)$ relating to the glucose concentration value at time $t - kT$ [i.e., $y(t - k)$], (2) the trend $(1 - z^{-T_m})e(t - kT)$ over the last $T_m = 15$ minutes, (3) the value of $y(t - kT)$, (4) the trend $(1 - z^{-T_m})y(t - kT)$ over the last $T_m = 15$ minutes, (5) the glucose rate of appearance at time t, i.e., $Ra(t)$ computed according to [2], and (6) the difference vector $[(1-z^{T_a}),(z^{T_a}-z^{2T_a}),(z^{2T_a}-z^{3T_a})]^T Ra(t)$, with $T_a = 10$ minutes for a prediction horizon of 30 minutes. Note that the model requires that the user should announce meal information at least kT minutes in advance. The weights and bias parameters of the network are trained based on the Levenberg–Marquardt back-propagation algorithm applied in a batch mode and with early-stopping (i.e., validation set). In addition, both network structure and inputs were determined by 10-fold crossvalidation over the training set. More specifically, the method was evaluated on 20 in silico subjects from the University of Virginia/Padova type 1 diabetes simulator [16] as well as on 15 subjects with type 1 diabetes monitored in free-living conditions within the DIAdvisor project [17]. Authors merged the data of all patients and, subsequently, properly divided them into training and test sets aiming at deriving a nonpersonalized predictive solution. The comparison with two state-of-the-art univariate glucose models, having a linear time-varying AR(1) [15] and a nonlinear FFNN structure [18], respectively, demonstrated, with regard to the real data and for a 30-minute prediction horizon, a RMSE almost identical to that of the FFNN (14.0 ± 4.1 vs 14.2 ± 4.5 mg/dL) accompanied by improved, comparable to those of the recursive AR(1) model, time gain (16.2 ± 3.7 vs 12.8 ± 1.6 minutes) and regularity indices (ESOD_{norm} 2.7 ± 1.6 vs 105.3 ± 52.8). It is worth noting that the predominance of the proposed by Zecchin et al. algorithm over the other two methods is more prominent in the case of simulated data.

Zecchin et al., in a subsequent study, simplified their glucose prediction algorithm by substituting a jump neural network for the abovementioned hybrid scheme and, in parallel, reducing the input complexity [3]. A jump neural network resembles a FFNN which inputs are connected to the first hidden layer and the output layer, as well. In particular, the s.c. glucose concentration at time t is predicted by feeding the jump neural network with (1) the glucose concentration value at time $t - kT$, i.e., $y(t - kT)$, (2) the difference $\Delta y(t - kT)$, (3) the rate of glucose appearance into plasma at time $t - kT$, i.e., $Ra(t - kT)$, and (4) the difference $\Delta Ra(t - kT)$. The connection of the input to the output introduces a term $w_{IO}^T [y(t-kT), \Delta y(t-kT), Ra(t-kT), \Delta Ra(t-kT), 1]^T$, where w_{IO} is the corresponding weight vector, which first two terms account for the linear glycemic dynamics and the last two capture the linear short-term effect of Ra on the s.c. glucose. The jump neural network comprises 1 hidden layer of $H = 5$ neurons with a tangent sigmoid activation function, and one output neuron with a linear function. As in the preceding study of Zecchin et al. [1], the model's parameters are optimized by the Levenberg–Marquardt back-propagation algorithm over the training set via crossvalidation. The method was evaluated on 20 subjects with type 1 diabetes, who were monitored over a 2–3 day period in real-life conditions; with the datasets of 10 patients forming the training and validation sets, and the remaining 10 datasets forming the test set. An average RMSE of 16.6 ± 3.1 mg/dL is obtained, whereas the predicted profile is characterized by a tolerable delay (time gain: 18.5 ± 3.4 minutes) and limited spurious oscillations (ESOD_{norm}: 9.6 ± 1.6). Moreover, besides its simpler structure, the jump neural network has on average a statistically comparable generalization performance to the reference model in [1].

Three different types of artificial neural networks (ANNs), i.e., a self-organizing map (SOM), a neuro-fuzzy network with wavelets as activation functions (wavelet fuzzy neural network,

WFNN), and a FFNN, were compared with respect to the prediction of the s.c. glucose concentration in type 1 diabetes over a 30-, 60-, and 120-minute horizon in [5]. The original SOM algorithm is modified in order to obtain multiple local linear models, which would allow its incorporation into a closed-loop glucose controller. Besides the glucose signal, information on the energy expenditure (EE) during daily physical activities is also exploited. In particular, the input vector comprises $y(t - kT)$, $\Delta y(t - kT)$ and the sum of EE within the 30-minute interval $[t - kT - 150, t - kT - 120]$, with a delay of 120 being imposed in the effect of the extra input such that predictions up to 120 minutes ahead being possible. Two input cases, i.e., Case 1 and Case 2, are defined to examine the contribution of information related to EE to the prediction performance. Data from 10 patients with type 1 diabetes observed for 6 days, in the framework of the EU-funded research project METABO, were used. All models were evaluated individually for each patient by 10-fold crossvalidation, whereas their hyper-parameters were either preselected or determined though 10-fold crossvalidation over each training set. In Case 1, SOM was found statistically more accurate than FFNN and WFNN in terms of the RMSE, the correlation coefficient (CC) and the mean absolute relative difference (MARD) for all horizons. Moreover, CG-EGA revealed its better performance in hypoglycemic and hyperglycemic ranges over the other models and for all horizons. Case 2 yielded a considerable improvement in predictive performance: (RMSE: -7%, -3%, -10%; CC: $+6\%$, $+5\%$, $+11\%$; MARD: -0.2%, $+0.1\%$, -1%, for SOM, WFNN and FFNN, respectively), whereas CG-EGA demonstrated that the beneficial effect of EE is more evident in the hypoglycemic range. SOM also outperformed the other models in Case 2, and, particularly in the hyperglycemic range according to CG-EGA.

6.3 Kernel-Based Regression Models

6.3.1 Basic Concepts of Kernel-Based Regression Models

A key feature of kernel methods is the ability to solve a nonlinear regression problem in the input space X as a linear one in a new feature space F. Kernel methods transform the input space X into a high-dimensional Reproducing Kernel Hilbert Space H through a mapping $\phi: X \rightarrow H$. A positive definite kernel function $\kappa: X \times X \rightarrow R$, such that $\kappa(x, x') = \phi(x) \, \phi(x')$, is utilized and all computations are expressed in terms of the inner product $\kappa(x, x') = \phi(x) \, \phi(x')$ avoiding working directly in the transformed feature space H [19–21]. The Representer Theorem ensures that the output of kernel methods lies in the span of the finite set of kernels centered at the input vectors x_i of the training set $Z_{train} = \{(x^i, y_i)\}_{i=1}^{N_{Z_{train}}}$ and it is expressed by a nonparametric function of the form [20]:

$$f(x) = \sum_{i=1}^{N_{Z_{train}}} a_i \kappa(x^i, x), \tag{6.9}$$

where $a = (a_1, \ldots, a_{N_{Z_{train}}})^T$ is the coefficient vector of the model. Since the number of adjustable parameters in Eq. (6.9) equals the size of the training dataset, some form of constraint should be imposed on the error function to avoid overfitting.

Gaussian Processes (GP) [22] and Support Vector Regression (SVR) [23] kernel-based methods are extensively applied to nonlinear system identification. In the case of GP, the output for a new point $x \in R^d$ is estimated from a Gaussian distribution with mean and covariance given by

$$m(x) = \sum_{i=1}^{N_{Z_{train}}} a_i \kappa(x, x^i), \quad \sigma^2(x) = \kappa(x, x) + \beta^{-1} - k^T C^{-1} k, \tag{6.10}$$

where a_j is the jth component of $C^{-1}y$, with C denoting the $N \times N$ covariance matrix and y the target vector $y = (y_1, y_2, \ldots, y_{N_{Z_{train}}})^T$, and the vector $k = \left[\kappa(x, x^1), \ldots, \kappa(x, x^{N_{Z_{train}}}) \right]^T$. The squared exponential kernel is the default one for GP regression. The noise on the observed values y is considered and it is further assumed to be Gaussian distributed with zero mean and constant variance β for all x^i. The latter contributes to the total variance of the predictive distribution given by (6.10). Note that the kernel function κ is evaluated for all possible pairs x^i and x^j resulting in a nonsparse model.

SVR obtains a sparse solution by utilizing an ε-insensitive loss function in which the error increases linearly with distance beyond the insensitive region. Errors larger than $\pm \varepsilon$ are treated by introducing the slack variables ξ_i and ξ_i^* for each data point x^i. The optimization problem is defined as

$$\text{Minimize} \quad C \sum_{i=1}^{N} (\xi_i + \xi_i^*) + \frac{1}{2} \|w\|^2,$$

$$\text{subject to} \quad \begin{cases} y_i \leq f(x^i) + \varepsilon + \xi_i \\ y_i \geq f(x^i) - \varepsilon - \xi_i^* \\ \xi_i, \xi_i^* \geq 0 \end{cases}. \tag{6.11}$$

The model's complexity is controlled by the regularization parameter C, which determines the tradeoff between the flatness of the SVR function f (i.e., small w) and the amount up to which deviations larger than ε are tolerated. Solving the optimization problem, it is found that the prediction for a new point $x \in R^d$ can be made using:

$$f(x) = \sum_{i=1}^{N_{Z_{train}}} (a_i - a_i^*) \kappa(x, x^i) + b, \tag{6.12}$$

where a_i and a_i^* ($a_i \geq 0$, $a_i^* \geq 0$) are the Lagrange multipliers introduced in the constrained optimization process. The corresponding Karush–Kuhn–Tucker conditions imply that $a_i a_i^* = 0$ for $i = 1, \ldots, N_{Z_{train}}$ and that all points lying inside the ε-tube have $a_i = a_i^* = 0$.

6.3.2 Glucose Prediction Applications

In [6], the problem of the s.c. glucose prediction in patients with type 1 diabetes was addressed in the context of SVR taking advantage of a multivariate dataset acquired under free-living conditions. Physiological models of the s.c. insulin absorption and the glucose absorption following oral ingestion are combined with a patient-specific predictive model of the s.c. glucose concentration. In particular, the s.c. glucose concentration at time t is given by an SVR function of the input $x \in R^d$ until time $t - kT$: (1) the s.c. glucose measurements within the last 30 minutes (y), (2) the plasma insulin concentration within the last 30 minutes with respect to the time of prediction t (I_p), (3) the rate of glucose appearance in plasma within the last 30 minutes with respect to the time of prediction t (Ra), (4) the cumulative amount of glucose that appeared in the systemic circulation with respect to t, calculated every 10 minutes over the last 90 minutes (SRa), (5) the cumulative amount of the energy consumed during physical activities or exercise, calculated every 10 minutes over the last 3 h (SEE), and (6) the hour of day (h) identifying the 24 hourly intervals within a day. Different inputs corresponding to combinations of the abovementioned variables are considered in order to elucidate their effect on the prediction accuracy of a regression technique. First, predictions are made using only past continuous measurements of the s.c. glucose concentration (Case 1). In order to model the glucose dynamics resulting from the insulin injections and the daily meals, the predictive model is enhanced with information regarding I_p and, either Ra alone (Case 2) or in combination with SRa (Case 3). The time of the day, h, is additionally used as a predictor of the 24-hour variation of glucose (Case 4). In addition to the inputs of the two previous cases, the energy consumed during daily physical activities, SEE, is utilized in Case 3 (to form Case 5) and in Case 4 (to form Case 6).

The evaluation of the method was based on a representative dataset from 27 patients with type 1 diabetes, following multiple-dose insulin therapy, which were collected in the framework of the METABO EU-funded research project [24]. Authors mentioned that data samples for which an event (i.e., food intake, insulin intake, moderate or intense exercise) occurs at the time interval $[t - kT, t]$ are not included into the final datasets, as they do not represent a rational mapping between the configured input and the output. This also ensures that for all samples, the upcoming values of Ra and I_p within $[t - kT, t]$ have been computed based only on the insulin and meal recordings until $t - kT$. Moreover, all input data are normalized between 0 and 1 prior to validation. The SVR model is built with a Gaussian radial basis function (RBF) kernel and the hyper parameters C, ε and the kernel parameter γ are optimized using the Differential Evolution (DE) algorithm, which objective function is defined as the average RMSE of the 10-fold cross validation process over each training set. The three-dimensional search space was set as $C \in [0.001, 1024]$, $\varepsilon \in [0.0001, 1]$, and $\gamma \in [0.00001, 8]$. The overall evaluation of the glucose predictive model was performed individually for each patient's dataset by 10-fold cross validation.

It was demonstrated that, in all cases, the short-term predictions (≤ 30 minutes) of the s.c. glucose concentration exhibit a low RMSE and a high degree of correlation with the observed ones, with Case 6 resulting in a 42% and 61% decrease in the average RMSE of 15- and 30-minute predictions, respectively, compared with Case 1. By introducing additional inputs, the 60- and 120-minute prediction accuracy was greatly improved and became clinically acceptable in both normal and critical glucose ranges (based on CG-EGA results). More specifically, the RMSE of 60- and 120-minute predictions in Case 4 reduced to 8.56 and 10.33 mg/dL (i.e., improved by 65% and 69% compared to Case 1), whereas it is reduced to

7.14 and 7.62 mg/dL (i.e., improved by 70% and 77%) in Case 6, respectively. Besides high performance over the full range of glucose values, more than 94% of both short-term (i.e., for 15 and 30 minutes) and medium- to long-term (i.e., for 60 and 120 minutes) hypoglycemic predictions were classified as clinically accurate or with benign errors according to the CG-EGA.

In a subsequent study, Georga et al. proposed feature ranking as a preprocessing step in the construction of patient-specific predictive models of the short-term s.c. glucose concentration in type 1 diabetes [9]. Two well-established feature ranking algorithms suitable for regression problems, i.e., Random Forests (RF) and RReliefF, were employed for assessing the set of features defined in [6] separately for each patient. RF is a prediction technique that incorporates feature ranking as part of the training process [25], while RRelief is a pure feature filtering algorithm based on the nearest neighbors approach [26]. Their main advantages which render them appropriate for the specific application are (1) the sensitivity to informative features as well as to the correlations among them, (2) the absence of assumptions about the (non)linearity of the underlying function, and (3) the low computational complexity [26,27].

The feature set $F = \{F_j\}$, with $j = 1, \ldots, d$, is evaluated individually for each subject by applying the RF or RReliefF algorithm on his/her dataset Z. In that way, each F_j is assigned an importance score W_j and a ranked list of features, R, is produced by sorting them in descending order by W_j. The generality and effectiveness of feature ranking for a specific subject is examined with respect to the predictive performance of a kernel-based regression model (SVR or GP) for the estimation of glucose concentration. A forward selection procedure is employed where features are sequentially added in decreasing order of importance based on RF or RReliefF ranking. To estimate the error rate of the prediction method, an external 10-fold crossvalidation is applied on the dataset Z with feature ranking following the resampling procedure itself. The latter ensures that the dataset used in the ranking process does not overlap with the test set and, therefore, reduces the selection bias in the estimates of the prediction error [28−31].

Both RF and RRelief highlighted how essential is the s.c. glucose signal itself for both prediction horizons and for all 15 patients. Of great interest is that the time at which the predictions are made (i.e., h) was systematically located in the first positions and its score is comparable to that of glucose. This reflects the existence of daily (24 hours) patterns in glucose time series which are imposed either by each patient's lifestyle or by circadian rhythms related to glucose homeostasis [32,33]. The contribution of the other features was also well demonstrated, with I_p features outweighing on average Ra, SRa, and SEE ones. The ranking of latter features, and especially of Ra and SRa, was characterized by substantial interpatient differences. In particular for SEE, its most recent values [i.e., $SSE(t - kT - 20)$, $SSE(t - kT - 10)$, $SSE(t - kT)$] belonged to the highly ranked features in more than 50% of the patients. In addition, both algorithms, and especially RF, revealed some rational attenuation trends over time in average scores of gl, Ra, and SEE [7,34−36]. The effect of I_p seems to be less immediate (since its scores tend to decrease as getting closer to the time of prediction t), which can be considered consistent with clinical evidence indicating inherent delays in peripheral and hepatic insulin action [37]. Short-term predictive modeling of the s.c. glucose concentration using SVR and GP further verified the quality of the resulting feature ranking. The behavior of the average RMSE curve and its convergence for almost $d/2$ features did confirm both feature ranking algorithms properly locate high in hierarchy the most predictive features of glucose concentration. The fact that the prediction performance did not degenerate by applying the average feature ranking reveals the generalizability and robustness of the results. In particular, individualized feature ranking was found to be more appropriate for 60-minute prediction, which may suggest personalized glucose predictive approaches are preferable as the prediction horizon increases. Moreover, the convergence of both error curves for a considerably smaller than $d = 46$ number of features, and the consequent reduction of the input size, is indeed of paramount importance for regression analysis. In particular, the average error of Case 4, in which the number of features is 28, can be obtained with much less features and, moreover, a better solution can be also achieved even when the 7 best features are used instead of Case 1.

6.4 Ensemble Methods

6.4.1 Basic Concepts of Ensemble Methods

A model combining multiple prediction models has the potential to produce significantly better predictions as compared with the individual ones. Bagging is one approach toward this direction according to which given the dataset Z and a model $f(x, \theta)$: (1) a number of datasets $Z_1, \ldots, Z_K$ is created by uniform sampling with replacement from Z, (2) $f(x, \theta)$ is trained on $Z_1, \ldots, Z_K$ resulting in K models $f_i(x, \theta)$ with $i = 1, \ldots, K$, and (3) the output of the final model for a new input x is computed by averaging the predictions of the individual models:

$$f_{\text{average}}(x, \theta) = \frac{1}{K} \sum_{i=1}^{K} f_i(x, \theta). \tag{6.13}$$

Averaging the output of multiple models trained on different versions of the same dataset Z has been shown to reduce the variance in the generalization error, i.e., the sensitivity of a predictive model on the training set Z. In particular, the generalization error of the average model in (6.13) will not exceed the average of the errors of the individual models [12]. For instance, RF is an ensemble of low correlated regression trees, which output is computed as the average of the individual predictions [25]. Each tree in the RF is constructed using an independent set of random vectors generated from a fixed probability distribution. Randomness is usually incorporated into the tree growing process by bootstrap resampling the original training set and randomly selecting the number of features to split a node.

Boosting is a much more powerful approach which differs from bagging in that the individual models are trained sequentially on datasets Z_i containing those samples which are not correctly learnt until iteration i. The predictions of the individual models are combined using weighted averaging, with weights reflecting the performance of f_i on Z_i and being computed as a function of the residuals errors. The generic gradient-based boosting method for regression computes the so-called pseudo-residuals, equal to the negative gradient of the loss function, and fits a base learner f_i to pseudo-residuals, i.e., the training set becomes $\{(x^n, r_n^{(i)}) \mid n = 1, \ldots, N\}$, where $r_n^{(i)}$ is the residual associated with the nth sample at ith iteration [38].

6.4.2 Glucose Prediction Applications

Let us denote with $\hat{y}_i^j$ the prediction of the s.c. glucose concentration at time $t_i = iT$ which is provided by the jth model M_j based upon information up to time $t_{i-k} = (i - k)T$, where k is the number of prediction steps and T the glucose sampling interval. The average prediction $\hat{y}_i^{\text{average}}$ is computed as the weighted sum of the individual predictions of each algorithm:

$$\hat{y}_i^{\text{average}} = \sum_j w_i^j \hat{y}_i^j = w_i^T \hat{y}_i. \tag{6.14}$$

In Ståhl et al. [10], the weight vector w_i is determined based on a sliding window Bayesian model averaging framework, where each component w_i^j is interpreted as the conditional probability $p(M_j | x^i)$. The dataset Z is assumed to be characterized by n dynamic modes $S_i \in S = [1, \ldots, n]$, with T'_{S_i} representing the time points corresponding to mode S_i. By introducing the latent variable $\theta_i \in \Theta = [1, \ldots, p]$ which represents the predictor modes and by assuming a one-to-one relationship between S and Θ (which in turn implies $n = p$), we obtain:

$$p(M_j | x^i) = \sum_q p(M_j | \theta_i = q, \ x^i) p(\theta_i = q | x^i) \Leftrightarrow$$

$$p(w_i) = [p(w_i | \theta_i = 1), \ldots, p(w_i | \theta_i = p)][p(\theta_i = 1 | x^i), \ldots, p(\theta_i = p | x^i)]^T. \tag{6.15}$$

Constrained optimization such that $\sum_j w_{i | \theta_i'} = 1$ is used on the training set to locate the optimal weights for every time point t_i (i.e., $\{w_{i | \theta_i = q}\}_{t_i \in T'_{S_q}}$ in the case of labeled training data and $\{w_{i | \theta_i = q}\}_{T'}$ in the case of unlabeled training data with time points T') and, subsequently, estimate the distribution $p(w_i | \theta_i = q)$ for $q = 1, \ldots, p$.

Starting from a nominal mode $\theta_i = 0$: $p(w_i | \theta_i = 0) \in N(1/m, I)$, the weight vector $w_{i | \theta_{i-1}}$ at each time point t_i is calculated based on the current active mode θ_{i-1}:

$$w_{i | \theta_{i-1}} = \arg\ \min \sum_{j=i-W}^{i-1} \mu^{i-j} L\left(y_j, w_{0 | \theta_{i-1}}^T \hat{y}_j\right) + \left(w_{i | \theta_{i-1}} - w_{i | \theta_{i-1}}\right) \Lambda_{\theta_{i-1}} \left(w_{i | \theta_{i-1}} - w_{0 | \theta_{i-1}}\right)^T,$$

$$\text{s.t.}\ \ \sum_j w_{i | \theta_{i-1}}^j = 1 \tag{6.16}$$

where the forgetting factor μ, the length of the evaluation period W and the regularization matrix Λ_{θ_i} balance the ensemble predictor's robustness and flexibility; Λ_{θ_i} is set equal to the covariance matrix $R_{\theta_k = i}$. Moreover, an asymmetric cost function is selected considering the absolute glucose value and the sign of the prediction error. A mode switch from θ_{i-1} to $\theta_i = q$ occurs according to the following rule:

$$p(\theta_i = q|w_i, x^i) > \lambda, \tag{6.17}$$

Since only one prediction mode θ_i is active at each t_i, (6.15) is condensed to $p(w_i) = p(w_i|\theta_i)$.

Simulated data (University of Virginia/Padova type 1 diabetes simulator) comprising two dynamic modes as well as real data from three clinical trials conducted within the DIAdvisor project [17] were used to demonstrate the efficacy of the averaging framework. Three linear state space models with input $u = [I_p, Ra]$ were first identified on the simulated data (Model I: trained on mode A data, Model II: trained on mode B data, Model III: trained on the entire dataset) and, subsequently, a k-step-ahead prediction model was evaluated using a Kalman filter supposing that $u(s)$ is known for $s \leq t - 1$. On the other hand, a state-space-based model [39], a recursive ARX model [40] and a kernel-based model [41] were identified on the real dataset. In both experiments, the RMSE of the average model was found comparable to that of the best individual model, which indicates the good tracking capability of the system dynamics achieved by the Bayesian model averaging framework.

An adaptive weighted average framework able to combine K different glucose prediction algorithms was proposed in [42]. Each algorithm is assigned an adaptive weight w_i^j, which is inversely proportional to the pertinent sum of squared prediction errors up to time t_i, i.e., $w_i^j \propto 1/SSE_i^j$. A forgetting factor $\alpha \in (0, 1)$ is also introduced in the instantaneous squared error $(e_i^j)^2$ aiming at controlling the contribution of past instances:

$$SSE_i^j = \sum_{n=1}^{i} a^{i-n} (e_n^j)^2, \quad j = 1, \ldots, K.. \tag{6.18}$$

All weights w_i^j are normalized such that:

$$w_i^j = \frac{1}{SSE_i^j} \Big/ \sum_{n=1}^{K} \frac{1}{SSE_i^n}, \quad j = 1, \ldots, K \tag{6.19}$$

Then, the value of $\hat{y}_i$ is given by the weighted sum of the individual predictions of each algorithm (6.14).

As an example, one linear and two nonlinear univariate models of s.c. glucose concentration, namely an autoregressive model AR(5), an ELM with 3 input and 25 hidden nodes, and a SVR ($C = 50$, $\varepsilon = 0.5$ and local optimization of kernel type and parameters), were combined according to (6.18)-(6.19) and evaluated on 10 subjects with type 1 diabetes randomly selected from a JDRF randomized clinical trial [39]. A $\sim 58\%$ of the dataset of each patient (which corresponds to the first 2500 minutes of CGM with a sampling interval $T = 5$ minute, i.e., 500 points) was used as the training set, and the remaining $\sim 42\%$ (which corresponds to the last 1800 minutes, i.e., 360 points) as the test set. The ensemble glucose prediction solution was systematically more accurate compared to the individual ones, in terms of the RMSE, the mean percentage error, the EGA and the J index, for prediction horizons ≤ 45 minutes and, moreover, provided improved robustness to glucose dynamics variations and prediction horizon increase.

6.5 Computational Experiments

The ability of linear regression schemes of the form (6.1) to predict the short-term glucose dynamics in type 1 diabetes is examined herein. A univariate time-invariant approach is followed according to which the k-step-ahead prediction of the s.c. glucose concentration comprises a fixed, trained in a batch mode, nonlinear FFNN- or SVR-based function of past sequences of the glucose signal within the last 30 minutes ($T = 5$ minute). Its generalization ability is tested under free-living dynamic conditions.

A short-term observational study was carried out in the framework of a national research project [43]. The study was approved by the Ethics Committees of the University Hospital of Ioannina (Greece) and all subjects provided written informed consent before enrollment. The glycemic profile of seven subjects with type 1 diabetes (5F/2M, Age: 49.0 ± 10.2 years, Body Mass Index: 26.5 ± 4.6 kg/m), following multiple-dose insulin therapy and without significant micro- and macrovascular complications, was recorded using the Medtronic IPro2 CGM system (Medtronic Minimed Inc.) in ambulatory conditions over a 2-week period. All subjects were obliged to abstain from any structured exercise program during the first week, whereas they had to perform a typical daily exercise program of ≥ 3 metabolic equivalents of task (METs) intensity during the second week. Women followed a 1400 kcal daily diet and men followed a 1600-kcal daily diet over the 2-week period. Table 6.3 presents the descriptive characteristics of the glucose dataset. The corresponding Ambulatory Glucose Profile report [44] of a typical subject (Subject #1) is portrayed in Fig. 6.1, where one can observe the glucose lowering effect of the exercise performed during the second week of the observational period.

Table 6.3 Descriptive Statistics of the Glucose Dataset

	Week #1	Week #2
Average glucose concentration (mg/dL)	154.79 ± 32.79	152.16 ± 41.10
Standard deviation (mg/dL)	52.82 ± 19.23	59.24 ± 26.77
Min glucose concentration (mg/dL)	56.29 ± 12.20	47.86 ± 7.65
Max glucose concentration (mg/dL)	312.43 ± 69.92	314.86 ± 75.55
% of hypoglycemic values[a]	2.44 ± 2.44	5.57 ± 2.33
% of hyperglycemic values[b]	50.03 ± 20.28	44.43 ± 23.09

Data are mean ± standard deviation values.
[a]A glucose concentration value ≤ 70 mg/dL is defined as hypoglycemic.
[b]A glucose concentration value ≥ 140 mg/dL is defined as hyperglycemic.

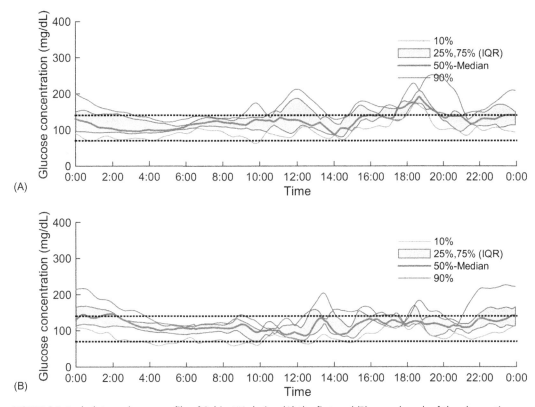

FIGURE 6.1 Ambulatory glucose profile of Subject#1 during (A) the first and (B) second week of the observation period. IQR denotes the interquartile range.

Both the SVR and the FFNN are trained on the first week of the observational period and they are tested on the second one. More specifically, the SVR is built with a Gaussian kernel and the hyper parameters C, ε and the kernel parameter γ are optimized using the DE algorithm, which fitness function is defined as the average RMSE of the fourfold cross validation process over the training set. The search space of the hyperparameters is set to $C \in [0.001, 1024]$, $\varepsilon \in [0.0001, 1]$, and $\gamma \in [0.00001, 8]$. The FFNN is comprised of one hidden layer with H neurons having a tangent sigmoid activation function, and one output layer with one neuron having a linear function. The weights and bias parameters of the network are trained based on the Levenberg–Marquardt back-propagation algorithm applied in a batch mode and with early-stopping (i.e., validation set). In addition, the value of H, in the range [5:5:30], minimizing the fourfold crossvalidation RMSE of the FFNN in the training set is selected, while multiple restarts are used to alleviate the local-minimum problem. The goodness of fit is assessed by: (1) the RMSE, (2) the FIT%, (3) the temporal gain (TG) [3], (4) the sensitivity (SNS) of predictions in the hypoglycemic range, and (5) the false positive rate (FPR) of predictions in the hypoglycemic range.

Table 6.4 presents the predictive performance of SVR over the second week of the observational period and for a prediction horizon of 15, 30, and 60 minutes. The RMSE of the 15-minute predictions as well as the associated FIT% values, ranging from 3.67 to 13.49 mg/dL and from 82.94 to 93.37 mg/dL, respectively, show a sufficiently accurate description of short-term glucose dynamics, which allow for a proactive time of 10 minutes. In addition, the corresponding SNS and FPR values (range: 0.51−0.91 and 0.04−0.15, respectively) demonstrate a reasonable predictive capacity in the hypoglycemic range. The increase of prediction horizon to 30 minutes results in an average RMSE of 17.49 ± 7.72 mg/dL and an average TG of 15.71 ± 1.89 minutes, whereas SNS and FPR of hypoglycemic predictions worsen significantly. The RMSE increases considerably (35.26 ± 12.86 mg/dL) for a prediction horizon of 60 minutes, with FIT% becoming lower than 50% though a 20-minute average time gain is preserved.

FFNN, as it is shown in Table 6.5, produces comparable RMSE and FIT% values for a prediction horizon of ≤ 30 minutes, with the exception of Subject #2 and Subject #5 for whom FFNN presumably falls into a local minimum. Nevertheless, FFNN tends to produce slightly higher RMSEs for 60-minute predictions, which is also translated to lower FIT% values. In addition, FFNN yields a less delayed glucose time series than SVR, which is balanced by a less smooth solution as compared with kernel-based learning. In particular, SVR exhibits highly regularized predictions, which is getting more apparent as horizon increases. In addition, FFNN is more sensitive to hypoglycemic predictions as compared with SVR, with the latter yielding less false positive predictions. Figs. 6.2 and 6.3 illustrate the measured vs the 30-minute-ahead predicted glucose time series for Subject #1 during two indicative days of the monitoring period (11th and 13th day, respectively), where we can observe that both nonlinear univariate solutions predict hyperglycemic excursions with an adequate accuracy but cannot track hypoglycemic ones. The fact that the examined herein univariate solutions cannot capture the variance of the full glucose signal for horizons ≥ 30 minutes, can be explained by the existence of unrepresented inputs (insulin therapy, food intake, exercise) and unmeasured disturbances.

6.6 Discussion and Conclusions

Linear regression models, which comprise linear combinations of adaptive nonlinear basis functions, have been effectively applied to the identification and prediction of the s.c. glucose in diabetes. In this chapter, we focused on neural networks and, mainly sparse, kernel-based learning algorithms, and, we provided a comprehensive overview of the relevant literature.

Both neural networks and kernel methods may approximate nonlinear functions of the input variables, such as glucose concentration, with a given accuracy, while controlling model's complexity to avoid overfitting. FFNNs yield a compact solution which universal approximation capabilities have been well studied; however, FFNNs involve a nonconvex loss function. On the other hand, the solution of kernel-based algorithms lies in the span of the finite set of kernels centered at the input vectors, which necessitates some form of

Table 6.4 Prediction Performance of the SVR Algorithm

| | Prediction Horizon | | | | | | | | | | | | | | | | | |
| | 15 min | | | | | | 30 min | | | | | | 60 min | | | | | |
	RMSE	FIT%	TG	ESOD$_{norm}$	SNS	FPR	RMSE	FIT%	TG	ESOD$_{norm}$	SNS	FPR	RMSE	FIT%	TG	ESOD$_{norm}$	SNS	FPR
Subject 1	3.95	86.95	10	8.84	0.81	0.04	11.25	62.84	15	14.38	0.46	0.12	22.28	26.46	15	9.25	0.11	0.14
Subject 2	3.67	88.86	10	7.93	0.91	0.08	8.43	74.42	20	15.11	0.75	0.23	24.46	25.83	40	129.29	0.21	0.52
Subject 3	6.00	90.93	10	8.95	0.51	0.15	17.10	74.16	15	15.60	0.17	0.50	34.87	47.26	20	13.36	0.11	0.61
Subject 4	8.50	82.94	10	6.88	0.87	0.15	25.02	49.92	15	13.85	0.72	0.40	48.33	3.62	15	14.34	0.33	0.64
Subject 5	13.49	84.70	10	7.72	0.81	0.11	29.87	66.12	15	15.42	0.52	0.29	55.95	36.56	20	20.75	0.18	0.66
Subject 6	4.52	89.32	10	10.43	0.79	0.10	12.39	70.55	15	14.36	0.42	0.05	24.88	40.17	10	9.21	0.23	0.27
Subject 7	6.75	93.37	10	7.50	0.69	0.04	18.34	82.00	15	12.17	0.35	0.14	36.04	64.70	20	15.48	0.18	0.41
Mean	6.70	88.15	10.00	8.32	0.77	0.10	17.49	68.57	15.71	14.41	0.48	0.24	35.26	34.94	20.00	30.24	0.19	0.46
SD	3.45	3.59	0.00	1.18	0.13	0.05	7.72	10.30	1.89	1.17	0.21	0.16	12.86	19.16	9.57	43.85	0.08	0.20

Table 6.5 Prediction Performance of the FFNN Algorithm

| | Prediction Horizon | | | | | | | | | | | | | | | | | |
| | 15 min | | | | | | 30 min | | | | | | 60 min | | | | | |
	RMSE	FIT%	TG	ESOD$_{norm}$	SNS	FPR	RMSE	FIT%	TG	ESOD$_{norm}$	SNS	FPR	RMSE	FIT%	TG	ESOD$_{norm}$	SNS	FPR
Subject 1	3.84	87.31	10	16.14	0.82	0.04	11.54	61.90	15	61.13	0.58	0.19	24.81	18.13	20	86.05	0.15	0.23
Subject 2	5.77	82.48	15	24.66	0.90	0.09	27.32	17.09	30	79.55	0.79	0.32	35.25	−6.90	60	103.64	0.34	0.62
Subject 3	5.32	91.96	10	28.66	0.67	0.08	15.82	76.09	20	115.61	0.50	0.33	36.40	44.95	25	134.07	0.13	0.19
Subject 4	8.09	83.76	15	15.30	0.89	0.13	23.00	53.97	20	60.59	0.59	0.42	47.70	4.88	20	112.39	0.29	0.68
Subject 5	36.96	58.07	15	22.05	0.80	0.12	27.37	68.96	15	70.64	0.53	0.28	77.39	12.25	30	270.12	0.15	0.83
Subject 6	4.60	89.13	10	26.92	0.67	0.14	12.24	70.93	15	74.76	0.25	0.14	25.57	38.51	20	67.87	0.00	1.00
Subject 7	5.97	94.13	10	18.15	0.83	0.13	18.77	81.59	15	70.21	0.58	0.36	51.92	49.15	20	185.12	0.33	0.76
Mean	10.08	83.84	12.14	21.70	0.80	0.10	19.44	61.50	18.57	76.07	0.55	0.29	42.72	22.99	27.86	137.04	0.20	0.61
SD	11.93	12.10	2.67	5.31	0.10	0.03	6.65	21.56	5.56	18.73	0.16	0.10	18.36	21.48	14.68	69.69	0.13	0.30

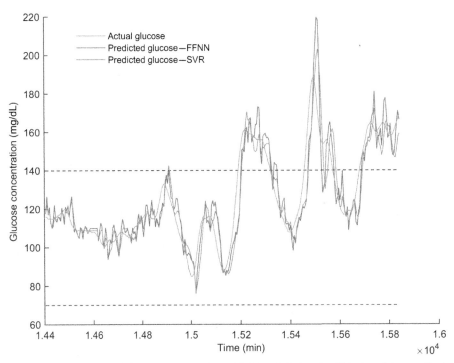

FIGURE 6.2 Predicted vs measured glucose concentration of Subject#1 during the 11th day of the monitoring period for a prediction horizon of 30 min.

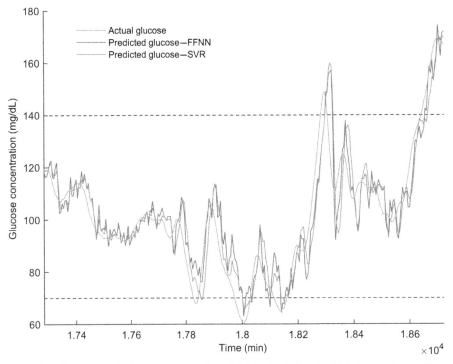

FIGURE 6.3 Predicted vs measured glucose concentration of Subject#1 during the 13th day of the monitoring period for a prediction horizon of 30 min.

sparsification to confine the structure of the underlying radial basis function network and, consequently, accomplish regularization. Particularly SVR, unlike GP, are able to produce regularized, global, sparse solutions to nonlinear regression problems, at the expense of a nonprobabilistic output. However, the procedure for optimizing the hyper-parameters in kernel machines introduces an additional computational cost compared to neural networks.

Literature suggests that nonlinear modeling of the short-term ($\leq$30 minutes) and mostly long-term ($>$30 minutes) s.c. glucose concentration is significantly more accurate as compared with linear, with respect to the input, approaches and, in addition, benefit from the utilization of particularly configured multivariate features sets. Ensemble modeling has also the potential to improve the generalization error of a glucose prediction scheme. Despite the fact that the majority of glucose prediction methods discussed in this chapter are personalized, it becomes evident that the efficient input customization and the representation of the spatio-temporal dependencies between the input variables and the glucose concentration is challenging. Given that linear regression methods are best suited for learning *a priori* defined and fixed memory mappings of input−output data in a stationary environment, techniques that can learn the different modes of the glucose system and represent its time-varying behavior are needed. This will be discussed in Chapter 8, Adaptive Glucose Prediction Models.

References

[1] Zecchin C, et al. Neural network incorporating meal information improves accuracy of short-time prediction of glucose concentration. IEEE Trans Biomed Eng 2012;59(6):1550−60.

[2] Dalla Man C, Camilleri M, Cobelli C. A system model of oral glucose absorption: validation on gold standard data. IEEE Trans Biomed Eng 2006;53(12 Pt 1):2472−8.

[3] Zecchin C, et al. Jump neural network for online short-time prediction of blood glucose from continuous monitoring sensors and meal information. Comput Methods Programs Biomed 2014;113(1):144−52.

[4] Zecchin C, et al. How much is short-term glucose prediction in type 1 diabetes improved by adding insulin delivery and meal content information to CGM data? A proof-of-concept study. J Diabetes Sci Technol 2016;10(5):1149−60.

[5] Zarkogianni K, et al. Comparative assessment of glucose prediction models for patients with type 1 diabetes mellitus applying sensors for glucose and physical activity monitoring. Med Biol Eng Comput 2015;53(12):1333−43.

[6] Georga EI, et al. Multivariate prediction of subcutaneous glucose concentration in type 1 diabetes patients based on support vector regression. IEEE J Biomed Health Inform 2013;17(1):71−81.

[7] Lehmann ED, Deutsch T. A physiological model of glucose−insulin interaction in type 1 diabetes mellitus. J Biomed Eng 1992;14(3):235−42.

[8] Tarin C, et al. Comprehensive pharmacokinetic model of insulin Glargine and other insulin formulations. IEEE Trans Biomed Eng 2005;52(12):1994−2005.

[9] Georga EI, et al. Evaluation of short-term predictors of glucose concentration in type 1 diabetes combining feature ranking with regression models. Med Biol Eng Comput 2015;53(12):1305−18.

[10] Ståhl F, Johansson R, Renard E. Ensemble glucose prediction in insulin-dependent diabetes. In: Marmarelis V, Mitsis G, editors. Data-driven modeling for diabetes: diagnosis and treatment. Berlin, Heidelberg: Springer Berlin Heidelberg; 2014. p. 37−71.

[11] Bishop CM. Neural networks for pattern recognition. Oxford University Press, Inc; 1995. p. 482.

[12] Bishop CM. Pattern recognition and machine learning (information science and statistics). Singapore: Springer-Verlag New York, Inc; 2006.

[13] Huang G, et al. Trends in extreme learning machines: a review. Neural Netw 2015;61:32−48.

[14] Wang X, Han M. Online sequential extreme learning machine with kernels for nonstationary time series prediction. Neurocomputing 2014;145(Supplement C):90−7.

[15] Sparacino G, et al. Glucose concentration can be predicted ahead in time from continuous glucose monitoring sensor time-series. IEEE Trans Biomed Eng 2007;54(5):931−7.

[16] Kovatchev BP, et al. In silico preclinical trials: a proof of concept in closed-loop control of type 1 diabetes. J Diabetes Sci Technol 2009;3(1):44−55.

[17] Poulsen JU, et al. A diabetes management system empowering patients to reach optimised glucose control: from monitor to advisor. Conf Proc IEEE Eng Med Biol Soc 2010;2010:5270−1.

[18] Perez-Gandia C, et al. Artificial neural network algorithm for online glucose prediction from continuous glucose monitoring. Diabetes Technol Ther 2010;12(1):81−8.

[19] Pillonetto G, et al. Kernel methods in system identification, machine learning and function estimation: a survey. Automatica 2014;50(3):657−82.

[20] Hofmann T, Scholkopf B, Smola AJ. Kernel methods in machine learning. Ann Stat 2008;36 (3):1171−220.

[21] Scholkopf B, Smola AJ. Learning with kernels: support vector machines, regularization, optimization, and beyond. Cambridge, Massachusetts: MIT Press; 2001. p. 632.

[22] Rasmussen CE, Nickisch H. Gaussian processes for machine learning (GPML) toolbox. J Mach Learn Res 2010;11:3011−15.

[23] Smola AJ, Scholkopf B. A tutorial on support vector regression. Stat Comput 2004;14(3):199−222.

[24] Georga E, et al. Data mining for blood glucose prediction and knowledge discovery in diabetic patients: the METABO diabetes modeling and management system. Conf Proc IEEE Eng Med Biol Soc 2009;2009:5633−6.

[25] Breiman L. Random forests. Mach Learn 2001;45(1):5−32.

[26] Robnik-Sikonja M, Kononenko I. Theoretical and empirical analysis of ReliefF and RReliefF. Mach Learn 2003;53(1−2):23−69.

[27] Strobl C, Malley J, Tutz G. An introduction to recursive partitioning: rationale, application, and characteristics of classification and regression trees, bagging, and random forests. Psychol Methods 2009;14 (4):323−48.

[28] Ambroise C, McLachlan GJ. Selection bias in gene extraction on the basis of microarray gene-expression data. Proc Natl Acad Sci USA 2002;99(10):6562−6.

[29] Krzanowski WJ. Discriminant-analysis and statistical pattern-recognition—McLachlan, GJ. J Classif 1993;10(1):128−30.

[30] Di Camillo B, Sanavia T, Martini M, Jurman G, Sambo F, Barla A. Effect of size and heterogeneity of samples on biomarker discovery: Synthetic and real data assessment. PLoS ONE 2012;7(3), 1-8, e32200. http://doi.org/10.1371/journal.pone.0032200.

[31] Furlanello C, et al. Entropy-based gene ranking without selection bias for the predictive classification of microarray data. BMC Bioinformatics 2003;4:1−20.

[32] Froy O. Metabolism and circadian rhythms—implications for obesity. Endocr Rev 2010;31(1):1−24.

[33] Huang W, et al. Circadian rhythms, sleep, and metabolism. J Clin Invest 2011;121(6):2133−41.

[34] Roy A, Parker RS. Dynamic modeling of exercise effects on plasma glucose and insulin levels. J Diabetes Sci Technol 2007;1(3):338−47.

[35] Kovatchev B, Clarke W. Peculiarities of the continuous glucose monitoring data stream and their impact on developing closed-loop control technology. J Diabetes Sci Technol 2008;2(1):158−63.

[36] Derouich M, Boutayeb A. The effect of physical exercise on the dynamics of glucose and insulin. J Biomech 2002;35(7):911−17.

[37] Miles PD, et al. Kinetics of insulin action in vivo. Identification of rate-limiting steps. Diabetes 1995;44 (8):947−53.

[38] Duffy N, Helmbold D. Boosting methods for regression. Mach Learn 2002;47(2−3):153−200.

[39] Ståhl F. Diabetes mellitus glucose prediction by linear and Bayesian ensemble modeling. Department of Automatic Control. Lund University Sweden, Lund; 2012.

[40] Estrada, G.C., et al. Innovative approach for online prediction of blood glucose profile in type 1 diabetes patients, In: Proceedings of the 2010 American control conference; 2010.

[41] Naumova V, Pereverzyev SV, Sivananthan S. A meta-learning approach to the regularized learning-case study: blood glucose prediction. Neural Netw 2012;33:181−93.

[42] Wang Y, Wu X, Mo X. A novel adaptive-weighted-average framework for blood glucose prediction. Diabetes Technol Ther 2013;15(10):792−801.

[43] Georga, E.I., et al. Development of a smart environment for diabetes data analysis and new knowledge mining, In: EAI 4th international conference on. 2014. Wireless Mobile Communication and Healthcare (Mobihealth); 2014.

[44] Bergenstal RM, et al. Recommendations for standardizing glucose reporting and analysis to optimize clinical decision making in diabetes: the Ambulatory Glucose Profile (AGP). Diabetes Technol Ther 2013;15(3):198−211.

Prediction Models of Hypoglycemia

7.1 Prediction of Hypoglycemic Events

The prevention of hypoglycemic events is of paramount importance in the daily management of insulin-treated diabetes. The use of short-term prediction algorithms of the subcutaneous (s.c.) glucose concentration may contribute significantly toward this direction. The literature suggests that, although the recent glucose profile is a prominent predictor of hypoglycemia, the overall patient's context greatly impacts its accurate estimation. This specific problem has been dealt with through linear, time-invariant or adaptive, autoregressive moving average (ARMA) models as well as batch or adaptive machine learning classification or regression algorithms, which exploit solely the recent continuous glucose monitoring (CGM) profile or in conjunction with information on medication (insulin therapy), behavior (e.g., meals, physical activity) or physiological signals linked to autonomic nervous system activation in response to a hypoglycemic excursion [1,2]. In particular, the hypoglycemia-induced changes in galvanic skin response (GSR), electrocardiogram (ECG) and electroencephalogram have been exploited toward hypoglycemia detection or prediction. Nevertheless, the nonspecificity of GSR- and ECG-related features to hypoglycemia (e.g., increase in perspiration or heart rate) as well as the effect of hypoglycemia-associated autonomic failure (HAAF) necessitate properly fusing them with blood or s.c. glucose data, aiming at reducing false-positive (FP) predictions.

An essential component of the evaluation or validation procedure of a glucose predictive modeling approach is the assessment of its predictive capacity in the hypoglycemic region, which is implemented either in a sample- or an event-based manner. As it has been described in Chapter 3, Methodology for Developing a Glucose Prediction Model, continuous glucose-error grid analysis (CG-EGA) enables the classification of predictions concerning hypoglycemic values as accurate readings (AR), benign errors (BE), or erroneous reading (ER) considering the result of the point-error and rate-error grid analyses as well as the clinical impact of the consequent treatment decisions. Individual glucose predictions can be also characterized as true-positive (TP) with regard to the corresponding actual glucose concentration value if both fall in the hypoglycemic region, which, in turn, allows the computation of classical statistical measures of the performance of a model (e.g., accuracy, sensitivity, specificity, FP rate) [3]. Table 7.1 defines TP, FP, true negative (TN), and false negative (FN) predictions considering hypoglycemic instances as positive and nonhypoglycemic instances as negative.

Table 7.1   Characterization of Predictions with Respect to Hypoglycemia

	Predicted Glucose Value	
Actual Glucose Value	Hypoglycemic	Nonhypoglycemic
Hypoglycemic	True positive (TP)	False negative (FN)
Nonhypoglycemic	False positive (FP)	True negative (TN)

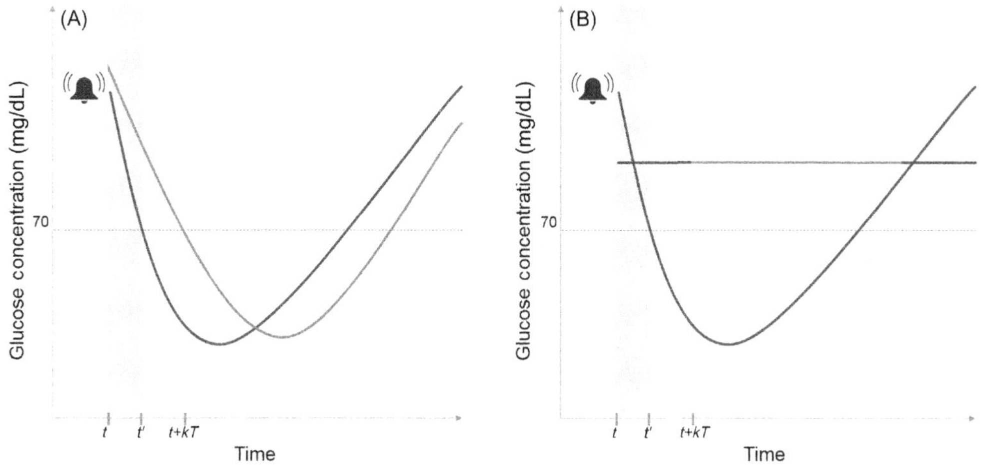

FIGURE 7.1 Prediction of a hypoglycemic event $t' - t$ min in advance based on: (A) Regression: The blue (gray in print versions) curve denotes the actual glucose time series and the red (black in print versions) curve denotes the predicted one, (B) Classification: The red and green lines denote "hypoglycemia" and "nonhypoglycemia" class, respectively, as predicted by the model. The dashed line represents the hypoglycemic threshold equal to 70 mg/dL.

On the other hand, the problem of hypoglycemic event prediction, which is related to the early prediction of the onset of the event, requires the detection of the hypoglycemic events in the actual glucose time series and the proper characterization of TP, FP, and FN hypoglycemic events in the predicted one [4,5]. We should recall that TN predictions cannot be applied, since nonhypoglycemic intervals cannot be considered as discrete events. The time of detection, defined as the time interval between the start of the alarm (or the start of the predicted hypoglycemic event) and the start of the actual hypoglycemic event, determines if an impeding event is truly preventable. Fig. 7.1 illustrates a typical scenario: (1) A glucose prediction algorithm, trained to produce k-step-ahead predictions, issues an alarm at time t for an impending hypoglycemic event at time $t + kT$, with T expressing the sampling interval of glucose concentration, (2) if the true event starts at time t', the time intervals $t' - t$ and $t + kT - t'$ denote the detection time and the time lag between the predicted and the actual glucose time series, respectively. The detection time or the time lag are commonly used to define TP predictions irrespective of whether a regression or classification approach is adopted. The process of building and validating a hypoglycemia prediction model is portrayed in Fig. 7.2 and described in the following sections.

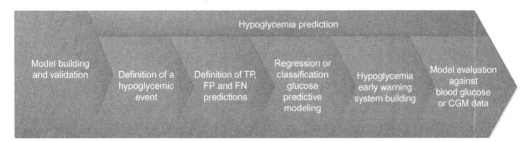

FIGURE 7.2 The process of developing a hypoglycemic event prediction model.

7.2 Hypoglycemia Prediction as a Regression Problem

Table 7.2 reports regression models which were evaluated with respect to their ability to predict single hypoglycemic concentration values. In Naumova et al. [6], data from a specially designed clinical trial was utilized enabling the evaluation of the proposed Tikhonov regularization learning algorithm against reference blood glucose samples by the Yellow Spring Instruments (YSI) analyzer. More specifically, the prediction-error grid analysis (PRED-EGA) characterized 90.89%, 90.82%, and 81.75% of predictions of blood glucose values ≤ 70 mg/dL, with reference to YSI, as accurate for a prediction horizon of 0, 10, and 20 minutes, respectively, slightly outperforming the DexCom CGM system which yielded 89.86% accurate predictions. In what follows, we focus on methods treating the problem of hypoglycemia prediction as an event prediction problem, which is solved through linear system identification or linear regression models of machine learning, mentioning which of them have been validated against blood glucose data (Table 7.3). In addition, we emphasize on the definition of the events, the inference of a predictive warning and the evaluation of TP event, whereas the technical specifications of the adopted linear or nonlinear glucose prediction models are discussed in Chapter 5, Linear Time Series Models of Glucose Concentration, Chapter 6, Nonlinear Models of Glucose Concentration, and Chapter 8, Adaptive Glucose Prediction Models.

7.2.1 Hypoglycemia Prediction Methods Based on Time Series Analysis

Weighted recursive least squares, with an adjustable forgetting factor, was used for the identification of ARMA models of s.c. glucose dynamics in type 2 diabetes [7]. Having set the hypoglycemic threshold to 60 mg/dL, a hypoglycemic event was defined as at least two consecutive (i.e., ≥ 10 minutes) blood glucose measurements ≤ 60 mg/dL, with its end being denoted by a reference glucose value > 65 mg/dL. In this context, three different methods were proposed to hypoglycemic alarm generation: (1) Absolute predicted value: A hypoglycemic alarm is issued at time t_i if the k-step-ahead prediction of s.c. glucose concentration $\hat{y}(t_{i+k}|\theta)$ is < 60 mg/dL, (2) Cumulative sum control chart (CUSUM): A hypoglycemic alarm is issued at time t_i if the lower control limit of the CUSUM $C_i^- = \max[0, (\mu_0 - K) - \hat{y}(t_{i+k}|\theta) + C_{i-1}^-]$, with $C_0^- = 0$, exceeds a certain threshold value $\approx 5\sigma$, where

Table 7.2 Hypoglycemia Prediction Methods Evaluated in a Sample-Based Mode

Study	Model	Input	Prediction Horizon	Evaluation Measures	Dataset	Prediction Performance	
Zarkogianni et al. [7]	Self-organizing map Hypoglycemic threshold: 70 mg/dL	CGM data Physical activity: energy expenditure	30, 60, 120 min	CG-EGA	Ten people with type 1 diabetes monitored in normal daily life conditions CGM device: Guardian RT, Medtronic Inc. Sampling interval: 5 min Monitoring period: 6 days	Case 1 *CG-EGA hypoglycemia* 30 min: AR 91.1% BE 2.4% ER 6.5% 60 min: AR 78.5% BE 2.5% ER 19.0% 120 min: AR 56.4% BE 2.1% ER 41.5%	Case2 *CG-EGA hypoglycemia* 30 min: AR 89.1% BE 0.9% ER 10.0% 60 min: AR 76.7% BE 1.2% ER 22.1% 120 min: AR 58.8% BE 1.2% ER 40.0%
Georga et al. [8]	SVR Hypoglycemic threshold: 70 mg/dL	CGM data Carbohydrate and insulin compartmental modeling Physical activity: energy expenditure Time of the day	5, 15, 30, 60, 120 min	CG-EGA	Fifteen people with type 1 diabetes monitored in normal daily life conditions CGM Device: Guardian RT, Medtronic Inc. Sampling interval: 5 min Monitoring period: 12.5 ± 4.6 days	Case 1 *CG-EGA hypoglycemia* 15 min: AR 95.3% BE 3.4% ER 1.3% 30 min: AR 81.9% BE 5.4% ER 12.6% 60 min: AR 42.6% BE 4.1% ER 53.3% 120 min: AR 16.2% BE 2.8% ER 81.0%	Case 6 *CG-EGA hypoglycemia* 15 min: AR 96.7% BE 2.4% ER 0.9% 30 min: AR 94.1% BE 2.9% ER 3.0% 60 min: AR 90.1% BE 3.9% ER 5.5% 120 min: AR 90.1% BE 6.3% ER 3.6%
Eren-Oruklu et al. [9]	ARMA Weighted recursive least squares with adaptive forgetting factor Hypoglycemic threshold: 70 mg/dL	CGM data	30 min	CG-EGA	Fourteen people with type 2 diabetes monitored in normal daily life conditions CGM Device: System Gold, Medtronic Inc. Sampling interval: 5 min Monitoring period: 2 days	*CG-EGA hypoglycemia* AR 92.94% BE 5.29% % ER 1.77%	

	Method	Data	Prediction horizon	Metrics	Study	Results
Eren-Oruklu et al. [10]	ARMAX Weighted recursive least squares with adaptive forgetting factor Hypoglycemic threshold: 60 mg/dL	CGM data Physiological data: energy expenditure, average longitudinal acceleration, heat flux, GSR, near-body temperature	30 min	Sensitivity False Discovery Rate ROC	Five people with type 2 diabetes monitored in normal daily life conditions CGM Device: MMT-7012, Medtronic Inc. Sampling interval: 5 min Monitoring period: 23.8 ± 2.4 days	*Sensitivity (%)* 74 *False discovery rate (%)* 31
Wang et al. [11,12]	Time-varying state-space model Extended Kalman filter Hypoglycemic Threshold: 70 mg/dL	CGM data FIR modeling of s.c. insulin absorption and meal absorption	30 min	Sensitivity False Discovery rate	Five people with type 1 diabetes using insulin pump monitored in normal daily life conditions CGM Device: Minimed CGM MMT-7102, Medtronic Inc. Sampling interval: 5 min Monitoring period: 60.4 ± 10.6 h	*Sensitivity (%)* 78.71 ± 7.26 *False discovery rate (%)* 35.60 ± 9.61 *Detection time (min)* 12.00 ± 10.37
Naumova et al. [6]	Regularized kernel learning Meta-learning approach to choosing a Kernel and a regularization parameter Hypoglycemic threshold: 70 mg/dL	CGM data	0, 10, 20 min	PRED-EGA (with reference to blood glucose measurements)	Six people with type 1 diabetes under a hospitalized setting CGM Device: DexCom CGM Sampling Interval: 5 min Blood Glucose Device: Yellow Springs Instrument BG sampling interval: 5–10 min for specific time periods resulting in 120 blood samples per patient Monitoring period: 3 days	*PRED-EGA* 0 min: AR: 90.89%, BE: 4.94%, ER: 4.17% 10 min: AR: 90.82%, BE: 5.16%, ER: 4.02% 20 min: AR: 81.75%, BE: 5.16%, ER: 13.09%

Table 7.3 Hypoglycemia Prediction Methods Evaluated in an Event-based Mode

Study	Model	Input	Prediction Horizon	Evaluation Measures	Dataset	Prediction Performance — Nocturnal Events: Case 1a	Nocturnal Events: Case 3a	Diurnal Events: Case 1	Diurnal Events: Case 2
Georga et al. [13]	SVR Hypoglycemic threshold: 70 mg/dL Event definition Start: ≥ 2 consecutive s.c. glucose concentration values below or equal to 70 mg/dL. End: >1 consecutive s.c. glucose concentration values above 70 mg/dL	CGM data Carbohydrate and insulin compartmental modeling Physical activity: energy expenditure Time of the day	30, 60 min	Sensitivity (SNS) Precision (PRC) Time lag (TL)	Fifteen people with type 1 diabetes monitored in normal daily life conditions CGM Device: Guardian RT, Medtronic Inc. Sampling interval: 5 min Monitoring period: 12.5 ± 4.6 days	SNS 30 min: 0.89 ± 0.21 60 min: 0.88 ± 0.20 PRC 30 min: 0.98 ± 0.06 60 min: 0.96 ± 0.12 TL (min) 30 min: 8.68 ± 8.73 60 min: 7.81 ± 10.39	SNS 30 min: 0.94 ± 0.10 60 min: 0.94 ± 0.10 PRC 30 min: 0.98 ± 0.08 60 min: 0.98 ± 0.08 TL (min) 30 min: 5.43 ± 7.11 60 min: 4.57 ± 5.47	SNS 30 min: 0.92 ± 0.12 60 min: 0.96 ± 0.14 PRC 30 min: 0.93 ± 0.13 60 min: 0.97 ± 0.10 TL (min) 30 min: 4.53 ± 5.30 60 min: 3.64 ± 4.72	SNS 30 min: 0.84 ± 0.23 60 min: 0.93 ± 0.17 PRC 30 min: 0.94 ± 0.16 60 min: 0.96 ± 0.14 TL (min) 30 min: 3.17 ± 4.65 60 min: 4.52 ± 5.97
Zhao et al [14,15]	ARX, Model migration Hypoglycemic threshold: 70 mg/dL Event definition Start: ≥ 3 consecutive s.c. glucose concentration values below or equal to 70 mg/dL. End: ≥ 3 consecutive s.c. glucose concentration values above 65 mg/dL.	CGM data Second-order transfer function models of insulin and meal intake [16]	30 min	Sensitivity Specificity Time lag	In silico data/University of Virginia/University of Padova Simulator Sampling Interval: 5 min	Sensitivity (%) Adolescents: 60.96 Adults: 58.84 Children: 74.92	Specificity (%) Adolescents: 99.65 Adults: 99.59 Children: 97.34	Time lag (samples) Adolescents: 4.71 ± 2.21 Adults: 5.00 ± 2.24 Children: 3.59 ± 2.45	
Eren-Oruklu et al [17]	ARMA Weighted recursive least squares with adaptive forgetting factor Hypoglycemic threshold: 60 mg/dL Event definition Start: ≥ 2 consecutive (10 min or more) blood glucose measurements below or equal to the threshold value. End: Blood glucose concentration rises above 65 mg/dL	CGM data	30 min	Sensitivity (SNS) Specificity (SPC) False positive rate (FPR) False discovery rate (FDR) Detection time (DT)	54 people with type 1 diabetes monitored in a hospital setting [18,19] CGM device: CGMS, Medtronic Inc. Sampling interval: 5 min Monitoring period: 1 day	Absolute predicted value SNS (%) 89.0 SPC (%) 67.0 FPR (%) 33.0 FDR (%) 15.0 DT (min) 30.00 ± 5.51	Cumulative sum SNS (%) 87.5 SPC (%) 74.0 FPR (%) 26.0 FDR (%) 12.5 DT (min) 25.80 ± 6.46	Exponentially weighted moving-average control chart SNS (%) 89.0 SPC (%) 78.0 FPR (%) 74.0 FDR (%) 22.0 DT (min) 27.7 ± 5.32	

Reference	Method	Input data	Prediction horizon	Metrics	Study details	Results
Turksoy et al. [20–22]	ARMAX in state-space form; Constrained recursive least squares; Real-time Kalman filtering; Hypoglycemic threshold: 70 mg/dL; Event definition; Start: ≥ 1 consecutive s.c. glucose concentration values below or equal to 70 mg/dL. End: ≥ 1 consecutive s.c. glucose concentration values above 70 mg/dL	CGM data; Insulin on-board; Energy expenditure and GSR	30 min	Sensitivity; False positive rate; Detection time	Fourteen people with type 1 diabetes monitored in normal daily life conditions; CGM Device: iPRO, Medtronic Inc.; Sampling interval: 5 min; Monitoring period: –	*Sensitivity* 0.78 ± 0.16; *False positive rate* 0.37 ± 0.06; *Detection time (min)* 32 ± 3.34
Bayrak et al. [23]	AR; Recursive partial least squares; Real-time Savitzky-Golay filter; Event definition; Start: ≥ 1 consecutive s.c. glucose concentration values below or equal to 70 mg/dL. End: ≥ 1 consecutive s.c. glucose concentration values above 70 mg/dL	CGM data	30 min	Sensitivity; False positives/day; Detection time	Seventeen people with type 1 diabetes; CGM Device: Guardian RT, Medtronic Inc.; Sampling interval: 5 min; Monitoring period: –	*Sensitivity* 0.86; *False positives/day* 0.42; *Detection time (min)* 25.25
Daskalaki et al. [24–25]	Ensemble modeling; ARX with output correction module; Recursive least squares; RNN—RTRL; Hypoglycemic threshold: 70 mg/dL; Event definition; Start: ≥ 2 consecutive s.c. glucose concentration values below or equal to 70 mg/dL	CGM data; Insulin infusion rate data	45 min	Correct warnings; Detection time; Daily false alarms	Twenty three people with type 1 diabetes under SAP therapy monitored in normal daily life conditions; CGM Device: Minimed CGM, Medtronic Inc.; CGM Sampling Interval: 5 min; Monitoring period: Training set 5.30 ± 1.40 days, Evaluation set 4.83 ± 1.80 days	*Correct warnings (%)* 100.0 (100.0—100.0)[a]; *Detection time (min)* 16.7 (10.0—25.0)[a]; *Daily false alarms* 0.8 (0.0—1.2)[a]

[a]Values are median (5th—95th percentiles)

$K = |\mu_1 - \mu_0|/2$, μ_0 and μ_1 are the target mean glucose value and the out-of-control mean glucose value which is going to be detected, respectively, and σ is the standard deviation of the glucose signal, and (3) Exponentially weighted moving average (EWMA) control chart: A hypoglycemic alarm is issued at time t_i if $z_i = \lambda \hat{y}(t_{i+k}|\theta) + (1 - \lambda)z_{i-1}$, with $z_0 = \mu_0$ and centerline equal to μ_0, crosses the lower control limit $\text{LCL}_i = \mu_0 - L\sigma\sqrt{\lambda/2 - \lambda[1 - (1-\lambda)^{2i}]}$, where the parameter L is the width of control limits and $0 \leq \lambda \leq 1$. The method was assessed on 54 subjects with type 1 diabetes during an insulin-induced hypoglycemia test (≤ 55 mg/dL) in their short-term (24 hours) admission to the hospital. Besides CGM, their reference blood glucose concentration was also measured at regular intervals, i.e., every 60 minutes during the day, every 30 minutes during the night and every 5 minutes during the hypoglycemic event. A TP prediction is considered when the alarm is issued 45 minutes at most before a true hypoglycemic event, as assessed by the reference blood glucose measurements, and an FP prediction is considered when an alarm is incorrectly issued during a nonhypoglycemic period or it is issued >45 minutes before the event. Eren-Oruklu et al. reported a sensitivity 89%, a precision rate (or equivalently positive predictive value) 78% and a detection time 27.7 minutes for the EWMA control chart method.

Physiological signals related to a subject's physical activity or emotional condition (i.e., energy expenditure, GSR) as well as information on insulin regime (i.e., insulin on-board) complemented the input of an ARMA model and, in conjunction with physiological constraints imposed to model parameters, led to stable accurate short-term (30-minute ahead) predictions of the s.c. glucose concentration [21]. Note that the CGM signal was smoothed prior to training of the ARMA model based on an online adaptive Kalman filter [27,28]. Turksoy et al. defined a hypoglycemic event as successive s.c. glucose concentration values ≤ 70 mg/dL, with sequences of hypoglycemic values being separated by ≥ 2 nonhypoglycemic values being two discrete events. An alarm is immediately issued when the current s.c. glucose concentration value or its 1-step-ahead (i.e., 5 minutes) prediction are below the defined threshold. Otherwise, the algorithm examines if the $k > 1$-step-ahead-predictions of glucose cross the hypoglycemic threshold and, accordingly, alerts the patient. The predictive alarm system becomes more sensitive to nocturnal or post exercise hypoglycemic events by increasing the threshold to 80 mg/dL based on information provided by the SenseWear Armband (BodyMedia Inc.) physical activity monitor. Similarly to [17], an alarm followed by a true event in the next 60 minutes signifies a TP prediction. On average, a sensitivity 0.78 ± 0.16 accompanied with a false discovery rate 0.37 ± 0.06 and a detection time 32.00 ± 0.06 minutes were obtained for a dataset of 14 subjects with type 1 diabetes who had been observed in real-life conditions.

7.2.2 Hypoglycemia Prediction Methods Based on Machine Learning

Machine-learning techniques may efficiently represent the linear or nonlinear effect of patient's contextual information (e.g., meals, insulin, exercise, sleep) on the s.c. glucose concentration, without requiring any a priori knowledge about the underlying glucose regulation dynamics, whereas they exhibit a very good generalization performance. Georga et al. [13]

extended their support vector regression-based (SVR) method to predict hypoglycemic events 30 and 60 minutes in advance using information on recent glucose profile, meals, insulin therapy and physical activities for a hypoglycemic threshold 70 mg/dL. A hypoglycemic event is defined as at least two consecutive s.c. glucose concentration values (i.e., 10 minutes or more) ≤70 mg/dL, whereas a s.c. glucose value rise above 70 mg/dL signifies the end of the event. In order to treat potential oscillations either in the predicted or in the actual glucose time series, consecutive hypoglycemic events which are ≤30 minutes away are considered as the same event. Considering that in type 1 diabetes hypoglycemia occurs most frequently at night during sleep and it is potentially fatal if untreated, the authors separated the hypoglycemic events into nocturnal and diurnal ones, where the sleep state is detected using the related information provided by the SenseWear Armband (BodyMedia Inc.) physical activity monitor. In particular for nocturnal events, new input variables were introduced, in addition to those defined in [29], with the aim of capturing the effect of HAAF on the incidence of a future hypoglycemic event (i.e., recent antecedent hypoglycemia, prior exercise and sleep). The method was evaluated on a dataset of 15 type 1 patients under free-living conditions. A prediction of a hypoglycemic event is considered TP when the start of the actual hypoglycemic either precedes the start of the predicted one by $\leq kT$ minutes or follows the start of the predicted one by $\leq kT$ minutes. Nocturnal hypoglycemic events were predicted with 94% sensitivity for both 30- and 60-minute horizons and with 5.43 and 4.57-minute time lag, respectively. As concerns the diurnal events, when physical activities were not considered, the sensitivity was 92% and 96% for 30- and 60-minute horizon, respectively, with both time lags being less than 5 minutes. However, when such information was introduced, the diurnal sensitivity decreased by 8% and 3%, respectively. Both nocturnal and diurnal predictions showed a high (>90%) precision.

Daskalaki et al. proposed an ensemble predictive modeling scheme linearly combining two online adaptive models, i.e., an autoregressive model with extra inputs (ARX) and a recurrent neural network (RNN) model with an output correction module, where the parameter $a \in [0, 1]$ (and $1 - a$), which balances their output, is selected such that the function $(TP^2 + \text{DetectionTime}^2)/(1 + FP^2)$ is maximized [24−26]. The input is formed by past sequences concerning the s.c. glucose concentration and the insulin infusion rate. The definition of an event encompasses ≥ 2 (i.e., ≥ 10 minutes) s.c. glucose measurements below 70 mg/dL with the maximum acceptable distance between the alarm and the start of the event, which also defines TP predictions, being set equal to the largest prediction horizon examined by the authors, i.e., 45 minutes. In the case where the following three rules apply then a hypoglycemic alarm is inferred: (1) the current glucose value is within the eyglycemic range, (2) the 15-minute-ahead or at least one of the 30- or 45-minute-ahead predictions are within the hypoglycemic range, and (3) the event is predicted for the first time. Both ARX and RNN models were individually trained and tested on data from 23 patients with type 1 diabetes under sensor-augmented pump therapy and during everyday living conditions; where the first half of the data was used in model identification and the second one in the model testing. The ensemble model exhibited on average 100% TP warnings with a detection time of 16.7 minutes and 0.8 daily false alarms.

7.3 Hypoglycemia Prediction as a Classification Problem

A retrospective analysis of CGM data, relying on support vector machines classification, has been proposed as a complementary procedure to CGM calibration algorithms, obviating the need for modeling the complex plasma-interstitial glucose dynamics [30,31]. In particular, Jensen et al. treated the problem of hypoglycemia detection as a 2-class problem, with hypoglycemia defined as a plasma glucose ≤ 70 mg/dL and nonhypoglycemia as a plasma glucose >70 mg/dL. A ≥ 30 minutes subsequent period with no plasma glucose ≤ 70 mg/dL signifies the end of the event. A candidate set of 2289 features, formed by using CGM measurements in the time interval $[t_i - 120, t_i + 120]$, is tested for its discriminative ability with respect to the classification of the s.c. glucose concentration at time t_i. A feature selection method based on principal component analysis is used to confine the input size, whereas SVR training is performed in parallel with a forward selection procedure in a leave-one-subject-out crossvalidation mode. In total, seven features were retained: (1) the current s.c. glucose concentration value, (2) the linear regression of CGM values in the interval $[t_i - 60, t_i + 5]$, (3) the kurtosis of CGM values in the interval $[t_i - 5, t_i + 115]$, (4) the time since last insulin injection, (5) the kurtosis of CGM values in the interval $[t_i - 50, t_i + 15]$, (6) the kurtosis of CGM values in the interval $[t_i - 70, t_i]$, and (7) the skewness of CGM values in the interval $[t_i - 120, t_i - 60]$. A minimum of four consecutive s.c. glucose values being classified as hypoglycemic define a detected event, whereas a TP prediction requires at least one of them be confirmed by a plasma glucose measurement ≤ 70 mg/dL. The study population consisted of 10 subjects with type 1 diabetes, who underwent an insulin-induced hypoglycemia test during which capillary blood samples were drawn every 10 minutes; otherwise, every 30–60 minutes. Moreover, patients were equipped with a CGM system (Guardian RT CGM, Medtronic). A 100% sensitivity with 1 FP showed a significant improvement over CGM alone (63% sensitivity with 0 FP) or an optimized calibration algorithm (89% sensitivity with 2 FP), which had been shown to improve the accuracy (i.e., mean absolute relative difference) of the Guardian RT CGM system in all glycemic ranges.

Cichosz et al. tested the hypothesis that the integration of ECG and CGM data could enhance the early detection of a hypoglycemic event as compared to a CGM system [32,33]. A two-class problem is defined, where each input vector x^i in the dataset $Z = \{(x^i, y_i)\}_{i=1}^{N}$ is classified as $y_i \in \{C_{nonhypo}, C_{hypo}\}$ based on the reference blood glucose measurement at time t_i. The RR intervals in the ECG signal are grouped in epochs of 5 minutes and the heart rate variability (HRV) in each epoch is analyzed using time domain, frequency domain and nonlinear measures. A number of features are extracted by combining HRV measures of different epochs prior to t_i using a set of typical statistical operators, i.e., differentiation, average, slope standard deviation, skewness, and ratio. In addition, a confined set of features are extracted from CGM measurements 0–30 minutes prior to t_i, i.e., the s.c. glucose concentration at $gl(t_i)$, the difference $gl(t_i) - gl(t_i - 30)$, the slope of all CGM measurements in the interval $[t_i - 30, t_i]$ and the slope relative to the current reading. The classification framework encompasses feature ranking, based on class seperability criteria [i.e., receiver operating characteristic (ROC) curve] and their intercorrelation, followed by a forward selection procedure in conjunction with a binary linear logistic regression classifier. Frequent blood glucose measurements (every 10 minutes) were obtained during an insulin-induced hypoglycemia test from ten patients with type 1 diabetes, who were continuously monitored (Guardian RT CGM, Medtronic Inc.; ECG Lead II) in a hospital setting for two days. A leave-one-patient-out crossvalidation showed that single blood glucose values below 70 mg/dL are predicted 1-step-ahead (i.e., 10 minutes) with a specificity comparable to that of the CGM (0.99 vs 0.98), a considerably higher sensitivity than CGM (0.79 vs 0.33) and a total area under the ROC curve (AUC) 0.98. In addition, hypoglycemic events, being defined as ≥ 2 consecutive low (<70 mg/dL) blood glucose concentration levels, are all correctly detected, compared to sensitivity 0.75 provided by CGM, without any FP predictions. Most importantly, the time difference between the onset of the detected event and the nadir blood glucose of a TP event is improved from 0 ± 11 to 22 ± 11 minutes. In a subsequent study, Cichosz et al. studied the performance of the developed algorithm in the detection of spontaneous hypoglycemic events in free-living conditions, using a dataset of 21 patients with type 1 diabetes collected over a 3-day monitoring period [33]. Single vein plasma glucose and self-monitoring blood glucose (SMBG) measurements below 70 mg/dL were used as reference hypoglycemic values in order to locate hypoglycemic events into CGM time series, which means that the precise start of the event is not known. Different prediction horizons were examined ranging from 0 to 30 minutes; for a prediction horizon of 20 minutes, the model yielded a ROC AUC 0.96 with sensitivity 100% and specificity 91%.

A novel approach to nocturnal hypoglycemia prediction consists in a data-driven aggregation of multiple hypoglycemia risk indices relying solely on SMBG data [34,35]. Let $x \in R^d$ denote the daily SMBG measurements. The risk of hypoglycemia during nocturnal sleep as it is assessed by the index I is given by

$$P^I(x) = \begin{cases} 1, & I(x) \geq c_I \\ -1, & I(x) < c_I \end{cases}, \tag{7.1}$$

where c_I is the discrimination threshold parameter related to index I, and $P^I(x) = 1$ (or $P^I(x) = -1$) means that nocturnal hypoglycemia is expected (or nocturnal hypoglycemia is not expected). Given a dataset $Z = \{(x^i, y_i)\}_{i=1}^N$ and an ensemble of L hypoglycemia indices $P^{I_l}(x), l = 1, \ldots, L$, a linear combination is learnt:

$$I^{ag}(x) = \sum_{l=1}^{L} c_l P^{I_l}(x), \tag{7.2}$$

which, similarly to (7.1), is associated with a threshold c_{ag}. The vector $c = (c_1, \ldots, c_L)^T$ is the solution of the linear system $Ac = b$, where $A = (a_{l,n})_{l,n=1}^L$ and $b = (b_1, \ldots, b_L)^T$ are formed such that

$$a_{l,n} = \frac{1}{N} \sum_{i=1}^{N} P^{I_l}(x^i) P^{I_n}(x^i), \tag{7.3}$$

$$b_l = \frac{1}{N^2} \sum_{i=1}^{N} P^{l_i}(x^i) \left((N-1)y_i - \sum_{\substack{j=1 \\ i \neq j}}^{N} y_j \right). \tag{7.4}$$

The theoretical framework behind (7.3) and (7.4) shows that the accuracy of (7.2) is at the level of accuracy of the best model $P^{l_i}(x) = 1, l = 1, \ldots, L$. In particular, the output of four hypoglycemia risk indices was aggregated to illustrate the efficacy of the method, i.e., the low blood glucose index, the hypoglycemic index, the glycemic risk assessment diabetes equation, and the quadratic risk factor associated with the last SMBG measurement before nocturnal sleep [36]. The threshold parameters of the individual predictors and the aggregated one were optimized based on the ROC curve. The aggregated classification scheme was trained and tested on a dataset including 150 days of SMBG (4 measurements per day) and 40 nocturnal hypoglycemia s by 34 patients with diabetes. A sensitivity of 80.0% and a specificity of 96.36% was achieved. An equally high performance was achieved (sensitivity 77.03%, specificity 83.46%) on a second dataset of 179 children with diabetes, where the method was applied without any tuning.

7.4 Computational Experiments

7.4.1 A Multivariate Support Vector Regression Model of Hypoglycemia

This section is devoted to the evaluation of the SVR-based glucose predictive model, which was presented in [13,29] and briefly described in Section 7.2.2, with respect to the prediction of hypoglycemic events for 30- and 60-minute time horizons. A multivariate dataset of 15 patients observed in free-living conditions (3 Female/12 Male; Age: 40.3 ± 13.5 years old; BMI: 25.2 ± 2.9 kg/m^2; HbA1c: $7.1 \pm 1.2\%$; Observation period: 12.5 ± 4.6 days) is utilized. Patients were equipped with the Guardian Real-Time CGM system (Medtronic Minimed Inc.) and the SenseWear Armband (BodyMedia Inc.) physical activity monitor. They also methodically recorded information on daily food intake and insulin regime. The descriptive characteristics of the s.c. glucose dataset are given in Table 7.4.

The SVR model is fed with three different cases of input. The reader is referred to the definition of variables gl, I_p, Ra, $SR\alpha$, SEE, and h in Section 6.3.2. In the first case, denoted as Case1$_{hypo}$ (corresponding to Case4 in [29]), the input consists of variables gl, I_p, Ra, $SR\alpha$, and h, while in the second case, namely Case2$_{hypo}$ (corresponding to Case6 in [29]), the variable SEE is additionally used. HAAF is mainly associated with hypoglycemic events that occur during sleep. Thus, in addition to the inputs of Case1$_{hypo}$, Case3$_{hypo}$ includes: (1) the total energy expenditure during day due to physical activities of intensity of <3 metabolic equivalents of task (METs) (EE$_{daily, <3METs}$), (2) the total energy expenditure during day due to physical activities of intensity ≥ 3 METs (EE$_{daily, \geq 3METs}$), (3) the time passed from the start of the sleep state (t_{sleep}), and (4) a Boolean variable describing the incidence or not of a hypoglycemic event

Table 7.4   Statistics of Glucose Dataset Per Patient

	Day	Night
Mean s.c. glucose concentration (mg/dL)	148.85 ± 23.41	140.75 ± 29.89
Min s.c. glucose concentration (mg/dL)	52.92 ± 11.96	60.79 ± 18.06
Max s.c. glucose concentration (mg/dL)	332.44 ± 47.81	281.12 ± 49.38
% of Hypoglycemic values	0.04 ± 0.04	0.05 ± 0.05
% of Hyperglycemic values	0.27 ± 0.15	0.22 ± 0.18
Hypoglycemic events per day/night	0.68 ± 0.48	0.35 ± 0.15
Duration per hypoglycemic event (min)	56.78 ± 28.31	75.98 ± 42.97

Information is given in the form mean ± standard deviation.
A glucose concentration value ≤ 70 mg/dL is defined as hypoglycemic.
A glucose concentration value ≥ 180 mg/dL is defined as hyperglycemic.

Table 7.5   Evaluation Results of SVR Model for Predicted Nocturnal Hypoglycemic Events

	Prediction Horizon					
	30 min			60 min		
	SNS	PRC	TL	SNS	PRC	TL
Case1$_{hypo}$	0.89 ± 0.21	0.95 ± 0.11	9.26 ± 9.78	0.86 ± 0.26	0.93 ± 0.12	14.39 ± 15.04
Case1a$_{hypo}$	0.89 ± 0.21	0.98 ± 0.06	8.68 ± 8.73	0.88 ± 0.20	0.96 ± 0.12	7.81 ± 10.39
Case2$_{hypo}$	0.88 ± 0.21	0.97 ± 0.10	7.50 ± 9.23	0.86 ± 0.23	0.90 ± 0.15	12.71 ± 15.07
Case2a$_{hypo}$	0.87 ± 0.20	0.97 ± 0.10	6.91 ± 9.54	0.86 ± 0.20	0.96 ± 0.12	8.13 ± 12.10
Case3$_{hypo}$	0.91 ± 0.23	0.98 ± 0.08	5.00 ± 6.85	0.90 ± 0.17	1.00 ± 0.00	6.18 ± 8.35
Case3a$_{hypo}$	0.94 ± 0.10	0.98 ± 0.08	5.43 ± 7.11	0.94 ± 0.10	0.98 ± 0.08	4.57 ± 5.47

SNS, sensitivity; *PRC*, precision; *TL*, time lag.

during the previous 24 hours (hypo). Note that the variable *SEE*, which concerns the energy expenditure during the last 3 hours, may only explain hypoglycemia shortly after exercise. However, exercise-related HAAF is exemplified by hypoglycemia that typically occurs several hours (6−15 hours) after exercise, and thus it is often nocturnal [37]. Provided that glucose levels change more gradually at night than during the day, one subcase (i.e., Case1a$_{hypo}$, Case2a$_{hypo}$, Case3a$_{hypo}$) is considered for each of the previous cases regarding the nocturnal events where the history of *gl* is set equal to 60 minutes. Case3$_{hypo}$ and Case3a$_{hypo}$ are defined only for nocturnal events, whereas Case1$_{hypo}$, Case1a$_{hypo}$, Case2$_{hypo}$, and Case2a$_{hypo}$ are applied to both the prediction of nocturnal and diurnal ones. This means that in Case3$_{hypo}$ and Case3a$_{hypo}$, the SVR model is trained to predict only the night glucose time series.

Tables 7.5 and 7.6 present the average sensitivity, precision and time lag regarding the prediction of nocturnal and diurnal hypoglycemic events, respectively. We recall that at least two consecutive s.c. glucose concentration values ≤ 70 mg/dL are needed to define a hypoglycemic event and a maximum time lag of $|kT|$ is allowed for TP events. Results suggest that the SVR method performs adequately well in all cases for both prediction horizons. In

Table 7.6   Evaluation Results of SVR Model for Predicted Diurnal Hypoglycemic Events

	Prediction Horizon					
	30 min			60 min		
	SNS	PRC	TL	SNS	PRC	TL
Case1$_{hypo}$	0.92 ± 0.12	0.93 ± 0.13	4.53 ± 5.30	0.96 ± 0.14	0.97 ± 0.10	3.64 ± 4.72
Case2$_{hypo}$	0.84 ± 0.23	0.94 ± 0.16	3.17 ± 4.65	0.93 ± 0.17	0.96 ± 0.14	4.52 ± 5.97

SNS, sensitivity; *PRC*, precision; *TL*, time lag.

Case1$_{hypo}$, the 30- and 60-minute nocturnal predictions are of satisfactory sensitivity and of high precision, but they are associated with relatively high time lags. Case2$_{hypo}$, as expected, does not induce significant changes in the number of TP and FP outcomes. The method's sensitivity and precision to nocturnal hypoglycemic events increases in Case3$_{hypo}$ as compared with Case1$_{hypo}$, which is also reflected to reduced time lags. In Fig. 7.3, we can see the actual onset of the nocturnal events of a patient and the predicted onset (with a 30-minute horizon) denoted by a vertical dashed line. The sensitivity of Case1$_{hypo}$ and Case2$_{hypo}$ is almost unaffected by increasing *gl* history from 30 to 60 minutes (Case1a$_{hypo}$ and Case2a$_{hypo}$), whereas there is a perceptible improvement in their precision rate. Nevertheless, it is obvious that *gl* history has a great influence on the time gain in the TP events for 60-minute prediction horizon. Regarding Case3a$_{hypo}$, it results in predicting correctly 94% of the events with 98% precision for both prediction horizons.

Regarding diurnal hypoglycemic events, Case1$_{hypo}$ predicts correctly 92% and 96% of the true hypoglycemic events 30 and 60 minutes in advance, respectively, with 93% and 97% of the positive predictions being indeed true. The time lag for both prediction horizons is less than 5 minutes. However, the sensitivity of the method is reduced when the variable SEE is additionally used in Case2$_{hypo}$, reaching 84% for 30-minute predictions and 93% for 60-minute predictions. In addition, there are no significant changes in precision rate compared to Case1$_{hypo}$, while the time lag is still less than 5 minutes. The output of Case1$_{hypo}$ and Case2$_{hypo}$ for a patient is illustrated in Fig. 7.4 where for the ninth hypoglycemic event we observe that Case2$_{hypo}$ generates a FN result contrary to Case1$_{hypo}$.

The authors note that a direct comparison of the results for 30 and 60 minutes should not be made since the set of hypoglycemic events upon which the methods are evaluated are different (i.e., the events for 60 minutes is a subset of the ones for 30 minutes). This stems from the fact that different datasets have been constructed for each horizon according to the method presented in [29] (e.g., instances at which meal, insulin or exercise events occurred within $[t, t + kT]$ were excluded).

7.5 Discussion and Conclusions

CGM enabled a high time-resolution description of the short-term glucose dynamics in the s.c. space, the awareness of which by both patients and physicians has been shown to

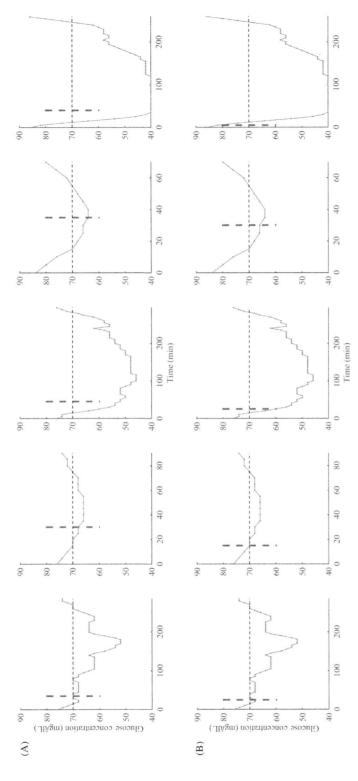

FIGURE 7.3 Prediction of nocturnal hypoglycemic events of a typical subject by (A) Case1$_{hypo}$ and (B) Case3$_{hypo}$ for a prediction horizon of 30 min. The onset of the predicted event is indicated by the vertical dashed line.

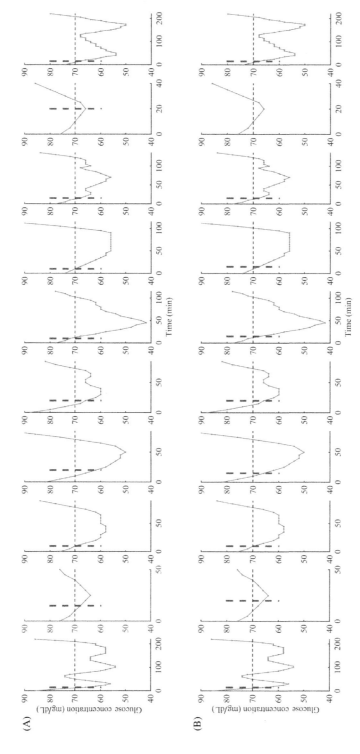

FIGURE 7.4 Prediction of diurnal hypoglycemic events of a typical subject by (A) Case1$_{hypo}$ and (B) Case2$_{hypo}$ for a prediction horizon of 30 min. The onset of the predicted event is indicated by the vertical dashed line.

improve the long-term glycemic control (i.e., HbA1c levels) in type 1 diabetes and facilitate the evaluation of the response to therapy, as compared to SMBG. The continuously improved accuracy of CGM effected its approval for making therapeutic decisions in Europe [38,39]. However, there is still room for improvements in the hypoglycemic range which, in conjunction with the lag time of interstitial fluid glucose relative to blood glucose, hinders the precise detection of hypoglycemia based merely on CGM data. In addition, only the combined use of CGM, continuous s.c. insulin infusion, and glucose predictive algorithms has been shown to reduce the incidence and duration of hypoglycemia, though it comes at a price of an increase in hyperglycemia [40,41]. In particular, the integration of low-glucose predictive alerts into today open- or semiclosed loop systems of glycemic control in diabetes is imperative toward minimizing the risk of hypoglycemia [1,42]. To this end, a considerable number of data-driven regression and classification approaches have been developed, aggregating CGM, behavioral and physiological information, aiming at an accurate robust predictive model of hypoglycemia in diabetes. These models have their predictive capability validated by hypoglycemic clamp studies or short-term observational studies under free-living conditions, with the former providing a more precise assessment of the method against reference blood glucose concentration data.

Herein, we replicated the results reported by Georga et al. [13] demonstrating that the prediction of nocturnal hypoglycemic events by a SVR model becomes more accurate when HAAF-related factors are additionally considered. Moreover, the increase of glucose history at night yields to considerably lower delays between the predicted and the actual glucose signal. The fact that the introduction of information on physical activity reduces the sensitivity of 30-minute predictions of diurnal events, as opposed to a feed-forward neural network and a Gaussian processes model which were trained on the same data and task, indicates that further evaluation is needed to encode the immediate effect of exercise on glucose within the overall patient's context. Additional descriptive characteristics could be derived for summarizing the daily physical activity for nocturnal hypoglycemic event prediction, and capturing the immediate effect of exercise on glucose concentration levels and the overall physiological changes triggered by hypoglycemia [43–45]. It is advised that the problem of hypoglycemia prediction should be handled differently for nocturnal and diurnal periods as regards input variables and interpretation of results.

References

[1] Howsmon D, Bequette BW. Hypo- and hyperglycemic alarms: devices and algorithms. J Diabetes Sci Technol 2015;9(5):1126−37.

[2] Cichosz SL, Johansen MD, Hejlesen O. Toward big data analytics: review of predictive models in management of diabetes and its complications. J Diabetes Sci Technol 2015;10(1):27−34.

[3] Palerm CC, Bequette BW. Hypoglycemia detection and prediction using continuous glucose monitoring —a study on hypoglycemic clamp data. J Diabetes Sci Technol 2007;1(5):624−9.

[4] Cameron F, et al. Statistical hypoglycemia prediction. J Diabetes Sci Technol 2008;2(4):612−21.

[5] Dassau E, et al. Real-time hypoglycemia prediction suite using continuous glucose monitoring: a safety net for the artificial pancreas. Diabetes Care 2010;33(6):1249–54.

[6] Naumova V, Pereverzyev SV, Sivananthan S. A meta-learning approach to the regularized learning-case study: blood glucose prediction. Neural Netw 2012;33:181–93.

[7] Zarkogianni K, et al. Comparative assessment of glucose prediction models for patients with type 1 diabetes mellitus applying sensors for glucose and physical activity monitoring. Med Biol Eng Comput 2015;53(12):1333–43.

[8] Georga EI, et al. Multivariate prediction of subcutaneous glucose concentration in type 1 diabetes patients based on support vector regression. IEEE J Biomed Health Inform 2013;17(1):71–81.

[9] Eren-Oruklu M, et al. Estimation of future glucose concentrations with subject-specific recursive linear models. Diabetes Technol Ther 2009;11(4):243–53.

[10] Eren-Oruklu M, et al. Adaptive system identification for estimating future glucose concentrations and hypoglycemia alarms. Automatica (Oxf) 2012;48(8):1892–7.

[11] Wang Q, et al. Personalized state-space modeling of glucose dynamics for type 1 diabetes using continuously monitored glucose, insulin dose, and meal intake: an extended kalman filter approach. J Diabetes Sci Technol 2014;8(2):331–45.

[12] Wang Y, Wu X, Mo X. A novel adaptive-weighted-average framework for blood glucose prediction. Diabetes Technol Ther 2013;15(10):792–801.

[13] Georga EI, et al. A glucose model based on support vector regression for the prediction of hypoglycemic events under free-living conditions. Diabetes Technol Ther 2013;15(8):634–43.

[14] Zhao C, Yu C. Rapid model identification for online subcutaneous glucose concentration prediction for new subjects with type I diabetes. IEEE Trans Biomed Eng 2015;62(5):1333–44.

[15] Zhao C, Sun Y, Zhao L. Interindividual glucose dynamics in different frequency bands for online prediction of subcutaneous glucose concentration in type 1 diabetic subjects. AIChE J 2013;59(11):4228–40.

[16] Grosman B, et al. Zone model predictive control: a strategy to minimize hyper- and hypoglycemic events. J Diabetes Sci Technol 2010;4(4):961–75.

[17] Eren-Oruklu M, Cinar A, Quinn L. Hypoglycemia prediction with subject-specific recursive time-series models. J Diabetes Sci Technol 2010;4(1):25–33.

[18] Accuracy of the GlucoWatch G2 Biographer and the continuous glucose monitoring system during hypoglycemia: experience of the Diabetes Research in Children Network. Diabetes Care, 2004; 27(3): 722-6.

[19] Tsalikian E, et al. GlucoWatch G2 Biographer alarm reliability during hypoglycemia in children. Diabetes Technol Ther 2004;6(5):559–66.

[20] Turksoy K, et al. Multivariable adaptive closed-loop control of an artificial pancreas without meal and activity announcement. Diabetes Technol Therap 2013;15(5):386–400.

[21] Turksoy K, et al. Hypoglycemia early alarm systems based on multivariable models. Ind Eng Chem Res 2013;52(35).

[22] Turksoy K, et al. Multivariable adaptive identification and control for artificial pancreas systems. IEEE Trans Biomed Eng 2014;61(3):883–91.

[23] Bayrak ES, et al. Hypoglycemia early alarm systems based on recursive autoregressive partial least squares models. J Diabetes Sci Technol 2013;7(1):206–14.

[24] Daskalaki E, et al. Real-time adaptive models for the personalized prediction of glycemic profile in type 1 diabetes patients. Diabetes Technol Ther 2012;14(2):168–74.

[25] Daskalaki E, et al. An early warning system for hypoglycemic/hyperglycemic events based on fusion of adaptive prediction models. J Diabetes Sci Technol 2013;7(3):689–98.

[26] Daskalaki E, Diem P, Mougiakakou S. *Adaptive algorithms for personalized diabetes treatment*, in *data-driven modeling for diabetes: diagnosis and treatment*In: Marmarelis V, Mitsis G, editors. Berlin, Heidelberg: Springer Berlin Heidelberg; 2014. p. 91−116.

[27] Bequette BW. Continuous glucose monitoring: real-time algorithms for calibration, filtering, and alarms. J Diabetes Sci Technol 2010;4(2):404−18.

[28] Facchinetti A, Sparacino G, Cobelli C. An online self-tunable method to denoise CGM sensor data. IEEE Trans Biomed Eng 2010;57(3):634−41.

[29] Georga E, et al. Multivariate prediction of subcutaneous glucose concentration in type 1 diabetes patients based on support vector regression. IEEE J Biomed Health Inform 2012. Available from: https://doi.org/10.1109/TITB.2012.2219876.

[30] Jensen MH, et al. Professional continuous glucose monitoring in subjects with type 1 diabetes: retrospective hypoglycemia detection. J Diabetes Sci Technol 2013;7(1):135−43.

[31] Jensen MH, et al. Evaluation of an algorithm for retrospective hypoglycemia detection using professional continuous glucose monitoring data. J Diabetes Sci Technol 2014;8(1):117−22.

[32] Cichosz SL, et al. A novel algorithm for prediction and detection of hypoglycemia based on continuous glucose monitoring and heart rate variability in patients with type 1 diabetes. J Diabetes Sci Technol 2014;8(4):731−7.

[33] Cichosz SL, et al. Combining information of autonomic modulation and CGM measurements enables prediction and improves detection of spontaneous hypoglycemic events. J Diabetes Sci Technol 2015;9 (1):132−7.

[34] Sampath S, et al. Glycemic control indices and their aggregation in the prediction of nocturnal hypoglycemia from intermittent blood glucose measurements. J Diabetes Sci Technol 2016;10(6):1245−50.

[35] Tkachenko P, et al. Prediction of nocturnal hypoglycemia by an aggregation of previously known prediction approaches: proof of concept for clinical application. Comput Methods Programs Biomed 2016;134:179−86.

[36] Rodbard D. Interpretation of continuous glucose monitoring data: glycemic variability and quality of glycemic control. Diabetes Technol Ther 2009;11(Suppl 1):S55−67.

[37] Cryer PE. Exercise-related hypoglycemia-associated autonomic failure in diabetes. Diabetes 2009;58 (9):1951−2.

[38] Rodbard D. Continuous glucose monitoring: a review of successes, challenges, and opportunities. Diabetes Technol Ther 2016;18(Suppl. 2):S3−13.

[39] Facchinetti A. *Continuous glucose monitoring sensors: past, present and future algorithmic challenges.* Sensors (Basel) 2016;16(12).

[40] Thabit H, Hovorka R. Coming of age: the artificial pancreas for type 1 diabetes. Diabetologia 2016;59 (9):1795−805.

[41] Kropff J, DeVries JH. Continuous glucose monitoring, future products, and update on worldwide artificial pancreas projects. Diabetes Technol Ther 2016;18(Suppl. 2):S253−63.

[42] Bequette BW. Hypoglycemia prevention using low glucose suspend systems. In: Marmarelis V, Mitsis G, editors. Data-driven Modeling for Diabetes: Diagnosis and Treatment. Berlin, Heidelberg: Springer Berlin Heidelberg; 2014. p. 73−89.

[43] Fabris C, et al. Hypoglycemia-related electroencephalogram changes assessed by multiscale entropy. Diabetes Technol Ther 2014;16(10):688−94.

[44] Christensen TF, et al. Hypoglycaemia and QT interval prolongation in type 1 diabetes–bridging the gap between clamp studies and spontaneous episodes. J Diabetes Complications 2014;28(5):723−8.

[45] Nuryani N, Ling SS, Nguyen HT. Electrocardiographic signals and swarm-based support vector machine for hypoglycemia detection. Ann Biomed Eng 2012;40(4):934−45.

8

Adaptive Glucose Prediction Models

8.1 Adaptive Learning

Assume a sequence of input–output pairs $Z = \{(x_i, y_i) | i = 1, \ldots, N\}$ where $(x_i, y_i) \in Z = X \times Y$, $X \subseteq R^d$ and $Y \subseteq R$, and a parametric class of functions $F = \{f_\theta : X \to Y, \theta \in R^m\}$. Each sample (x_i, y_i) associates the input vector x_i corresponding to observations up to time $t_i - kT$ with the observed subcutaneous (s.c.) glucose concentration y_i at time t_i, where k is the prediction step and T is the sampling interval of glucose concentration. For ease of notation we will assume $t_{i+1} - t_i = T$. Moreover, for consistency, throughout this Chapter, the input x^i at time t_i is expressed as x_i. Adaptive learning builds sequentially a continuous input–output mapping $f : X \to R$, minimizing a certain error function $E(\theta)$ on Z, such that f_i (the estimate at iteration i) is updated on the basis of the last estimate f_{i-1} and the prediction error $e_i = y_i - f_{i-1}(x_i)$ on the current sample (x_i, y_i).

The adaptive learning process is outlined in Table 8.1. At each time instant t_i, the error e_i between the actual output y_i and the estimated output $\hat{y}_i = f_{i-1}(x_i)$ is computed, and the new solution f_i is obtained based on e_i and according to the employed algorithm. We recall that the input vector x_i comprises previous input–output data up to time $t_i - kT$ which is used to predict the observed glucose at time t_i, i.e., y_i. The prediction performance of the glucose model is evaluated as it is being constructed. In particular, the updated model f_i is tested on the prediction of glucose at time $t_i + kT$ using an input information up to the current time t_i. The prediction error of f_i on the corresponding sample (x_{i+k}, y_{i+k}) is given by $e_{i+k}^{\text{test}} = y_{i+k} - f_i(x_{i+k})$, with $e_j^{\text{test}} = 0$ for $1 \leq j \leq k$, and it is actually computed at time $t_i + kT$ when y_{i+k} is observed. The learning curve of the model is calculated using e_i (i.e., the loss incurred on the data pair (x_i, y_i)), whereas the prediction curve is calculated using e_i^{test}. In the case of 1-step-ahead predictions, the two curves are identical; however, for $k > 1$, e_i is calculated using f_{i-1} whereas e_i^{test} is calculated using f_{i-k}. We expect that both error curves will be very similar with a time delay between them.

8.2 Linear Adaptive Models

8.2.1 Least Mean Square Algorithm

The least mean square (LMS) algorithm assumes a linear model of the form $f(x) = \theta^T x$, with $\theta \in R^d$, and a mean squared error loss function $E(\theta) = E[e_i^2]$ [1,2]. It is based on the stochastic gradient descent method, thereby, at each time instant $t_i, i = 1, \ldots, N$, the instantaneous error function $E_i(\theta) = 1/2 e_i^2$ is minimized, with respect to θ, via the following update rule:

$$\theta_i = \theta_{i-1} - \eta \nabla E_i(\theta) = \theta_{i-1} + \eta x_i(y_i - \theta_{i-1}^T x_i) = \theta_{i-1} + \eta e_i x_i, \tag{8.1}$$

Personalized Predictive Modeling in Type 1 Diabetes. DOI: http://dx.doi.org/10.1016/B978-0-12-804831-3.00008-X

Table 8.1   Adaptive Learning

Input: $\{(x_i, y_i) | x_i \in R^d, y_i \in R\}, i = 1, 2, \ldots$
Computation:
while (x_i, y_i) is available
    Predict output $\hat{y}_i = f_{i-1}(x_i)$
    Compute error $e_i = y_i - \hat{y}_i$
    Update solution f_i based on e_i
    Predict output $\hat{y}_{i+k} = f_i(x_{i+k})$.
    Compute test error $e_i^{\text{test}} = y_i - f_{i-k}(x_i)$
end while
Output: f_i

---

where the gradient of $E_i(\theta)$ equals $\nabla E_i(\theta) = -x_i(y_i - \theta_{i-1}^T x_i)$. The step-size parameter η defines the learning rate of the algorithm and provided that $0 < \eta < 1/\lambda_{\max}$, with $\lambda_{\max}$ being the largest eigenvalue of the correlation matrix $R = E[x_i x_i^T]$, the mean square error of the LMS algorithm converges to a constant value as $i \to \infty$:

$$E\left[e_i^2\right] \to \text{constant as} \ \ i \to \infty, N \to \infty. \tag{8.2}$$

However, in practice, $0 < \eta < 1/tr(R)$ needs to be satisfied, where $tr(R)$ is the trace of R. The parameter η should be properly chosen as it is also involved in the estimation of the misadjustment parameter $M = (E_\infty - E_{\min})/E_{\min}$, which provides a measure of the proximity of $E_\infty = \lim_{i \to \infty} E\left[e_i^2\right]$ to the optimal mean squared error $E_{\min}$:

$$M = \frac{\eta}{2} \sum_{i=1}^{L} \lambda_i \approx \frac{\eta}{2} tr(R). \tag{8.3}$$

The output of LMS at iteration i for a new input x is given by:

$$f_i(x) = \theta_i^T x = \eta \sum_{j=1}^{i} e_i x_i^T x. \tag{8.4}$$

The LMS algorithm is summarized in Table 8.2, with the parameter vector being typically initialized to zero (i.e., $\theta_0 = 0$). Its computational complexity is $O(d)$.

8.2.2 Recursive Least Squares Algorithm

The recursive least squares (RLS) algorithm adopts also a linear parametric model. However, unlike LMS, RLS, at each iteration i, locates $\theta_i \in R^d$ minimizing a regularized loss function accounting for the sum of squared errors up to the current time t_i:

$$\arg \min_{\theta} E(\theta) = \arg \min_{\theta} \sum_{j=1}^{i} \left| y_j - \theta^T x_j \right|^2 + \lambda \|\theta\|^2 \Rightarrow \theta_i = (X_i X_i^T + \lambda I)^{-1} X_i Y_i, \tag{8.5}$$

Table 8.2   Least Mean Squares

Input: $\{(x_i, y_i) | x_i \in R^d, y_i \in R\}, i = 1, 2, \ldots$
Initialization:
Choose $\eta > 0$
$\theta_0 = 0$
Computation:
while (x_i, y_i) is available
$\quad e_i = y_i - \theta_{i-1}^T x_i$
$\quad \theta_i = \theta_{i-1} + \eta e_i x_i$
end while
Output: θ_i

---

where $X_i = [x_1, \ldots, x_i] \in R^{d \times i}$, $Y_i = [y_1, \ldots, y_i]^T$, I is the $d \times d$ identity matrix and $\lambda > 0$ is the regularization parameter [2,3]. The inversion of the matrix $P_i = (X_i X_i^T + \lambda I)^{-1}$ is eliminated by using the matrix inversion lemma $(A + BCD)^{-1} = A^{-1} - A^{-1}B(C^{-1} + DA^{-1}B)^{-1}DA^{-1}$:

$$P_i^{-1} = P_{i-1}^{-1} + x_i x_i^T \Rightarrow P_i = P_{i-1} - \frac{P_{i-1} x_i x_i^T P_{i-1}}{1 + x_i^T P_{i-1} x_i}. \tag{8.6}$$

with $P_{i-1} \rightarrow A, x_i \rightarrow B, 1 \rightarrow C, x_i^T \rightarrow D$. Then, θ_i in Eq. (8.5) is computed recursively as follows:

$$
\begin{aligned}
\theta_i &= P_i X_i Y_i \\
&= \left[P_{i-1} - \frac{P_{i-1} x_i x_i^T P_{i-1}}{1 + x_i^T P_{i-1} x_i} \right] \left[X_{i-1} Y_{i-1} + x_i y_i \right] \\
&= P_{i-1} X_{i-1} Y_{i-1} - \frac{P_{i-1} x_i x_i^T}{1 + x_i^T P_{i-1} x_i} P_{i-1} X_{i-1} Y_{i-1} + P_{i-1} x_i y_i - \frac{P_{i-1} x_i x_i^T P_{i-1} x_i y_i}{1 + x_i^T P_{i-1} x_i} \\
&= \theta_{i-1} - \frac{P_{i-1} x_i x_i^T \theta_{i-1}}{1 + x_i^T P_{i-1} x_i} + P_{i-1} x_i y_i - \frac{P_{i-1} x_i x_i^T P_{i-1} x_i y_i}{1 + x_i^T P_{i-1} x_i} \\
&= \theta_{i-1} - \frac{P_{i-1} x_i x_i^T \theta_{i-1}}{1 + x_i^T P_{i-1} x_i} + \frac{P_{i-1} x_i x_i^T}{1 + x_i^T P_{i-1} x_i} \\
&= \theta_{i-1} - \frac{P_{i-1} x_i}{1 + x_i^T P_{i-1} x_i} \left(y_i - x_i^T \theta_{i-1} \right) \\
&= \theta_{i-1} - \frac{P_{i-1} x_i}{1 + x_i^T P_{i-1} x_i} e_i.
\end{aligned}
\tag{8.7}
$$

The RLS algorithm is summarized in Table 8.3. Its computational complexity is $O(d^2)$ featuring, however, an order of magnitude higher convergence rate than the LMS algorithm.

Table 8.3   Recursive Least Squares

Input: $\{(x_i, y_i) | x_i \in R^d, y_i \in R\}, i = 1, 2, \ldots$

Initialization:

Choose $\lambda > 0$

$\theta_0 = 0$

$P_0 = \lambda^{-1}I$

Computation:

while (x_i, y_i) is available

$\quad r_i = 1 + x_i^T P_{i-1} x_i$

$\quad k_i = P_{i-1} x_i / r_i$

$\quad e_i = y_i - \theta_{i-1}^T x_i$

$\quad \theta_i = \theta_{i-1} + k_i e_i$

$\quad P_i = P_{i-1} - k_i k_i^T r_i$

end while

Output: θ_i

8.2.2.1 Exponentially Weighted Recursive Least Squares

Exponentially weighted recursive least squares (EW-RLS) [2,3] introduces a forgetting factor $0 \ll \beta \leq 1$ into Eq. (8.5) such that:

$$\arg \min_{\theta} E(\theta) = \arg \min_{\theta} \sum_{j=1}^{i} \beta^{i-j} |y_j - \theta^T x_j|^2 + \beta^i \lambda \|\theta\|^2 \Rightarrow \theta_i = (X_i B_i X_i^T + \beta^i \lambda I)^{-1} X_i B_i Y_i. \qquad (8.8)$$

The error of the linear model on more recent samples, with respect to the current time t_i, is emphasized through the term β^{i-j}, whereas the effect of regularization is attenuated as i increases (through β^i). B_i is a diagonal matrix with elements $(\beta^{i-1}, \beta^{i-2}, \ldots, 1)$. Similar to RLS, Eq. (8.8) is written recursively as:

$$\theta_i = \theta_{i-1} - \frac{\beta^{-1} P_{i-1} x_i}{1 + \beta^{-1} x_i^T P_{i-1} x_i} e_i, \qquad (8.9)$$

where $P_i = (X_i B_i X_i^T + \beta^i \lambda I)^{-1}$ (Table 8.4).

8.2.3 Glucose Prediction Applications

Table 8.5 presents the main linear adaptive approaches to s.c. glucose concentration prediction in diabetes. The feasibility of a recursive in time solution to predict the short-term s.c. glucose dynamics in type 2 diabetes has been demonstrated in [4,5]. In particular, weighted recursive least squares (WRLS) with an adjustable forgetting factor, according to the variation of model parameters, was used to identify both autoregressive moving average (ARMA) and autoregressive moving average with extra inputs (ARMAX) models of the s.c. glucose concentration. It was shown that a multivariate ARMAX model including physiological signals

Table 8.4   Exponentially Weighted Recursive Least Squares

Input: $\{(x_i, y_i) | x_i \in R^d, y_i \in R\}, i = 1, 2, \ldots$
Initialization:
Choose $\lambda > 0$ and $0 \ll \beta < 1$
$\theta_0 = 0$
$P_0 = \lambda^{-1} I$
Computation:
while (x_i, y_i) is available

$\quad r_i = 1 + \beta^{-1} x_i^T P_{i-1} x_i$
$\quad k_i = \beta^{-1} P_{i-1} x_i / r_i$
$\quad e_i = y_i - \theta_{i-1}^T x_i$
$\quad \theta_i = \theta_{i-1} + k_i e_i$
$\quad P_i = \beta^{-1} P_{i-1} - k_i k_i^T r_i$

end while
Output: θ_i

---

related to a subject's physical activity and emotional condition outperforms a univariate model as applied to type 2 diabetes.

Similarly, constrained WRLS with a time-varying forgetting factor provided a stable 30-minute-ahead ARMAX prediction model of glucose concentration in patients with type 1 diabetes in which parameters related to the insulin on-board and physical activity follow physiological constraints [6]. Its incorporation into a generalized predictive insulin controller allowed the accurate prediction of hypoglycemic events and led to the prevention of postexercise hypoglycemia [7].

8.3 Nonlinear Adaptive Models

8.3.1 Kernel Adaptive Filters

Kernel adaptive filters (KAF) combine the universal approximation property of neural networks (for universal kernels) with the convexity of least squares problems. KAF accomplish a nonlinear regularized function by expressing all operations in terms of inner products in the reproducing kernel Hilbert space (RKHS) and sparsifying the solution online to confine the structure of the underlying network [2,8]. Nonlinear modeling is achieved by transforming the input space X into a high-dimensional RKHS H through the mapping φ: Chi; $\rightarrow H$, where $\varphi(x) = \kappa(x, \cdot)$ and $\kappa: X \times X \rightarrow R$ a positive definite kernel function and, then, by performing linear adaptive filtering in H. A useful property of RKHS, which is widely exploited in the formulation of nonlinear adaptive filtering algorithms, expresses the inner product between $\varphi(x)$ and $\varphi(x')$ in the high-dimensional feature space (infinite in the case of the Gaussian kernel) as the kernel of x and x' in the original space X:

$$\varphi(x)^T \varphi(x') = \kappa(x, x').$$
(8.10)

Table 8.5 Adaptive Linear Glucose Predictive Models

Study	Model	Input	Prediction Horizon	Evaluation Measures	Dataset	Prediction Performance		
Sparacino et al. [9]	AR weighted recursive least squares Forgetting factor 0.5	CGM data	30, 45 min	Mean Squared Prediction Error ESOD Time Lag	Twenty eight people with type 1 diabetes CGM device: Glucoday Sampling interval: 3 min Monitoring period: 48 h	*MSPE (10%, 90% percentiles)* 30 min: 353 (146, 924) 45 min: 1200 (480, 3690)	*ESOD (10%, 90% percentiles)* 30 min: 35925 (6675, 302,364) 45 min: 90780 (14,543, 917,982)	*Time lag (min)* *Positive trends* 30 min: 2.15 ± 15.63 45 min: 8.09 ± 19.37 *Negative trends* 30 min: 2.35 ± 13.03 45 min: 7.42 ± 15.27
Finan et al. [10]	ARX weighted recursive least squares	CGM, Meal and insulin modeling Model Gains	30–90 min	FIT% RMSE	Six people with type 1 diabetes monitored in normal daily life conditions. They were administered Prednisone for 3 days. CGM Device: CGMS, Medtronic Minimed Inc. Sampling Interval: 5 min Monitoring Period: 2–8 days without the prednisone medication. 3 additional days with the prednisone medication	*FIT (%)* 30 min: 65 60 min: 40 90 min: 19		*RMSE (mg/dL)* 30 min: 27 60 min: 45 90 min: 61
Eren-Oruklu et al. [4]	ARMA weighted recursive least squares with adaptive forgetting factor	CGM data	30 min	RAD (%) Sum of Squares of the Glucose Prediction Error (SSGPE)	Fourteen people with type 2 diabetes monitored in normal daily life conditions CGM device: System Gold, Medtronic Inc. Sampling interval: 5 min Monitoring period: 48 h	*SSGPE (%)* 5.56 ± 2.38 *RAD (%)* 3.83 + 1.63 *Hypoglycemia* Accurate readings 92.94% Benign errors 5.29%	*CG-EGA* *Euglycemia* Accurate readings 91.50% Benign errors 7.87%	*Hyperglycemia* Accurate readings 89.79% Benign errors 8.70%

Reference	Method	Input data	Prediction horizon	Metrics	Dataset	Univariate model	RAD (%)	Multivariate model	RAD (%)
Eren-Oruklu et al. [5]	ARMAX weighted recursive least squares with adaptive forgetting factor	CGM data Physiological data: Energy expenditure, average longitudinal acceleration, heat flux, galvanic skin response, near-body temperature	30 min	RAD (%) Sum of Squares of the Glucose Prediction Error (SSGPE)	Five people with type 2 diabetes monitored in normal daily life conditions CGM device: MMT-7012, Medtronic Inc. Sampling Interval: 5 min Monitoring Period: 23.8 ± 2.4 days	SSGPE (%) 8.81	5.77 ± 7.18	SSGPE (%) 7.43	4.24 ± 5.14
Turksoy et al. [6,7,11]	ARMAX in state-space form Constrained recursive least squares Real-time Kalman filtering	CGM data Insulin on board Energy expenditure and galvanic skin response	15, 30, 60 min	RMSE sum of squares of the Glucose prediction error (SSGPE)	Fourteen people with type 1 diabetes monitored in normal daily life conditions CGM device: iPRO, Medtronic Inc. Sampling Interval: 5 min Monitoring Period: -	RMSE (mg/dL) 15 min: 7.18 30 min: 18.55 60 min: 48.93		SSGPE (%) 15 min: 3.84 30 min: 9.91 60 min: 26.08	
Bayrak et al. [12]	AR recursive partial least squares Real-time Savitzky–Golay filter	CGM data	10, 20, 30, 40, 50 min	RMSE Sum of Squares of the Glucose Prediction Error (SSGPE)	Seventeen people with type 1 diabetes CGM device: Guardian RT, Medtronic Inc. Sampling Interval: 5 min Monitoring Period: -	RMSE (mg/dL) 10 min: 1.78 20 min: 4.32 30 min: 7.79 40 min: 11.84 50 min: 15.92		SSGPE (%) 10 min: 1.66 20 min: 4.06 30 min: 7.35 40 min: 11.22 50 min: 15.19	

For instance, kernel least mean square (KLMS) [13] and kernel recursive least squares (KRLS) [3] algorithms constitute a generalization of the respective linear adaptive filters, i.e., LMS and RLS, in the RKHS H, having expressed all of their operations in terms of inner products in the RKHS H. The Representer Theorem ensures that the minimizer $f \in H$ at iteration i lies in the span of the finite set of kernels centered at the input vectors $x_1, x_2, \ldots, x_i$ and it is expressed as:

$$f_i(x) = \sum_{j=1}^{i} a_j^i \kappa(x_j, x), \tag{8.11}$$

where a_j^i denotes the jth component of the coefficient vector at iteration i, i.e., $a^i = \left[a_1^i, \ldots, a_i^i\right]^T$. As the size of the expansion (8.11) increases linearly with the number of training data, sequential online sparsification criteria are elaborately combined with KAF in order to derive an informative set $C \subset X$ resulting in a model of improved complexity and, in parallel, of equivalent accuracy.

8.3.1.1 Kernel Least-Mean-Square Algorithm

KLMS considers a linear parametric model $f(x) = \theta^T \varphi(x)$ in a high-dimensional feature space H where the input space X is mapped to and which is associated with a positive definite kernel κ [1,13]. The parameters θ_i, minimizing the instantaneous squared error e_i^2 in H, are updated at each iteration i by the stochastic gradient descent:

$$\theta_i = \theta_{i-1} + \eta e_i \varphi(x_i), \tag{8.12}$$

where $e_i = y_i - \theta_{i-1}^T \varphi(x_i)$. Even though KLMS solves a nonregularized least squares problem, it has been shown that the norm of the KLMS solution, i.e., $\|\theta\|^2$, is constrained which ensures its generalization capacity and overall stability. Provided that φ is only implicitly known, as the eigenfunctions of the kernel κ, Eq. (8.10) is exploited in order to express all operations in terms of the kernel function κ. In particular, assuming $\theta_0 = 0$ and by repeatedly applying Eq. (8.12) we obtain:

$$\theta_i = \eta \sum_{j=1}^{i} e_j \varphi(x_j). \tag{8.13}$$

Thus, the output $f_i(x)$ of KLMS is given by:

$$f_i(x) = \theta_i^T \varphi(x) = \left(\eta \sum_{j=1}^{i} e_j \varphi(x_j)^T\right) \varphi(x) = \eta \sum_{j=1}^{i} e_j \kappa(x_j, x) \Rightarrow f_i(x) = f_{i-1}(x) + \eta e_i \kappa(x_i, x), \tag{8.14}$$

with $e_i = y_i - f_{i-1}(x_i)$. In line with Eq. (8.11), the set of kernel centers at iteration i is augmented by x_i, i.e., $C(i) = \{x_1, \ldots, x_i\}$, and the corresponding coefficient vector equals

Table 8.6   Kernel Least Mean Square

Input: $\{(x_i, y_i) | x_i \in R^d, y_i \in R\}, i = 1, 2, \ldots$
Initialization:
Choose $\eta > 0$ and kernel κ
$a_1^1 = \eta y_1$
$C_1 = \{x_1\}$
$f_1 = a_1^1 \kappa(x_1, \cdot)$
Computation:
while (x_i, y_i) is available

$\quad f_{i-1}(x_i) = \eta \sum_{j=1}^{i-1} a_j^{i-1} \kappa(x_i, x_j)$
$\quad e_i = y_i - f_{i-1}(x_i)$
$\quad a_i^i = \eta e_i$
$\quad C_i = \{C_{i-1}, x_i\}$
end while
Output: C_i, a_i

$a_i = [\eta e_1, \ldots, \eta e_i]^T$. Table 8.6 presents the KLMS algorithm, where we can observe that its time and space complexity are both of order $O(i)$.

As in the case of LMS, an upper bound for the step-size parameter η can be determined by means of the eigenvalues λ_j of the input data autocorrelation matrix in H:

$$0 < \eta < \frac{1}{\lambda_{\max}} \Leftrightarrow 0 < \eta < \frac{1}{tr(R_\Phi)} = \frac{N}{tr(K_\Phi)} = \frac{N}{\sum_{j=1}^N \kappa(x_j, x_j)}, \quad (8.15)$$

where $\Phi = [\varphi(x_1), \ldots, \varphi(x_N)]$, $R_\varphi = (1/N)\Phi\Phi^T$ is its autocorrelation matrix, and $K_\Phi = \Phi^T\Phi$ is the Gram matrix. Let σ_A denote the spectrum of matrix A. It holds that $\sigma_{R_\Phi} = N\sigma_{K_\Phi}$, with all eigenvalues of positive semidefinite matrices R_Φ and K_Φ being nonnegative. In addition, according to Eq. (8.3), the misadjustment M of KLMS is proportional to η and it is estimated as:

$$M = \frac{\eta}{2} tr(R_\Phi) = \frac{\eta}{2N} tr(K_\Phi). \quad (8.16)$$

8.3.1.2 Kernel Recursive Least Squares Algorithm
KRLS minimizes at each iteration i the sum of squared errors:

$$\arg\min_\theta E(\theta) = \arg\min_\theta \sum_{j=1}^i |y_j - \theta^T \varphi(x_j)|^2 + \lambda \|\theta\|^2 \Rightarrow \theta_i = (\Phi_i \Phi_i^T + \lambda I)^{-1} \Phi_i Y_i, \quad (8.17)$$

where $\Phi_i = [\varphi(x_1), \ldots, \varphi(x_i)]$ and $Y_i = [y_1, \ldots, y_i]^T$ [3]. Regularization is imposed by the high-dimensionality of the feature space H. The matrix inversion lemma is utilized in order to rearrange $(\Phi_i \Phi_i^T + \lambda I)^{-1} \Phi_i$ to $\Phi_i (\Phi_i^T \Phi_i + \lambda I)^{-1}$ and introduce the Gram matrix $K_i = \Phi_i^T \Phi_i$ into Eq. (8.17):

$$\theta_i = \Phi_i (\Phi_i^T \Phi_i + \lambda I)^{-1} Y_i. \tag{8.18}$$

Let $a_i = (\Phi_i^T \Phi_i + \lambda I)^{-1} Y_i$ and $Q_i = (\Phi_i^T \Phi_i + \lambda I)^{-1}$. A recursive method for the computation of a_i is developed to overcome the need for matrix inversion. The inverse of Q_i can be written as:

$$Q_i^{-1} = \begin{bmatrix} Q_{i-1}^{-1} & h_i \\ h_i^T & \lambda + \varphi(x_i)^T \varphi(x_i) \end{bmatrix}, \tag{8.19}$$

where $h_i = \Phi_{i-1}^T \varphi(x_i)$. Applying the matrix inversion lemma:

$$\begin{bmatrix} A & B \\ C & D \end{bmatrix}^{-1} = \begin{bmatrix} (A - BD^{-1}C)^{-1} & -A^{-1}B(D - CA^{-1}B)^{-1} \\ -D^{-1}C(A - BD^{-1}C)^{-1} & (D - CA^{-1}B)^{-1} \end{bmatrix}, \tag{8.20}$$

we obtain the following expression of Q_i:

$$Q_i = r_i^{-1} \begin{bmatrix} Q_{i-1} r_i + z_i z_i^T & -z_i \\ -z_i^T & 1 \end{bmatrix}, \tag{8.21}$$

where $z_i = Q_{i-1} \Phi_{i-1}^T \varphi(x_i)$ and $r_i = \varphi(x_i)^T \varphi(x_i) - z_i^T \Phi_{i-1}^T \varphi(x_i)$. Hence:

$$a(i) = Q_i Y_i = \begin{bmatrix} Q_{i-1} + z_i z_i^T r_i^{-1} & -z_i r_i^{-1} \\ -z_i^T r_i^{-1} & r_i^{-1} \end{bmatrix} \begin{bmatrix} Y_{i-1} \\ y_i \end{bmatrix} = \begin{bmatrix} a(i-1) - z_i r_i^{-1} e_i \\ r_i^{-1} e_i \end{bmatrix}. \tag{8.22}$$

where $z_i = Q_{i-1} \Phi_{i-1}^T \varphi(x_i)$ and $r_i = \varphi(x_i)^T \varphi(x_i) - z_i^T \Phi_{i-1}^T \varphi(x_i)$. From Eq. (8.22), we observe that KRLS at each iteration i updates not only the coefficient associated with x_i, i.e., $a_i^i = r_i^{-1} e_i$, as it is the case for KLMS, but also all the previous coefficients a_j^i by $-z_i r_i^{-1} e_i$ and with $j = 1, \ldots, i - 1$. The output of KRLS at iteration i is derived as:

$$f_i(x) = \varphi(x)^T \theta_i = \varphi(x)^T \Phi_i a_i = [\kappa(x_1, x), \ldots, \kappa(x_i, x)]^T a_i = \sum_{j=1}^{i} a_j^i \kappa(x_j, x). \tag{8.23}$$

Notice the growing set of kernel centers C_i which at iteration i comprises $C_i = \{x_1, \ldots, x_i\}$. In addition, by substituting Eq. (8.22) into Eq. (8.23), we obtain the following sequential rule for the computation of f_i:

$$f_i = f_{i-1} + r_i^{-1} \left[\kappa(x_i, \cdot) - \sum_{j=1}^{i-1} z_j^i \kappa(x_j, \cdot) \right] e_i, \tag{8.24}$$

with $e_i = y_i - f_{i-1}(x_i)$. The KRLS algorithm is presented in Table 8.7. The time and space complexity increases to the order of $O(i^2)$ for KRLS.

Table 8.7   Kernel Recursive Least Squares

Input: $\{(x_i, y_i) | x_i \in R^d, y_i \in R\}, i = 1, 2, \ldots$
Initialization:
Choose $\lambda > 0$ and kernel κ
$Q_1 = (\lambda + \kappa(x_1, x_1))^{-1}$
$C(1) = \{x_1\}$
$a(1) = Q_1 y_1$
Computation:
while (x_i, y_i) is available

$\quad h_i = [\kappa(x_i, x_1), \ldots, \kappa(x_i, x_{i-1})]^T$
$\quad z_i = Q_{i-1} h_i$
$\quad r_i = \lambda + \kappa(x_i, x_i) - z_i^T h_i$
$\quad Q_i = r_i^{-1} \begin{bmatrix} Q_{i-1} r_i + z_i z_i^T & -z_i \\ -z_i^T & 1 \end{bmatrix}$
$\quad e_i = y_i - h_i^T a_{i-1}$
$\quad a_i = \begin{bmatrix} a_{i-1} - z_i r_i^{-1} e_i \\ r_i^{-1} e_i \end{bmatrix}$
$\quad C_i = \{C_{i-1}, x_i\}$
end while
Output: C_i, a_i

8.3.1.3 Sparse Kernel Adaptive Filters

KAF typically employ a sequential process in order to attain a sparse and, in parallel, regularized solution. A representative set $C \subset X$ is sequentially built in which content at iteration i is denoted by $C_i = \{c_j^i | j = 1, \ldots, m_i\}$ and m_i is its cardinality. The set C is called the dictionary. Given a new input $x \in R^d$, the output $f_i(x)$ at time t_i is expressed as follows:

$$f_i(x) = \sum_{j=1}^{m_i} a_j^i \kappa(c_j^i, x), \tag{8.25}$$

where a_j^i denotes the jth component of the coefficient vector a_i. The quantized kernel least mean square (QKLMS) algorithm [14] and the approximate linear dependency kernel recursive least squares algorithm (KRLS-ALD) [15] are presented in the following subsections.

8.3.1.3.1 QUANTIZED KERNEL LEAST MEAN SQUARES

Vector quantization is performed in the input space X according to which a new input vector x_i is inserted into the current dictionary $C_i = C_{i-1} \cup \{x_i\}$ if the minimum distance of x_i from C_{i-1} is larger than the quantization size ε_x:

$$\min_{1 \le j \le m_{i-1}} \| x_i - c_j^{i-1} \| > \varepsilon_x. \tag{8.26}$$

Table 8.8   Quantized Kernel Least Mean Square

Input: $\{(x_i, y_i) | x_i \in R^d, y_i \in R\}, i = 1, 2, \ldots$
Initialization:
Choose $\eta > 0$, $\varepsilon_x > 0$, and kernel κ
$C_1 = \{x_1\}$
$a_1 = [\eta y_1]$
Computation:
while (x_i, y_i) is available

$\qquad f_{i-1}(x_i) = \sum_{j=1}^{m_i} a_j^{i-1} \kappa(c_j^{i-1}, x_i)$

$\qquad e_i = y_i - f_{i-1}(x_i)$
$\qquad dis(x_i, C_{i-1}) = \min_{1 \le j \le m_{i-1}} \left\| x_i - c_j^{i-1} \right\|$
$\qquad j^* = \arg\min_{1 \le j \le m_{i-1}} \left\| x_i - c_j^{i-1} \right\|$
$\qquad$ if $dis(x_i, C_{i-1}) \le \varepsilon_x$
$\qquad\qquad C_i = C_{i-1}$
$\qquad\qquad a_{j^*}^i = a_{j^*}^{i-1} + \eta e_i$
$\qquad$ else
$\qquad\qquad C_i = \{C_{i-1}, x_i\}$
$\qquad\qquad a_i = [a_{i-1}, \eta e_i]$
$\qquad$ end if
end while
Output: C_i, a_i

Otherwise, the dictionary is kept unchanged, i.e., $C_i = C_{i-1}$, and x_i is quantized to the closest vector $c_{j^*}^{i-1}$, where $j^* = \arg\min_{1 \le j \le m_{i-1}} \left\| x_i - c_j^{i-1} \right\|$. QKLMS relies on the stochastic gradient descent and, similar to KLMS, at each iteration i, updates only the coefficient of the new center:

$$a_{m_i}^i = \eta e_i, \tag{8.27}$$

or quantizes a redundant sample to its nearest center $c_{j^*}^{i-1}$:

$$a_{j^*}^i = a_{j^*}^{i-1} + \eta e_i. \tag{8.28}$$

The QKLMS algorithm is summarized in Table 8.8.

8.3.1.3.2   KERNEL RECURSIVE LEAST SQUARES WITH APPROXIMATE LINEAR DEPENDENCY

The approximate linear dependency (ALD) criterion is not only an effective sparsification approach, with its proven relationship to kernel principal components analysis, but also improves the stability of the KRLS algorithm. KRLS-ALD ensures that the centers of the dictionary at each iteration i are approximately linearly independent in the RKHS H:

$$\delta_i = \min_b \left\| \sum_{j=1}^{m_{i-1}} b_j \varphi(c_j) - \varphi(x_i) \right\|^2 \le v, \tag{8.29}$$

with the parameter $v > 0$ determining the level of sparsity. Assuming that the $m_{i-1} \times m_{i-1}$ Gram matrix $\tilde{K}_{i-1}$ is invertible and setting $\mathbf{k}_i = [\kappa(x_i, c_1), \ldots, \kappa(x_i, c_{m_{i-1}})]^T$, the optimal b_i is the solution of $\tilde{K}_{i-1} b_i = \mathbf{k}_i$

$$b_i = \tilde{K}_{i-1}^{-1} \mathbf{k}_i \tag{8.30}$$

and, correspondingly, the ALD condition becomes

$$\delta_i = \kappa(x_i, x_i) - \mathbf{k}_i^T b_i = \kappa(x_i, x_i) - \mathbf{k}_i^T \tilde{K}_{i-1}^{-1} \mathbf{k}_i \leq v. \tag{8.31}$$

In the case where $\delta_i > v$ then the dictionary is expanded such that $C(i) = C(i-1) \cup \{x_i\}$. Provided that v is sufficiently small, each $\varphi(x_i)$ up to time t_i can be approximated by:

$$\varphi\left(x_i\right) \approx \sum_{j=1}^{m_i} b_j^i \varphi(c_j), \tag{8.32}$$

which is equivalent to

$$K_i \approx B_i \tilde{K}_i B_i^T, \tag{8.33}$$

where $B_i = [b_1, \ldots, b_i]^T$ and $B_{i,j} = 0$ for all $j > i$. KRLS-ALD minimizes, at each iteration i, the sum of squared errors over the current dictionary and, similar to KRLS, we have:

$$E(\theta) = \left\| \Phi_i^T \theta - y_i \right\|^2 \Leftrightarrow E(a) = \left\| K_i a - y_i \right\|^2 \overset{(8.33)}{=} \left\| B_i \tilde{K}_i B_i^T a - y_i \right\|^2 \overset{\tilde{a} \overset{\text{def}}{=} B_i^T a}{\Leftrightarrow} E(\tilde{a}) = \left\| B_i \tilde{K}_i \tilde{a} - y_i \right\|^2. \tag{8.34}$$

The solution of the modified minimization problem is given by:

$$\tilde{a}_i = (B_i \tilde{K}_i)^\dagger y_i = \tilde{K}_i^{-1} (B_i^T B_i)^{-1} B_i^T y_i. \tag{8.35}$$

Two cases are defined depending on the value of δ_i: (i) Case 1: $\delta_i \leq v$ and (ii) Case 2: $\delta_i > v$.

CASE 1: If $\delta_i \leq v$, $C_i = C_{i-1}$, $m_i = m_{i-1}$, $\tilde{K}_i = \tilde{K}_{i-1}$ and B_i is modified as follows:

$$B_i = [B_{i-1}^T, b_i]^T, \tag{8.36}$$

where b_i is given by Eq. (8.30). Therefore,

$$B_i^T B_i = B_{i-1}^T B_{i-1} + b_i b_i^T, \tag{8.37}$$

and

$$B_i^T y_i = B_{i-1}^T y_{i-1} + b_i y_i. \tag{8.38}$$

Defining $P_i = (A_i^T A_i)^{-1}$ and by applying the matrix inversion lemma, we obtain a recursive formula for P_i:

$$P_i = P_{i-1} - \frac{P_{i-1} b_i b_i^T P_{i-1}}{1 + b_i^T P_{i-1} b_i}. \tag{8.39}$$

Then, substituting Eqs. (8.38) and (8.39) into Eq. (8.35) and denoting $q_i = P_{i-1} b_i / 1 + b_i^T P_{i-1} b_i$, we derive the following recursive update rule for $\tilde{a}_i$:

$$
\begin{aligned}
\tilde{a}_i &= \tilde{K}_i^{-1} P_i B_i^T y_i \\
&= \tilde{K}_i^{-1} (P_{i-1} - q_i b_i^T P_{i-1})(B_{i-1}^T y_{i-1} + b_i y_i) \\
&= \tilde{a}_{i-1} + \tilde{K}_i^{-1} (P_i b_i y_i - q_i b_i^T \tilde{K}_i \tilde{a}_{i-1}) \\
&= \tilde{a}_{i-1} + \tilde{K}_i^{-1} q_i (y_i - \mathbf{k}_i \tilde{a}_{i-1})
\end{aligned}
\tag{8.40}
$$

where $\mathbf{k}_i = \tilde{K}_i b_i$.

CASE 2: If $\delta_i > v$, $C_i = C_{i-1} \cup \{x_i\}$, $m_i = m_{i-1} + 1$, and $\tilde{K}_i$ and B_i are modified as follows:

$$\tilde{K}_i = \begin{bmatrix} \tilde{K}_{i-1} & \mathbf{k}_i \\ \mathbf{k}_i^T & \kappa(x_i, x_i) \end{bmatrix} \Rightarrow \tilde{K}_i^{-1} = \frac{1}{\delta_i} \begin{bmatrix} \delta_i \tilde{K}_{i-1} + b_i b_i^T & -b_i \\ -b_i^T & 1 \end{bmatrix}, \tag{8.41}$$

$$B_i = \begin{bmatrix} B_{i-1} & 0 \\ 0^T & 1 \end{bmatrix}, B_i^T B_i = \begin{bmatrix} B_{i-1}^T B_{i-1} & 0 \\ 0^T & 1 \end{bmatrix}, P_i = (B_i^T B_i)^{-1} = \begin{bmatrix} P_{i-1} & 0 \\ 0^T & 1 \end{bmatrix}. \tag{8.42}$$

Substituting Eqs. (8.41) and (8.42) into Eq. (8.35), we obtain the following update rule for $\tilde{a}_i$:

$$\tilde{a}(i) = \tilde{K}_i^{-1} (B_i^T B_i)^{-1} B_i^T y_i = \tilde{K}_i^{-1} \begin{bmatrix} (B_{i-1}^T B_{i-1})^{-1} B_{i-1}^T y_{i-1} \\ y_i \end{bmatrix} = \begin{bmatrix} \tilde{a}_{i-1} - \dfrac{b_i}{\delta_i} \left(y_i - \mathbf{k}_i^T \tilde{a}_{i-1} \right) \\ \dfrac{1}{\delta_i} \left(y_i - \tilde{\mathbf{k}}_i^T \tilde{a}_{i-1} \right) \end{bmatrix}, \tag{8.43}$$

where $\mathbf{k}_i^T = b_i^T \tilde{K}_{i-1}$.

KRLS-ALD, at each iteration i, updates the coefficient associated with the new center, i.e., $\tilde{a}_{m_i}^i$, and all previous coefficients, i.e., $\tilde{a}_j^i$, with $j = 1, \ldots, m_{i-1}$, as well. The KRLS-ALD algorithm is presented in Table 8.9. The dependence of KRLS-ALD on the Gram matrix $\tilde{K}_{i-1}$ defined on C_{i-1} increases its time and space complexity from $O(m_i)$ in the case of QKLMS to $O(m_i^2)$.

8.3.2 Glucose Prediction Applications

Table 8.10 reports the state-of-the-art studies employing nonlinear dynamical models to the short-term prediction of s.c. glucose concentration in diabetes. A discrete-time nonlinear

Table 8.9   Approximate Linear Dependency Kernel Recursive Least Squares

Input: $\{(x_i, y_i) | x_i \in R^d, y_i \in R\}, i = 1, 2, \ldots$

Initialization:

Choose $v > 0$ and kernel κ

$\tilde{K}_1 = [\kappa(x_1, x_1)]$

$\tilde{K}_1^{-1} = [1/\kappa(x_1, x_1)]$

$\tilde{a}_1 = y_1/\kappa(x_1, x_1)$

$P_1 = [1]$

$m_1 = 1$

Computation:

while (x_i, y_i) is available

    $b_i = \tilde{K}_{i-1}^{-1} \mathbf{k}_i$

    $\delta_i = \kappa(x_i, x_i) - \mathbf{k}_i^T b_i$

    if $\delta_i > v$

    $C_i = \{C_{i-1}, x_i\}$

$$\tilde{K}_i^{-1} = \frac{1}{\delta_i} \begin{bmatrix} \delta_i \tilde{K}_{i-1} + b_i b_i^T & -b_i \\ -b_i^T & 1 \end{bmatrix}$$

$$P_i = \begin{bmatrix} P_{i-1} & 0 \\ 0^T & 1 \end{bmatrix}$$

$$\tilde{a}(i) = \begin{bmatrix} \tilde{a}_{i-1} - \dfrac{b_i}{\delta_i}(y_i - \mathbf{k}_i^T \tilde{a}_{i-1}) \\ \dfrac{1}{\delta_i}(y_i - \mathbf{k}_i^T \tilde{a}_{i-1}) \end{bmatrix}$$

    $m_i = m_{i-1} + 1$

    else

    $C_i = C_{i-1}$

    $q_i = \dfrac{P_{i-1} b_i}{1 + b_i^T P_{i-1} b_i}$

    $P_i = P_{i-1} - \dfrac{P_{i-1} b_i b_i^T P_{i-1}}{1 + b_i^T P_{i-1} b_i}$

    $\tilde{a}_i = \tilde{a}_{i-1} + \tilde{K}_i^{-1} q_i (y_i - \mathbf{k}_i \tilde{a}_{i-1})$

    end if

end while

Output: $C_i, \tilde{a}_i$

dynamic system of glucose in type 1 diabetes, whose state as well as time-varying coefficients were estimated by an extended Kalman filter (EKF) and, in which the effect of food intake and s.c. insulin delivery was modeled through normalized finite impulse response filter functions, was found to outperform a recursively identified ARX having a similar configuration [16]. However, EKF-identified state-space models provide a solution to nonlinear problems which is suboptimal [17,18].

The fusion of real-time adaptive models, i.e., a recurrent neural network (RNN) with real-time recurrent learning (RTRL) and an autoregressive (AR) model, resulted in 100%

Table 8.10 Adaptive Nonlinear Glucose Predictive Models

Study	Model	Input	Prediction Horizon	Evaluation Measures	Dataset	Prediction Performance
Daskalaki et al. [19-21]	Ensemble modeling (1) ARX with output correction module (cARX) Recursive least squares (2) RNN with RTRL	CGM data Insulin infusion rate data	15, 30, 45 min	RMSE Time Lag (TL) Correlation Coefficient (CC)	Twenty three people with type 1 diabetes under SAP therapy monitored in normal daily life conditions CGM device: Minimed CGM, Medtronic Inc. CGM sampling interval: 5 min Monitoring period: Training set: 5.30 ± 1.40 days Evaluation set: 4.83 ± 1.80 days	cARX RMSE (mg/dL) 15 min: 16.8 30 min: 27.7 45 min: 37.0 TL (min) 15 min: 5 30 min: 15 45 min: 30 CC 15 min: 0.96 30 min: 0.90 45 min: 0.82 RNN RMSE (mg/dL) 15 min: 11.9 30 min: 18.9 45 min: 26.1 TL (min) 15 min: 5 30 min: 10 45 min: 20 CC 15 min: 0.98 30 min: 0.94 45 min: 0.90
Naumova et al. [22]	Regularized kernel learning Meta-learning approach to choosing a kernel and a regularization parameter	CGM data	30, 60, 75 min	Clarke Error Grid Analysis (EGA) Prediction Error Grid Analysis (PRED-EGA) with reference to blood glucose measurements	Six people with type 1 diabetes under a hospitalized setting CGM device: DexCom CGM sampling interval: 5 min Blood glucose device: Yellow Springs Instrument	Clarke EGA Zone A (%) 30 min: 91.3 60 min: 75.14 75 min: 68.77 Zone B (%) 30 min: 8.51 60 min: 24.13 75 min: 29.97 Zone D (%) 30 min: 0.19 60 min: 0.54 75 min: 0.82 PRED-EGA Hypoglycemia: Accurate readings (%) 10 min: 90.82 20 min: 81.75 Benign errors (%) 10 min: 5.16 20 min: 5.16 Euglycemia: Accurate readings (%) 10 min: 82.96 20 min: 82.11 Benign errors (%) 10 min: 13.05 20 min: 16.08 Hyperglycemia: Accurate readings (%) 10 min: 90.52 20 min: 90.81 Benign errors (%) 10 min: 4.14 20 min: 1.33

Wang et al. [16]	Time-varying state-space model Extended Kalman Filter	CGM data FIR modeling of s.c. insulin absorption and meal absorption	30 min	R^2 RAD Time gain	Five people with type 1 diabetes using insulin pump monitored in normal daily life conditions CGM device: Minimed CGM MMT-7102, Medtronic Inc. Sampling interval: 5 min Monitoring period: 60.4 ± 10.6 hours	R^2 0.71 ± 0.19	RAD (%) 20.31 ± 10.44	Time gain (min) 12.00 ± 10.37	J 377.93 ± 644.32

prediction accuracy of hypoglycemic events for patients under sensor-augmented pump (SAP) therapy during everyday living conditions [20,21]. An alternative approach to the problem of glucose prediction than that of recursive model identification and purely subject-dependent solutions has been proposed by Naumova et al. [22]. They presented a meta-learning subject-independent optimization procedure for adjusting the hyperparameters of an iterated Tikhonov regularization learning algorithm (i.e., the regularization parameter and the parameters of the kernel generating the associated RKHS) to each new input. Both 30-minute and 60-minute predictions of that regularized scheme, with input previous, but not-necessarily equi-sampled, CGM measurements were significantly better compared to the two state-of-the-art glucose prediction methods [23,24].

In this context, novel nonlinear recursive frameworks to the online identification and prediction of the dynamic glucose system in type 1 diabetes, taking advantage of KAF, can be evaluated. Targeting at a real-time autoregressive or multivariate model, special emphasis should be placed on their time and space complexity in combination with their convergence behavior and generalization capacity.

8.4 Computational Experiments

A nonlinear recursive predictive model of the dynamic glucose system in type 1 diabetes is presented. Nonlinear regression is performed in a RKHS by the KRLS-ALD algorithm [24], such that a sparse model structure is accomplished. All simulations were performed using the Kernel Adaptive Filtering MATLAB Toolbox [25]. The method is evaluated on seven people with type 1 diabetes observed in free-living conditions, where a change in glycemic dynamics is forced by increasing the level of physical activity in the middle of the observational period [26]. A comprehensive description of the glucose dataset is provided in Chapter 6, Nonlinear Models of Glucose Concentration. We speculate that a sparse KAF, as implemented by the KRLS-ALD, can adapt to changing environmental conditions, and, thus, perform more efficiently than time-invariant linear regression models.

KRLS-ALD is evaluated individually for each patient. A Gaussian kernel has been selected, with σ denoting its bandwidth. For each patient, the values of the free parameters (i.e., σ, v) minimizing the root mean squared error (RMSE) over the period starting from the third day of monitoring are selected by grid search. The goodness of fit is assessed by (1) the RMSE, (2) the FIT (%), (3) the time gain (TG) [27], (4) the normalized energy of the second order differences $ESOD_{norm}$ [27], and (5, 6) the sensitivity (SNS) and false positive rate (FPR) of predictions in the hypoglycemic range.

Table 8.11 presents the predictive performance of KRLS-ALD over the second week of the observational period and for a prediction horizon of 15, 30, and 60 minutes. The RMSE of the 15-minute predictions as well as the associated FIT values, ranging from 2.65 to 8.99 mg/dL and from 85.74 to 94.50, respectively, show a highly accurate description of short-term glucose dynamics, which allow for a $\sim$11-minute proactive time. In addition, the corresponding SNS and FPR values (range: $0.75-0.91$ and $0.07-0.18$, respectively) demonstrate

Table 8.11 Prediction Performance of KRLS-ALD Algorithm

	PH 15 min						PH 30 min						PH 60 min					
	RMSE	FIT (%)	TG	ESOD$_{norm}$	SNS	FPR	RMSE	FIT (%)	TG	ESOD$_{norm}$	SNS	FPR	RMSE	FIT (%)	TG	ESOD$_{norm}$	SNS	FPR
Subject 1	3.58	88.16	10	19.31	0.84	0.07	10.54	65.21	TG	52.06	0.65	0.20	21.42	29.09	20	57.34	0.47	0.27
Subject 2	2.65	91.97	10	21.74	0.91	0.08	7.42	77.48	15	74.74	0.72	0.23	16.57	49.74	25	88.19	0.46	0.44
Subject 3	4.89	92.61	10	23.13	0.83	0.13	14.99	77.33	20	62.11	0.55	0.25	33.45	49.26	20	105.82	0.28	0.40
Subject 4	7.00	85.74	15	13.76	0.85	0.14	21.73	55.88	15	61.07	0.59	0.38	43.74	11.59	20	48.89	0.07	0.71
Subject 5	8.99	89.80	10	16.87	0.80	0.09	23.82	72.98	20	58.24	0.48	0.28	46.03	47.84	20	87.16	0.11	0.67
Subject 6	4.17	90.08	10	28.11	0.75	0.18	11.73	71.85	15	85.92	0.48	0.23	24.31	40.09	15	27.94	0.10	0.50
Subject 7	5.60	94.50	10	21.29	0.86	0.10	16.33	84.00	15	42.65	0.68	0.25	36.02	64.82	20	69.26	0.19	0.58
Mean	5.27	90.41	10.71	20.60	0.83	0.11	15.22	72.10	17.14	62.40	0.59	0.26	31.65	41.78	20.00	69.23	0.24	0.51
SD	2.16	2.92	1.89	4.60	0.05	0.04	5.95	9.21	17.14	14.27	0.09	0.06	11.26	17.14	2.89	26.71	0.17	0.16

a high-predictive capacity in the hypoglycemic range. The increase of prediction horizon to 30-minute results in an average RMSE 15.22 ± 5.95 mg/dL and an average TG 17.14 ± 2.67 minutes, whereas SNS and FPR of hypoglycemic predictions remain sufficient. Nevertheless, the RMSE increases considerably for longer prediction horizons, where FIT becomes lower than 0.5 though a 20-minute TG is preserved. Figs. 8.1−8.7 illustrate the prediction error curves of KRLS-ALD regarding Subject#1−Subject#7, respectively, where we can observe the progressive adaptation of the KRLS-ALD model as well as the considerable dependence of model's performance on each patient's glycemic dynamics. Figs. 8.8 and. 8.9 portray the measured versus the 30-minute-ahead predicted glucose time series for Subject #1 during two indicative days of the monitoring period (11th and 13th day, respectively), where we can observe that the solution obtained by KRLS-ALD is closer to that of SVR.

Comparing the performance of KRLS-ALD with that of SVR and TDNN, which were presented in Chapter 6, Nonlinear Models of Glucose Concentration, we perceive that SVR tends to produce slightly higher RMSEs, which is also translated to lower FIT values, and comparable TG values. KRLS-ALD is also more sensitive to hypoglycemic predictions as compared with SVR, with the latter yielding less false positive predictions especially for a horizon of

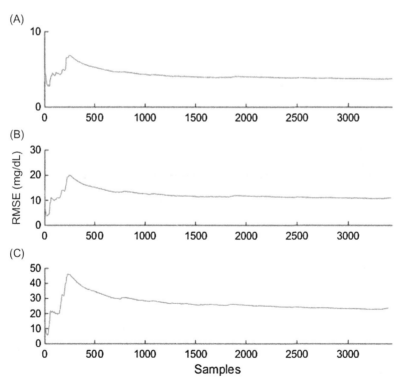

FIGURE 8.1 Convergence curves of KRLS-ALD regarding Subject #1 for each prediction horizon, i.e., 15, 30, and 60 min (A−C).

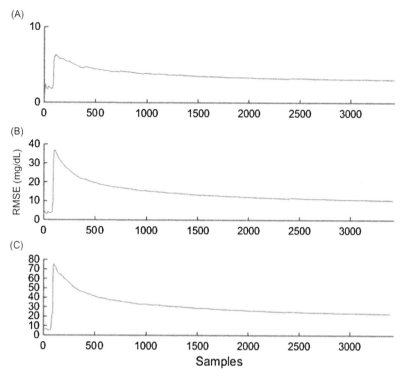

FIGURE 8.2 Convergence curves of KRLS-ALD regarding Subject #2 for each prediction horizon, i.e., 15, 30, and 60 min (A−C).

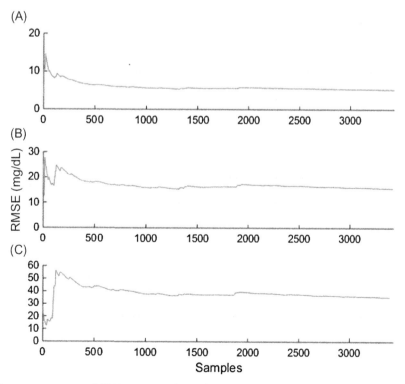

FIGURE 8.3 Convergence curves of KRLS-ALD regarding Subject #3 for each prediction horizon, i.e., 15, 30, and 60 min (A−C).

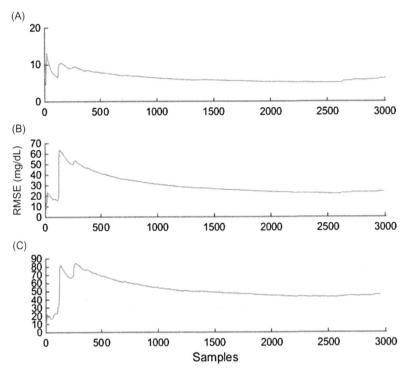

FIGURE 8.4 Convergence curves of KRLS-ALD regarding Subject #4 for each prediction horizon, i.e., 15, 30, and 60 min (A−C).

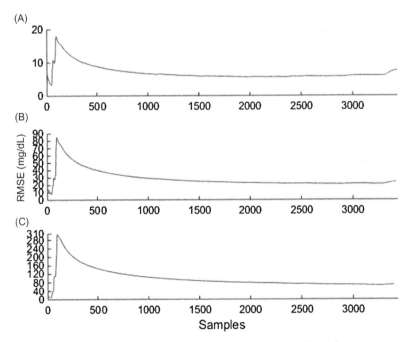

FIGURE 8.5 Convergence curves of KRLS-ALD regarding Subject #5 for each prediction horizon, i.e., 15, 30, and 60 min (A−C).

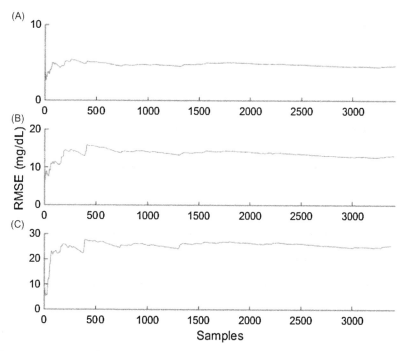

FIGURE 8.6 Convergence curves of KRLS-ALD regarding Subject #6 for each prediction horizon, i.e., 15, 30, and 60 min (A−C).

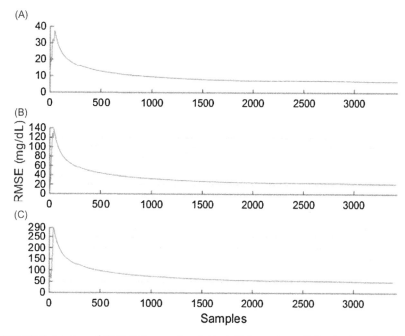

FIGURE 8.7 Convergence curves of KRLS-ALD regarding Subject #7 for each prediction horizon, i.e., 15, 30, and 60 min (A−C).

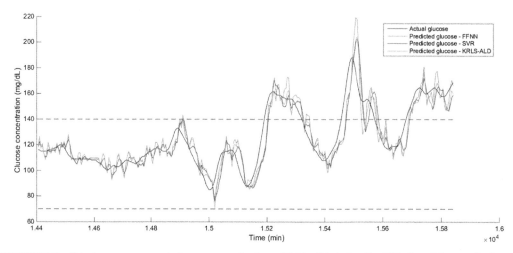

FIGURE 8.8 Predicted versus measured glucose concentration of Subject#1 during the 11th day of the monitoring period for a prediction horizon of 30 min.

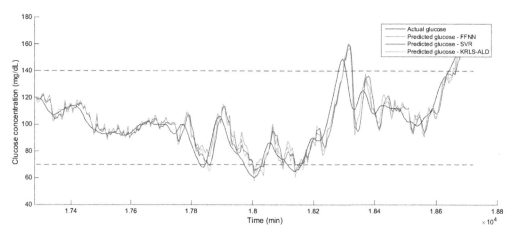

FIGURE 8.9 Predicted versus measured glucose concentration of Subject#1 during the 13th day of the monitoring period for a prediction horizon of 30 min.

60 minutes. Similarly, KRLS-ALD outperforms the TDNN in terms of RMSE and FIT, whereas their capacity is comparable in the hypoglycemic range for horizons $\leq$ 30 minutes. However, TDNN yields, on average, a less delayed glucose time series than both KRLS-ALD and SVR. In addition, $ESOD_{norm}$ reveals that kernel-based learning is associated with smoother predictions, with SVR, followed by KRLS-ALD, exhibiting highly regularized predictions.

8.5 Discussion and Conclusions

The requirement for an individualized recursively identified glucose prediction model is imposed by the high inter- and intrapatient variability of glucose dynamics in response to exogenous inputs due to biological (e.g., variations in insulin sensitivity or body mass) or environmental (e.g., variations in the level of physical activity which is the case in the present study) variations. In this chapter, increased emphasis was placed on KAF-based algorithms which are proposed to the recursive nonlinear identification and prediction of the glucose system. Their efficiency consists in the expressive power of the RKHS and the convexity of linear adaptive LMS and RLS models. Nevertheless, in a nonstationary context, consideration should be given to the specification of their hyperparameters which largely affect the generalization ability of KAF. For instance, adaptive learning of kernel bandwidth has been shown to improve the prediction accuracy of KLMS significantly [26].

The benefit of an adaptive nonlinear glucose predictive modeling scheme over a time-invariant one, during everyday living conditions, was demonstrated through the direct comparison of a univariate kernel-based recursive model, i.e., KRLS-ALD, with univariate SVR or TDNN models trained in a batch mode. KRLS-ALD results in a sparse regularized solution in a RKHS, featuring also a high-convergence rate. The univariate input allows for short-term ($\leq$30 minutes) predictions with KRLS-ALD reaching an average RMSE of 15.22 ± 5.95 mg/dL and an average time lag of 17.14 ± 2.67 minutes for a horizon of 30 minutes. Nevertheless, the presence of unmodeled inputs and unmeasured disturbances greatly confounds the accurate prediction of glucose concentration particularly for horizons $\geq$ 30 minutes. The dependence of KRLS-ALD on the Gram matrix increases its computational complexity to $O(m_i^2)$, being, however, lower than the time complexity of SVR, which scales superlinearly with the size of the training set. As we had hypothesized, KRLS-ALD outperformed both SVR and TDNN, whereas its generalization ability, for horizons $\leq$30 minutes, compares well to that of multivariate recursively identified ARMAX model and nonlinear approaches (i.e., RNNs) found in the literature [21,23].

As we have stated in Chapter 5, Linear Time Series Models of Glucose Concentration, and Chapter 6, Nonlinear Models of Glucose Concentration, linear time-invariant functions suffice to model low-frequency glycemic dynamics associated with circadian or ultradian rhythms, whereas nonlinear dynamical functions may learn the time-varying effect of exogenous inputs and endogenous processes. To this end, contemporary system identification and prediction approaches, which may express more efficiently temporal input−output relationships (e.g., state-space models in the RKHS [28]), should be evaluated with respect to glucose prediction in diabetes.

References

[1] Liu W, Príncipe JC, Haykin S. Kernel least-mean-square algorithm. Kernel adaptive filtering. Hoboken, New Jersey: John Wiley & Sons, Inc., Published simultaneously in Canada; 2010. p. 27−68.

[2] Slavakis K, Bouboulis P, Theodoridis S. Chapter 17—Online learning in reproducing kernel Hilbert spaces. In: Paulo JAKSRC, Diniz SR, Sergios T, editors. Academic Press library in signal processing. Waltham, USA: Elsevier, Oxford, UK; 2014. p. 883−987.

[3] Liu W, Príncipe JC, Haykin S. Kernel recursive least-squares algorithm. Kernel adaptive filtering. Hoboken, New Jersey: John Wiley & Sons, Inc., Published simultaneously in Canada; 2010. p. 94−123.

[4] Eren-Oruklu M, et al. Estimation of future glucose concentrations with subject-specific recursive linear models. Diabetes Technol Ther 2009;11(4):243−53.

[5] Eren-Oruklu M, et al. Adaptive system identification for estimating future glucose concentrations and hypoglycemia alarms. Automatica (Oxf) 2012;48(8):1892−7.

[6] Turksoy K, et al. Hypoglycemia early alarm systems based on multivariable models. Ind Eng Chem Res 2013;52:35.

[7] Turksoy K, et al. Multivariable adaptive identification and control for artificial pancreas systems. IEEE Trans Biomed Eng 2014;61(3):883−91.

[8] Liu W, Príncipe JC, Haykin S. Background and preview. Kernel adaptive filtering. Hoboken, New Jersey: John Wiley & Sons, Inc., Published simultaneously in Canada; 2010. p. 1−26.

[9] Sparacino G, et al. Glucose concentration can be predicted ahead in time from continuous glucose monitoring sensor time-series. IEEE Trans Biomed Eng 2007;54(5):931−7.

[10] Finan DA, et al. Experimental evaluation of a recursive model identification technique for type 1 diabetes. J Diabetes Sci Technol 2009;3(5):1192−202.

[11] Turksoy K, et al. Multivariable adaptive closed-loop control of an artificial pancreas without meal and activity announcement. Diabetes Technol Ther 2013;15(5):386−400.

[12] Bayrak ES, et al. Hypoglycemia early alarm systems based on recursive autoregressive partial least squares models. J Diabetes Sci Technol 2013;7(1):206−14.

[13] Liu W, Pokharel PP, Principe JC. The Kernel least-mean-square algorithm. IEEE Trans Signal Process 2008;56(2):543−54.

[14] Chen BD, et al. Quantized Kernel Least Mean Square Algorithm. IEEE Trans Neural Netw Learn Syst 2012;23(1):22−32.

[15] Engel Y, Mannor S, Meir R. The kernel recursive least-squares algorithm. IEEE Trans Signal Process 2004;52(8):2275−85.

[16] Wang Q, et al. Personalized state-space modeling of glucose dynamics for type 1 diabetes using continuously monitored glucose, insulin dose, and meal intake: an extended Kalman filter approach. J Diabetes Sci Technol 2014;8(2):331−45.

[17] Picard J. Efficiency of the extended Kalman filter for nonlinear systems with small noise. SIAM J Appl Math 1991;51(3):843−85.

[18] Wan EA, Merwe RVD. The unscented Kalman filter for nonlinear estimation. In: Proceedings of the IEEE 2000 adaptive systems for signal processing, communications, and control symposium (Cat. No.00EX373), 2000.

[19] Daskalaki E, et al. Real-time adaptive models for the personalized prediction of glycemic profile in type 1 diabetes patients. Diabetes Technol Ther 2012;14(2):168−74.

[20] Daskalaki E, et al. An early warning system for hypoglycemic/hyperglycemic events based on fusion of adaptive prediction models. J Diabetes Sci Technol 2013;7(3):689−98.

[21] Daskalaki E, Diem P, Mougiakakou S. Adaptive algorithms for personalized diabetes treatment. In: Marmarelis V, Mitsis G, editors. Data-driven modeling for diabetes: diagnosis and treatment. Berlin, Heidelberg: Springer Berlin Heidelberg; 2014. p. 91−116.

[22] Naumova V, Pereverzyev SV, Sivananthan S. A meta-learning approach to the regularized learning-case study: blood glucose prediction. Neural Netw 2012;33:181−93.

[23] Reifman J, et al. Predictive monitoring for improved management of glucose levels. J Diabetes Sci Technol 2007;1(4):478−86.

[24] Pappada SM, et al. Neural network-based real-time prediction of glucose in patients with insulin-dependent diabetes. Diabetes Technol Ther 2011;13(2):135−41.

[25] Vaerenbergh SV, Santamaría I. A comparative study of kernel adaptive filtering algorithms. In: 2013 IEEE Digital signal processing and signal processing education meeting (DSP/SPE). 2013.

[26] Georga EI, et al. Development of a smart environment for diabetes data analysis and new knowledge mining. In: 2014 EAI 4th international conference on wireless mobile communication and healthcare (Mobihealth), 2014.

[27] Zecchin C, et al. Jump neural network for online short-time prediction of blood glucose from continuous monitoring sensors and meal information. Comput Methods Programs Biomed 2014;113(1):144−52.

[28] Li K, Principe JC. The Kernel adaptive autoregressive-moving-average algorithm. IEEE Trans Neural Netw Learn Syst 2016;27(2):334−46.

Existing and Potential Applications of Glucose Prediction Models

9.1 Closed-Loop Control of Glucose in Type 1 Diabetes

The most vital and challenging issue for people with type 1 or advanced type 2 diabetes is the achievement and maintenance of euglycemia overtime in a safe manner. Intensive insulin therapy, implemented by either multiple daily injections (MDI) or continuous subcutaneous insulin infusion (CSII), could be the remedy for hyperglycemia in type 1 diabetes should it did not increase the risk of hypoglycemia [1]. The effective integration of continuous glucose monitoring (CGM) and CSII technologies into one system, i.e., sensor-augmented pump (SAP), allows for improvements in glycemic control of type 1 diabetes when compared with MDI therapy or the individual components alone [2−4]; however, the problem of severe hypoglycemia and, in particular, nocturnal hypoglycemia is not solved. CGM enabled a high time-resolution description of the short-term glucose dynamics in the subcutaneous space, the awareness of which by both patients and physicians has been shown to improve the long-term glycemic control (i.e., HbA1c levels) in type 1 diabetes and facilitate the evaluation of the response to therapy, as compared to SMBG. The continuously improved accuracy of CGM effected its approval for making therapeutic decisions in Europe [5,6]. However, there is still room for improvement in the hypoglycemic range which, in conjunction with the lag time of interstitial fluid glucose relative to blood glucose, hinders the precise detection of hypoglycemia based merely on CGM data. In addition, only the combined use of CGM, CSII, and glucose predictive algorithms has been shown to reduce the incidence and duration of hypoglycemia, though it may come at a price of an increase in hyperglycemia [7,8]. In particular, the integration of low-glucose predictive alerts into today open- or hybrid closed-loop systems of glycemic control in diabetes is imperative toward minimizing the risk of hypoglycemia [9,10]. To this end, more proactive and sensitive to overall patient's context glucose predictive algorithms may result in tighter glycemic control minimizing the risk of hypoglycemia, while set the appropriate circumstances for closing the loop during the day.

9.1.1 Components of Artificial Pancreas Systems

CGM, CSII, and control algorithms constitute the backbone technologies of current systems of closed-loop control of glucose concentration in type 1 diabetes or, the so-called artificial pancreas (AP) systems, being meticulously combined to emulate the feedback glucose-responsive functionality of beta-cells in normal physiology of glucose metabolism [7]. Fig. 9.1 illustrates the main components of an AP system. Interstitial glucose concentration measurements are the main input of the controller which, depending on the underlying algorithm,

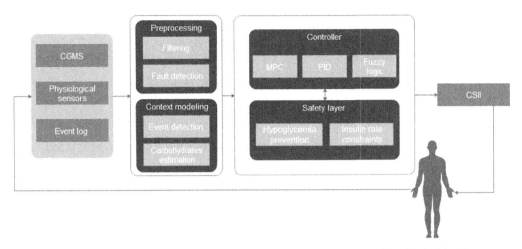

FIGURE 9.1 Components of closed-loop controller of glucose in type 1 diabetes based on the double subcutaneous route (CGM, CSII).

determines the insulin delivery rate such that euglycemia is safely achieved and maintained. Additional bio- and physiological signals (e.g., galvanic skin response, heart rate variability, skin temperature, energy expenditure), predictive or reflective of glycemia as well as patient's physiological, emotional, and behavioral status, may be exploited in order to adjust the operating mode of the controller [11,12].

The main algorithmic approaches to closed-loop control in type 1 diabetes rely on proportional-integral-derivative (PID) control and model predictive control (MPC), where the proper tuning of the control algorithm's parameters determines its sensitivity to hypoglycemic or hyperglycemic excursions [13,14]. In addition, fuzzy logic theory [15,16] and mathematical models of β-cell physiology [17] have been also successfully applied to regulating blood glucose. Most importantly, the degree of system's automation, and subsequently, the sophistication of the overall control algorithm, depends on the management of external disturbances to the glucose system (e.g., meals, exercise) [11,12]. For instance, the hybrid closed-loop approach employs meal announcement or manual prandial insulin bolus delivery, which may lessen the effect of the intrinsic delays imposed by the double subcutaneous route and, therefore, mitigate the risk of postprandial hyperglycemia or late-onset postprandial hypoglycemia [18]. More elaborate AP approaches may involve automatic food recognition and quantification of the nutrient content of meals by properly combining image processing, computer vision and machine-learning technologies [19,20]. Moreover, the functionality of the controller may be supported by hypoglycemia risk minimizing modules, i.e., threshold-based insulin pump interruption or predictive low-glucose-insulin suspension [21]. A three-layer modular architecture for closed-loop control in type 1 diabetes has been proposed which separates functionalities assuring patient's safety (e.g., hypoglycemia prevention) from real-time customizable (e.g., body weight, insulin-to-carbohydrate ratio, and basal insulin delivery) MPC of basal insulin rate [22]. To this end, bihormonal AP systems adopt a more holistic approach, regulating glucose homeostasis by subcutaneously delivering both insulin and glucagon hormones aiming at hypoglycemia prevention or counterregulation [7,23,24].

9.1.2 Algorithmic Approaches to Closed-Loop Control of Glucose

The classical PID control algorithm modulates insulin delivery rate reactively by considering three functions of the error $e(t) = y(t) - r(t)$ between the actual (i.e., $y(t)$) and the reference (i.e., $r(t)$) subcutaneous glucose concentration at time t: (1) the first is directly proportional to the error (the proportional component, P), (2) the second is proportional to the integral of the error (the integral component, I), and (3) the third is proportional to the derivative of the error (the derivative component, D) [18,25-28]. The PID controller proposed by Steil et al. included a feedback of a model-predicted insulin profile, which allows the PID algorithm to reduce insulin delivery rate in response to rising plasma insulin levels [25,27]. The PID algorithm with insulin feedback is represented mathematically as follows:

$$P(t) = K_p e(t) \tag{9.1}$$

$$I(t) = I(t-1) + \frac{K_p}{T_1} e(t) \tag{9.2}$$

$$D(t) = K_p T_D \frac{dy(t)}{dt} \tag{9.3}$$

$$PID(t) = P(t) + I(t) + D(t) \tag{9.4}$$

$$\hat{I}_p(t) = K_0 u(t-1) + K_1 \hat{I}_p(t-1) - K_2 \hat{I}_p(t-2) \tag{9.5}$$

$$u(t) = (1 + \gamma)PID(t) - \gamma \hat{I}_p(t-1) \tag{9.6}$$

where $dy(t)/dt$ denotes the rate of change of $y(t)$, $\hat{I}_p(t)$ is the estimated plasma insulin concentration, and $u(t)$ is the manipulated insulin infusion rate. Tuning of model parameters was performed as follows: (1) the gain parameter $K_p = I_{DIR}/135$ was set proportional to subject's daily insulin requirements I_{DIR} (U/kg), (2) the integration time T_1 and the derivative time T_D were set to 450 and 90 min during the day (06:00-22:00h), whereas the corresponding values were reduced to $T_1 = 150$min and $T_D = 60$min during the night, and (3) the parameters of the pharmacokinetic model of insulin were set to $K_1 = 1.966308$, $K_2 = 0.966584$, $K_0 = 1 - K_1 + K_2$, and $\gamma = 0.5$. The I component and both $I_p(t-1)$ and $I_p(t-2)$ were initialized to the subject's overnight basal rate. Finally, a maximum value was specified for the integral component I:

$$I_{MAX} = \begin{cases} K_P(r - y_{RESET}), & y < y_{RESET} \\ 3I_b, & otherwise \end{cases} \tag{9.7}$$

where $y_{\text{RESET}} = 60$ mg/dL and I_b is the subject's 06:00h open-loop basal insulin infusion rate.

MPC, a more proactive and sensitive to patient's context approach compared with PID, may result in tighter glycemic control minimizing the risk of hypoglycemia, while increasing the efficacy of closed-loop control during the day by acceptably accommodating delays associated with CGM and CSII [7,29,30]. MPC is where mechanistic models of the glucose-insulin system or linear/nonlinear dynamical predictive regression models of subcutaneous glucose dynamics reside. The estimation of short-term glucose trajectory, on the basis of recent history of glucose concentration and current/future insulin infusion rate as well as more comprehensive inputs aggregating behavioral and physiological information, drives the computation of the optimal insulin infusion rate such that glucose concentration is maintained within the therapeutic range or/and a reference glucose level is achieved [31−35]. More specifically, MPC, at each time instance t, selects the sequence of control actions $u(t + k|t)$, $k = 1, \ldots, N$ minimizing an objective function of the deviations between the predicted subcutaneous glucose concentration trajectory $\hat{y}(t + k|t)$, $k = 1, \ldots, N$ and a reference glucose profile $r(t + k|t)$, $k = 1, \ldots, N$ over a finite horizon N, subject to maximum and minimum constraints on the manipulated input u (i.e., insulin infusion rate) [28]. Only the first control action of the optimal solution to the system is applied, which corresponds to the estimated insulin infusion rate. Similarly, zone MPC defines a target range for glucose concentration (e.g., 70−180 mg/dL) and costs only control actions yielding a diverging glucose trajectory [36-38].

The objective function of an exemplar of nonlinear MPC, which was proposed by Hovorka et al. [29], considers both the adherence of the predicted glucose $\hat{y}$ to the target trajectory r as well as the variation in the control sequence u over an N-step-ahead prediction horizon:

$$\underset{0 \le u(t+1),\ldots,u(t+N) \le 4}{\text{argmin}} \left\{ \sum_{i=1}^{N} \left[\hat{y}(t+i|t) - r(t+i) \right]^2 + \frac{1}{k_{\text{agr}}} \sum_{i=1}^{N} [u(t+i) - u(t+i-1)]^2 \right\} \tag{9.8}$$

The parameter k_{agr} determines the aggressiveness of the controller balancing the contribution of the two terms. Estimations of subcutaneous glucose concentration are obtained by a nonlinear physiological model of glucose and insulin kinetics, which adopts a recursive Bayesian optimization to address inter- as well as intrapatient variability of glycemic dynamics. Having set the target glucose concentration equal to 6 mmol/L, the target trajectory is linearly declining with a maximum decrease of 2 mmol/L/h when the current glucose measurement, $y(t)$, is above the target value; otherwise, a faster exponential normalization of glucose values is specified to prevent an impending hypoglycemia. Note that the insulin infusion rate was limited to $u(t) \le 4\ U/h$ due to technical limitations of insulin pumps.

The targeted breakthrough of MPC approaches consists in (1) efficient learning of the effect of insulin therapy and overall patient's context (e.g., meals, physical activities, stress) on subsequent glucose dynamics under normal daily life conditions and, (2) producing adaptive solutions that explain the intrapatient and interpatient variability (e.g., accounting for variable insulin sensitivity). In this context, personalized, adaptive, real-time, data-driven computational models of glucose are needed with a view to developing accurate robust solutions of glucose concentration, and in turn precise insulin delivery. Generalized predictive control belongs to adaptive control techniques, which adjust their parameters to the dynamic behavior of the glucose system [11,39,40]. For instance, a generalized predictive insulin controller accompanied with constrained weighted recursive least squares with a time-varying forgetting factor, which parameters related to the exogenous inputs (i.e., insulin on-board and physical activity) conform to physiological constraints, provided a stable 30-minute-ahead autoregressive moving average prediction model of glucose concentration in patients with type 1 diabetes and led to the prevention of postexercise hypoglycemia [40].

9.1.3 Clinical Evaluation of Current Paradigms of Closed-Loop Control of Glucose

The safety and efficacy of current paradigms of overnight closed-loop control of glucose concentration in type 1 diabetes has been well-demonstrated in numerous, mainly randomized controlled, clinical trials, with all studies consistently concluding that AP approaches, implemented by PID, MPC or fuzzy logic, can reduce nocturnal hypoglycemia and improve overall nocturnal glycemic control both in an inpatient and an outpatient setting. Today, research groups focus on multicenter, long-term, large-scale trials of the safety and efficacy of day and night closed-loop control for children, adolescents and adults under free-living conditions. There is now considerable evidence that 24 h closed-loop glucose control in outpatient setting results in an increase in the percentage of time in the target range which is accompanied by less hypoglycemic and hyperglycemic excursions as compared with sensor-augmented insulin pump therapy, with the nocturnal period being associated with better glycemic outcomes than the 24 h period [7,23,41−44]. The first step toward the adoption of AP systems in type 1 diabetes daily care was taken on September 28, 2016, when the first hybrid closed-loop system, namely the Medtronic's MiniMed 670G System, has been approved by the US Food and Drug Administration [18].

A recent systematic review and meta-analysis of randomized controlled trials comparing AP systems (insulin only or insulin plus glucagon) with conventional CSII therapy or SAP therapy in adults and children with type 1 diabetes confirmed: (1) a 12.59% higher time in target (3.9−10 or 3.9−8 mmol/L) with AP systems (95% CI 9.02−16.16; $P < 0.0001$), (2) a greater improvement in time in target range with dual-hormone AP systems compared with single-hormone systems (19.52% [95% CI 15.12−23.91] vs 11.06% [6.94 to 15.18]; $P = 0.006$), (3) a 2.45% lower time in hypoglycemia (<3.9 mmol/L) with AP systems (95% CI 1.11−3.79; $P < 0.0001$), which is equivalent to a relative risk reduction of 50%, with remote monitoring enhancing differences in reduction in hypoglycemia (-3.92 vs -0.63%; P value for subgroup differences $= 0.01$), and (4) whilst no significantly differences were observed, the predominance of MPC and fuzzy logic control algorithms vs PID ones with respect to time in target range, which is consistent with the findings of a trial directly comparing PID and MPC [23,45]. The main clinical outcomes of current research approaches to overnight and 24 h AP are presented in Tables 9.1 and 9.2, respectively.

Table 9.1 List of Studies on Overnight Closed-Loop Control of Glucose in Type 1 Diabetes

Study	Study Population (n)	Study Setting (Study Duration)	Closed-Loop Control Algorithm	Target Range	Time (%) in Hypoglycemia	Time (%) in Range	Time (%) in Hyperglycemia
Brown et al., 2015 [46]	Adults (n = 10) Age (years): 46.4 (8.5) HbA1c (%): 7.03 (1.05)	Two-center randomized crossover trial Supervised overnight closed-loop control in an outpatient setting vs sensor-augmented insulin pump therapy of the same duration at home. (5 nights)	Diabetes Assistant (DiAs) system Modular range control algorithm [22] Safety supervision module [47]	80–140 mg/dL	<70 mg/dL: 0.55 (0–0) vs 1.56 (0–0)	54.5 (36.5–74.7) vs 32.2 (7.8–54.7)	>180 mg/dL: 14.1 (0–28.4) vs 39.4 (0–69.8) >250 mg/dL: 0.9 (0–0) vs 10.1 (0–11.5)
Del Favero et al., 2015 [32]	Adults (n = 13) Age (years): 45 (14) HbA1c (%): 7.4 (0.9)	Nonrandomized outpatient 42-h experiment which included two evening meals and overnight periods Supervised closed-loop control during second dinner & night period vs sensor-augmented pump therapy during first dinner & night period	Diabetes Assistant (DiAs) system Modular range control algorithm [22,48] Safety supervision module [47]	3.9–10 mmol/L	<3.9 mmol/L: 1.96 (4.56) vs 12.76 (15.84)	83.56 (14.02) vs 62.43 (29.03)	>10 mmol/L: 14.48 (14.66) vs 24.81 (31.69)
Hovorka et al., 2014 [49]	Adolescents (n = 16) Age (years): 15.6 (2.1) HbA1c (%): 8.0 (0.9)	Open-label, randomized, crossover study Unsupervised overnight closed-loop insulin delivery vs sensor-augmented pump therapy in free-living conditions (3 weeks)	MPC (FlorenceD2A closed-loop system)Safety mechanisms: Maximum insulin infusion constraint; Insulin delivery suspension at sensor glucose at or less than 4.3 mmol/L, or when sensor glucose was rapidly decreasing	70–180 mg/dL	<70 mg/dL: 1.4 (0.4, 5.0) vs 0.9 (0.0, 9.7) <63 mg/dL: 0.4 (0.1, 1.9) vs 0.3 (0.0, 4.4) <54 mg/dL: 0.1 (0.0, 0.4) vs 0.0 (0.0, 1.1)	85 (68, 94) vs 69 (42, 87)	>144 mg/dL: 30.1 (15.6, 51.8) vs 42.6 (15.4, 81.8) >180 mg/dL: 9.5 (1.9, 27.8) vs 16.2 (2.2, 53.2) >300 mg/dL: 0.0 (0.0, 0.1) vs 0.0 (0.0, 0.9)
Kropff et al., 2015 [50]	Adults (n = 32) Age (years): 47.0 (11.2) HbA1c (%): 8.2 (0.6)	Multinational, randomized, crossover open-label study Supervised closed-loop control from dinner to waking up plus SAP during the day vs 24 h SAP only under free-living conditions (2 months)	Diabetes Assistant (DiAs) system Modular range control algorithm [22] Safety supervision module [47]	3.9–10.0 mmol/L	<3.9 mmol/L: 1.7 (0.8, 2.5) vs 3.0 (1.6, 4.9) <2.8 mmol/L: 0.1 (0.0, 0.2) vs 0.3 (0.1, 0.6)	4.4–7.8 mmol/L: 37.7% (9.1) vs 31.2% (6.0) 3.9–10 mmol/L: 66.7% (10.1) vs 58.1% (9.4)	>10 mmol/L: 31.6% (9.9) vs 38.5% (9.7)
Ly et al., 2014, [51]	Children and adolescents (n = 20)	Participants were randomized to either closed-loop control or sensor-augmented therapy for the first night and then crossed over every other night to the other therapy Overnight closed-loop control vs sensor-augmented therapy in a diabetes camp setting (5–6 days)	Diabetes Assistant (DiAs) system Modular range control algorithm [22] Safety supervision module [47]	70–150 mg/dL	—	73 (50, 89) vs 52 (24, 83)	—

Study	Population	Intervention	Target range	Intention-to-Treat Analysis
Ly et al., 2016 [52]	Adolescents and adults (n = 21) Age (years): 14.7 (3.9) HbA1c (%): 7.9 (1.4)	PID with insulin feedback Safety modules: Individualized constraint on the maximal insulin delivery rate Participants were randomized to either closed-loop control or sensor-augmented pump therapy for the first night and then crossed over on alternate nights to the other treatment arm over the course of the 5–6-day camp session Overnight supervised closed-loop control vs sensor-augmented pump therapy (5–6 days)	70–180 mg/dL	<70 mgdL⁻¹: 5.4 (30) vs. 19.5 (3.1) — 70–180 mgdL⁻¹: 79.9 (3.8) vs. 60.0 (4.0) — >150 mgdL⁻¹: 28.4 (4.7) vs. 30.2 (4.8) <60 mgdL⁻¹: 2.6 (2.4) vs. 11.2 (2.5) — 70–150 mgdL⁻¹: 66.4 (4.2) vs. 50.6 (4.3) — >180 mgdL⁻¹: 14.8 (3.8) vs. 20.6 (3.9) <50 mgdL⁻¹: 0.4 (1.5) vs. 5.6 (1.5) — >250 mgdL⁻¹: 1.7 (1.3) vs. 5.2 (1.3) <70 mg/dL: 0.1 (2.3) vs 11.0 (2.5) — 70–180 mg/dL: 88.1 (4.6) vs 60.5 (5.1) — >150 mg/dL: 24.5 (5.9) vs 41.20 (6.5) <60 mg/dL: −0.6 (1.2) vs 4.8 (1.4) — 70–150 mg/dL: 75.5 (5.4) vs. 47.6 (6.0) — >180 mg/dL: 12.4 (5.0) vs 28.9 (5.5) <50 mg/dL: 0.0 (0.2) vs 0.3 (0.2) — >250 mg/dL: 1.5 (1.8) vs 6.4 (2.0)
Nimri et al., 2014 [53]	Children, adolescents and adults (n = 24) Age (years): 21.2 (8.9) HbA1c (%):7.5 (0.8)	MD-Logic System—Fuzzy Logic Single-center, crossover, randomized trial Supervised overnight MD-Logic closed-loop control vs sensor-augmented pump therapy in real-life conditions (6 weeks)	70–140 mg/dL	*Intention-to-treat analysis (n = 19)* <70 mg/dL: 2.53 (1.33, 3.78) vs 5.16 (2.03, 7.32) — >240 mg/dL: 5.01 (2.63, 7.77) vs 8.82 (5.94, 19.23) <50 mg/dL: 2.53 (1.33, 3.78) vs 5.16 (2.03, 7.32) — 47.41 (35.13, 55.86) vs 36.36 (30.76, 40.90) *Per-protocol analysis (n = 18)* <70 mg/dL: 2.09 (0.90, 2.67) vs 4.72 (1.97, 7.43) — >240 mg/dL: 3.83 (2.52, 5.07) vs 8.71 (5.52, 18.07) <50 mg/dL: 0.07 (0.00, 0.34) vs 0.51 (0.11, 1.12) — 49.14 (36.48, 57.42) vs 36.21 (29.99, 41.30)

(Continued)

Table 9.1 (Continued)

Study	Study Population (n)	Study Setting (Study Duration)	Closed-Loop Control Algorithm	Target Range	Time (%) in Hypoglycemia	Time (%) in Range	Time (%) in Hyperglycemia
Phillip et al., 2013 [54]	Adolescents (n = 56) Age(years): 13.8 (1.8) HbA1c (%):8.0 (0.7)	Multicenter, multinational, randomized, crossover trial Supervised overnight closed-loop control vs sensor-augmented insulin pump therapy at a diabetes camp (2 consecutive overnight sessions)	MD-Logic System—Fuzzy Logic Safety modules: Real-time alarms of impending hypoglycemia and long-standing hyperglycemia	70–140 mg/dL	<70 mg/dL: 0 vs 10.4 (0 to 79.7)[a] <63 mg/dL: 0 vs 0 (0 to 42.5)[a]	4.4 (2.8 to 6.7) vs 2.8 (1.5 to 4.4)[b]	>140 mg/dL: 146.2 (58.4 to 231.1) vs 233.8 (13.4 to 327.5)[a] >180 mg/dL: 0 (0 to 65.4) vs 28.4 (0 to 177)[a] >250 mg/dL: 0 vs 0 (0 to 66.2)[a]
Sharifi et al., 2016 [55]	Adolescents (n = 12) Age(years): 15.2 (1.6) HbA1c (%):7.8 (0.5) Adults (n = 16) Age(years): 42.1 (9.6) HbA1c (%): 7.3 (0.6)	Open-label, prospective, randomized crossover study Supervised overnight hybrid closed-loop system vs sensor-augmented pump with low-glucose suspend function in an outpatient setting (4 nights)	PID with insulin feedback Meal Announcement	72–144 mg/dL	<72 mg/dL: 0.0 (0.0, 0.0) vs 1.8 (0.1, 7.9) <50 mg/dL: 0.0 (0.0, 0.0) vs 0.0 (0.0, 2.0) <72 mg/dL: 0.0 (0.0, 0.4) vs 0.8 (0.0, 3.9) <54 mg/dL: 0.0 (0.0, 0.0) vs 0.0 (0.0, 0.7)	61.7 (17.6) vs 64.9 (15.7) 57.7 (18.6) vs 44.5 (14.5)	> 144 mg/dL: 38.1 (17.6) vs 31.5 (16.7) > 144 mg/dL: 42.0 (18.7) vs 52.6 (16.5)
Stewart et al., 2016 [56]	Pregnant women (n = 16) Age (years): 34.1 (4.6) HbA1c (%):6.8 ± 0.6	Open-label, randomized, crossover study Supervised overnight closed-loop therapy vs sensor-augmented pump therapy (4 weeks)	MPC Meal announcement: Manually administered prandial insulin boluses	63–140 mg/dL	<63 mg/dL: 1.9 vs 1.3 <50 mg/dL: 0.6 vs 0.3	59.5 vs 74.7	>140 mg/dL: 38.6 vs 24.0 >180 mg/dL: 15.7 vs 7.4
Thabit et al., 2014, [57]	Adults (n = 24) Age (years): 43 (12) HbA1c (%): 8.1 (0.8)	Multicenter crossover study design Overnight closed loop vs insulin pump therapy in which participants used real-time display of continuous glucose monitoring independent of their pumps as control (4 weeks)	MPC (FlorenceD2A closed-loop system) Safety mechanisms: Maximum insulin infusion constraint; Insulin delivery suspension at sensor glucose at or less than 4.3 mmol/L, or when sensor glucose was rapidly decreasing	3.9–8.0 mmol/L	<3.9 mmol/L: 1.8 (0.6, 3.6) vs 2.1 (0.7, 3.9) <3.5 mmol/L: 0.7 (0.3, 1.4) vs 0.7 (0.3, 2.0) <2.8 mmol/L: 0.2 (0.0, 0.7) vs 0.2 (0.0, 1.3)	3.9–8.0 mmol/ L: 52.6 (10)· vs 39.1 (12.8) 3.9–10.0 mmol/ L: 73.2 (9.0) vs 61.2 (13.7)	>8.0 mmol/L: 44.3 (11.9) vs 57.1 (15.6) >16.7 mmol/L: 1.1 (0.0, 2.8) vs 1·5 (0.1, 3.4)

Values are mean (SD) and median (25th, 75th percentile).

[a]Median time at glucose level (25th, 75th percentile)—min.

[b]Median time within range (25th, 75th percentile)—h.

Table 9.2 List of Studies on Day and Night Closed-Loop Control of Glucose in Type 1 Diabetes

Study	Study Population (n)	Study Setting (Study Duration)	Closed-Loop Control Algorithm	Target Range	Time (%) in Hypoglycemia	Time (%) in Range	Time (%) in Hyperglycemia
Anderson et al., 2017 [58]	Adults (n = 30) Age (years): 44 (18–66) HbA1c (%): 7.3 (7.1, 7.7)	2-Weeks baseline sensor-augmented pump period followed by 2 weeks of overnight only closed-loop control and 2 weeks of 24 h closed-loop control at home Supervised 24 h closed-loop control vs sensor-augmented pump therapy Supervised overnight closed-loop control vs sensor-augmented pump therapy (2 weeks)	Diabetes Assistant (DiAs) system Modular range control algorithm [22] Safety supervision module [47] Meals announcement	70–180 mg/dL	24 h Closed-loop control <70 mg/dL: 1.7 (1.1, 2.7) vs 4.1 (2.0, 7.8) Overnight closed-loop control <70 mg/dL: 1.1 (0.2, 1.6) vs 3.0 (1.1, 6.3)	73 (68, 76) vs 65 (59, 69) 75 (69, 80) vs 61 (53, 73)	>180 mg/dL: 25 (22, 28) vs 32 (25, 36) >180 mg/dL: 24 (19, 28) vs 37 (24, 45)
Bally et al., 2017 [59]	Adults (n = 29) Age (years): 41 (13) HbA1c (%): 6.9 (0.5)	Open-label, randomized, crossover study Unsupervised 24 h hybrid closed-loop control vs usual pump therapy under free-living conditions (4 weeks)	MPC (FlorenceD2A closed-loop system) Safety mechanisms: maximum insulin infusion constraint; insulin delivery suspension at sensor glucose at or less than 4.3 mmol/L, or when sensor glucose was rapidly decreasing Manual administration of prandial insulin bolus	3.9–10.0 mmol/L	<3.9 mmol/L: 2.9 (2.3, 4.0) vs 5.3 (3.5, 10.0) <3.5 mmol/L: 1.3 (0.8, 2.3) vs 3.4 (1.9, 7.2) <2.8 mmol/L: 0.3 (0.1, 0.5) vs 1.0 (0.5, 2.6)	76.2 (6.4) vs 65.6 (8.1)	>10.0 mmol/L: 20.4 (6.3) vs 27.4 (9.6) >13.9 mmol/L: 3.8 (2.6) vs 6.9 (3.9) >16.7 mmol/L: 0.9 (0.8) vs 2.1 (1.8)
Bergenstal et al., 2016 [18]	Adults and adolescents (n = 124) Age (years): 37.8 (16.5) HbA1c (%): 7.4 (0.9)	Multicenter before and after study with a 2-week run-in period (baseline) 24 h hybrid closed-loop control in an outpatient setting vs open-loop control (3 months)	PID with insulin feedback [60] Meals announcement: Carbohydrate estimation	71–180 mg/dL	≤70 mg/dL: 3.3 (2.0) vs 5.9 (4.1) ≤50 mg/dL: 0.6 (0.6) vs 1.0 (1.1)	72.2 (8.8) vs 66.7 (12.2)	>180 mg/dL: 24.5 (9.2) vs 27.4 (13.7) >300 mg/dL: 1.7 (1.9) vs 2.3 (4.2)
de Bock et al., 2015 [61]	Adults (n = 4) Age (years): 30–40 Adolescents (n = 8) Age (years): 13–18 HbA1c (%): 7.5 (0.6)	Open-label randomized crossover trial Supervised outpatient feasibility study comparing 24 h Medtronic MiniMed hybrid closed-loop to sensor-augmented pump therapy with low-glucose suspend (5 days)	PID with insulin feedback Primary safety mechanism: Upper limit of allowable insulin delivery Meals announcement: Carbohydrate estimation and capillary blood glucose measurement	4.0–9.9 mmol/L	<3.3 mmol/L: 0.54 (0.6) vs 1.13 (1.5) 3.3–3.9 mmol/L: 1.15 (1.0) vs 1.98 (2.0)	4.0–9.9 mmol/L: 67.41 (9.8) vs 60.97 (16.4)	10.0–14.9 mmol/L: 26.44 (9.1) vs 30.17 (12.9) ≥15 mmol/L: 4.46 (3.1) vs 5.75 (6.2)
de Bock et al., 2017 [62]	Adults and adolescents (n = 8) Age (years): 18 (14–36) HbA1c (%): 7.9 (6.3–8.8)	In-clinic observational study 24 h Medtronic MiniMed hybrid closed-loop control challenged with hypoglycemic stimuli: exercise and an overreading glucose sensor [4 days (and 3 nights)]	PID with insulin feedback Primary safety mechanism: Upper limit of allowable insulin delivery Meals announcement: Carbohydrate estimation and capillary blood glucose measurement	72–144 mg/ dL72–180 mg/dL	<72 mg/dL: 1.5 (1.4)	72–144 mg/ dL: 50.9 (11.6) 72–180 mg/ dL: 75.2 (10.3)	180–270 mg/dL: 22.0 (10.5) >270 mg/dL: 1.3 (1.6)

(Continued)

Table 9.2 (Continued)

Study	Study Population (n)	Study Setting (Study Duration)	Closed-Loop Control Algorithm	Target Range	Time (%) in Hypoglycemia	Time (%) in Range	Time (%) in Hyperglycemia
Del Favero et al., 2016 [63]	Children (n = 30) Age (years): 7.6 (1.2) HbA1c (%): 7.3 (0.9)	Open-label, randomized, crossover trial in a supervised outpatient setting 24 h closed-loop control was compared with parent-managed sensor-augmented pump (3 days)	Modular MPC [22,48]	70–180 mg/dL	<70 mg/dL: 2.0 (1.2, 4.5) vs 6.7 (2.3, 11.5) <50 mg/dL: 0.1 (0.0, 0.4) vs 0.9 (0.0, 2.2)	70–180 mg/dL: 56.8 (13.5) vs 63.1 (11.0)	—
Garg et al., 2017 [64]	Adolescents (n = 30) Age (years): 16.5 (2.29) HbA1c (%): 7.7 (0.84)	Multicenter pivotal trial with a 2 week run-in phase 24 h outpatient Medtronic MiniMed hybrid closed-loop control vs sensor-augmented pump therapy (3 months)	PID with insulin feedback	71–180 mg/dL	≤70 mg/dL: 2.8 (1.3) vs 4.3 (2.9) ≤50 mg/dL: 0.5 (0.5) vs 0.7 (0.6)	67.2 (8.2) vs 60.4 (10.9)	>180 mg/dL: 30.0 (8.0) vs 35.3 (11.4) >300 mg/dL: 2.8 (2.0) vs 3.8 (4.3)
	Adults (n = 94) Age (years): 44.6 (12.79) HbA1c (%): 7.3 (0.91)				≤70 mg/dL: 3.4 (2.1) vs 6.4 (4.3) ≤50 mg/dL: 0.6 (0.6) vs 1.1 (1.2)	73.8 (8.4) vs 68.8 (11.9)	>180 mg/dL: 22.8 (8.9) vs 24.9 (13.5) >300 mg/dL: 1.3 (1.7) vs 1.8 (4.1)
Kovatchev et al., 2014 [65]	Adults Age (years): 46 (10) HbA1c (%): 7.4 (0.7)	Nonblinded, randomized crossover design Closed-loop control vs open-loop sensor-augmented insulin pump therapy in a supervised outpatient setting	**Diabetes Assistant (DiAs) system** Modular range control algorithm [22] Safety supervision module [47] Meals announcement	70–180 mg/dL	<70 mg/dL: 0.70 vs 1.25	66.1 vs 70.7	>180 mg/dL: 33.1 vs 28.0
Kovatchev et al., 2017 [66]	Adults (14) Age (years): 45 (34, 51) HbA1c (%): 7.2 (0.6)	5-month trial with a 1-month run-in phase (Semi)Supervised 24/7 closed-loop control vs sensor-augmented pump therapy during free-living conditions (5 months)	**Diabetes Assistant (DiAs) system** Modular range control algorithm [22] Safety supervision module [47] Meals announcement	3.9–10.0 mmol/L	<3.9 mmol/L: 1.3 (0.6, 1.7) vs 4.1 (2.9, 7.5) <3.3 mmol/L: 0.3 (0.2, 0.6) vs 2.2 (1.5, 3.4) <2.8 mmol/L: 0.1 (0.0, 0.2) vs 1.0 (0.8, 1.3)	77 (73–81) vs 66 (59–69)	>10 mmol/L: 22 (19, 27) vs 31 (23, 38) >13.9 mmol/L: 3 (2, 6) vs 6 (3, 11) >16.7 mmol/L: 0 (0, 1) vs 2 (0, 3)
Leelarathna et al., 2014 [67]	Adults (n = 17) Age (years): 34 (9) HbA1c (%): 7.6 (0.8)	Open-label prospective multinational three-center randomized crossover design Unsupervised day and night closed-loop control vs sensor-augmented insulin pump therapy under free-living conditions (7 days)	MPC (FlorenceD2A closed-loop system) Safety mechanisms: Maximum insulin infusion constraint; Insulin delivery suspension at sensor glucose at or less than 4.3 mmol/L, or when sensor glucose was rapidly decreasing Meals announcement: Carbohydrate estimation and meal bolus calculation for meals >30 g carbohydrates	3.9–10.0 mmol/L	<3.9 mmol/L: 3.7 (2.2, 7.9) vs 5.0 (2.3, 8.5) <2.8 mmol/L: 0.3 (0.2, 1.1) vs 0.6 (0.2, 1.6)	3.9–10.0 mmol/L: 74.5 (61.1, 78.9) vs 61.8 (53.3, 70.1) 3.9–8.0 mmol/L: 54.9 (42.2, 58.3) vs 43.3 (33.0, 49.1)	>10.0 mmol/L: 21.9 (16.7, 32.3) vs 30.5 (24.3, 41.4) >16.7 mmol/L: 1.5 (0.5, 3.5) vs 3.3 (1.4, 5.0)

Study	Population	Study design	Control algorithm / mechanisms	Target range	Glucose metrics
Ly et al., 2015 [26]	Adolescents and adults (n = 21) Age (years): 18.6 (3.7) HbA1c (%): 8.6 (1.5)	Randomized, stratified by HbA1c, study design Day and night supervised Medtronic MiniMed hybrid closed-loop control vs a sensor-augmented pump therapy with insulin suspension (Medtronic MiniMed 530G) in a diabetes camp setting (6 days)	PID with insulin feedback and safety constraints Meal announcement: Carbohydrate estimation; Premeal insulin bolus calculation Safety mechanisms: Adaptive, individualized constraint on the maximal insulin delivery rate	70–180 mg/dL	<70 mg/dL: 2.1 (0.4) vs 2.4 (0.6) <60 mg/dL: 0.5 (0.3) vs 0.7 (0.4) <50 mg/dL: 0.1 (0.1) vs 0.1 (0.1) 70–180 mg/dL: 69.9 (3.3) vs 73.1 (5.0) 70–150 mg/dL: 51.8 (4.1) vs 58.0 (6.2) >180 mg/dL: 28.4 (3.5) vs 24.8 (5.2) >250 mg/dL: 8.2 (1.9) vs 6.3 (2.8)
Renard et al., 2016 [35]	Adults (n = 20) Age (years): 46.3 (11.0) HbA1c (%): 8.2 (0.7)	1-Month single-arm nonrandomized extension study of a multinational initially randomized crossover open-label study in patients with type 1 diabetes investigating evening-and-night use of an AP at home vs patient-managed SAP therapy [50] Day and night supervised closed-loop control (nonrandomized) under free-living conditions vs evening-and-night use of an AP at home vs patient-managed SAP therapy (1 month)	Diabetes assistant (DiAs) system Modular range control algorithm [22] Safety supervision module [47] Meals announcement	3.9–10 mmol/L	*Intention-to-treat analysis* <3.9 mmol/L: 1.9 (1.1) vs 2.1 (1.3) vs 3.2 (1.8) <2.8 mmol/L: 0.2 (0.1, 0.3) vs 0.1 (0.0, 0.3) vs 0.3 (0.1, 0.5) 70–180 mg/dL: 64.7 (7.6) vs 63.6 (9.9) vs 59.7 (9.6) >10 mmol/L: 33.3 (7.3) vs 34.2 (10.0) vs 37.0 (10.2)
Russell et al., 2014 [33]	Adolescents (n = 32) Age (years): 16 (3) HbA1c (%): 8.2 (1.0) Adults (n = 20) Age (years): 40 (16) HbA1c (%): 7.1 (0.8)	Random-order, crossover design Supervised 24 h bihormonal "bionic" pancreas vs insulin pump therapy under unrestricted outpatient conditions (5 days)	MPC Meal announcement	70–180 mg/dL	<70 mg/dL: 3.1 (2.7) vs 4.9 (5.1) <60 mg/dL: 1.3 (1.7) vs 2.2 (3.6) 70–180 mg/dL: 75.9 (7.9) vs 64.5 (14.1) 70–120 mg/dL: 42.0 (7.7) vs 30.0 (11.8) <70 mg/dL: 4.1 (3.5) vs 7.3 (4.7) <60 mg/dL: 1.5 (1.7) vs 3.7 (3.3) 70–180 mg/dL: 79.5 (8.3) vs 58.8 (14.6) 70–120 mg/dL: 47.7 (10.5) vs 30.8 (15.7) >180 mg/dL: 21.0 (7.0) vs 30.6 (15.4) >250 mg/dL: 5.9 (4.1) vs 10.8 (9.1) >180 mg/dL: 16.5 (7.9) vs 33.8 (16.4) >250 mg/dL: 4.9 (3.7) vs 12.3 (9.9)
Russell et al., 2016 [68]	Preadolescents (n = 19) Age (years): 9.8 (1.6) HbA1c (%): 7.8 (0.8)	Randomized, open-label, crossover study Supervised 24 h bihormonal "bionic" pancreas vs insulin pump therapy under unrestricted outpatient conditions (5 days)	MPC Meal announcement	3.9–10.0 mmol/L	<3.3 mmol/L: 1.2 (1.1) vs 2.8 (1.2) 80.6 (7.4) vs 57.6 (14.0) >10 mmol/L: 16.5 (6.4) vs 36.3 (15.7)
Stewart et al., 2016 [56]	Pregnant women (n = 16) Age (years): 34.1 (4.6) HbA1c (%): 6.8 (0.6)	Open-label, randomized, crossover study Supervised day and night closed-loop therapy vs sensor-augmented pump therapy (4 weeks)	MPC	63–140 mg/dL	<63 mg/dL: 1.9 vs 1.8 <50 mg/dL: 0.4 vs 0.3 66.3 vs 56.8 >140 mg/dL: 31.6 vs 40.9 >180 mg/dL: 12.6 vs 17.3

(Continued)

Table 9.2 (Continued)

Study	Study Population (n)	Study Setting (Study Duration)	Closed-Loop Control Algorithm	Target Range	Time (%) in Hypoglycemia	Time (%) in Range	Time (%) in Hyperglycemia
Tauschmann et al., 2016 [69]	Adolescents (n = 12) Age (years): 15.4 (2.6) HbA1c (%): 8.3 (0.9)	Open-label, randomized, free-living, crossover study design Day-and-night hybrid closed-loop insulin delivery under free-living conditions without remote monitoring or supervision (7 days)	MPC (FlorenceD2A closed-loop system) Safety mechanisms: maximum insulin infusion constraint; insulin delivery suspension at sensor glucose at or less than 4.3 mmol/L, or when sensor glucose was rapidly decreasing Meals announcement: Carbohydrate estimation and meal bolus calculation for meals >30 g carbohydrates	3.9–10.0 mmol/L	<3.9 mmol/L: 2.9 (1.8, 4.8) vs 1.7 (0.9, 5.1) <2.8 mmol/L: 0.2 (0.0, 0.6) vs 0.1 (0.0, 0.6)	72 (59, 77) vs 53 (46, 59)	>10.0 mmol/L: 26 (21,35) vs 43 (38, 52)
Tauschmann et al., 2016 [70]	Adolescents (n = 12) Age (years): 14.6 (3.1) HbA1c (%): 8.5 (0.7)	Open-label, randomized, two-period crossover design Day-and-night hybrid closed-loop insulin delivery vs sensor-augmented insulin pump therapy under free-living conditions without remote monitoring or supervision (21 days)	MPC (FlorenceD2A closed-loop system) Safety mechanisms: maximum insulin infusion constraint; insulin delivery suspension at sensor glucose at or less than 4.3 mmol/L, or when sensor glucose was rapidly decreasing Meals announcement: carbohydrate estimation and meal bolus calculation for meals >30 g carbohydrates	3.9–10.0 mmol/L	<3.9 mmol/L: 4.3 (1.4, 5.2) vs 2.4 (0.3, 5.7) <2.8 mmol/L: 0.3 (0.0, 0.5) vs 0.1 (0.0, 0.7)	66.6 (7.9) vs 47.7 (14.4)	>10.0 mmol/L: 29.7 (9.2) vs 49.1 (16.5) >16.7 mmol/L: 5.1 (0.8, 5.6) vs 8.0 (1.9, 17.4)
Thabit et al., 2015 [34]	Adults (n = 33) Age (years): 40.0 (9.4) HbA1c (%): 8.5 (0.7) Children and adolescents (n = 25) Age (years): 12.0 (3.4) HbA1c (%): 8.1 (0.9)	Two multicenter, crossover, randomized, controlled studies Closed-loop insulin delivery vs sensor-augmented pump therapy under free-living home conditions. The closed-loop system was used day and night by adults and overnight by children and adolescents (12 weeks)	MPC treat-to-target algorithm Meal announcement: Carbohydrate estimation and fingerstick capillary glucose measurements	70–180 mg/dL 70–145 mg/dL	<70 mg/dL: 2.9 (1.4,4.5) vs 3.0 (1.8,6.1) <50 mg/dL: 0.3 (0.1,0.7) vs 0.4 (0.1,0.9) <70 mg/dL: 2.4 (1.1,3.7) vs 4.0 (1.8,5.8) <50 mg/dL: 0.3 (0.1,0.6) vs 0.4 (0.2,1.2)	67.7 (10.6) vs 56.8 (14.2) 59.1 (9.5) vs 39.4 (13.3)	> 180 mg/dL: 29.2 (11.4) vs 38.9 (16.6) > 145 mg/dL: 38.0 (9.4) vs 55.6 (15.8)

Values are mean (SD) and median (25th, 75th percentile).

9.2 Mobile Cognitive Systems in Diabetes

The ever-increasing computational power of smartphones, the rise of mobile health devices and the improved wireless communication technologies have contributed altogether to the development of remarkable mobile tools for diabetes self-management [71]. Contemporary paradigms offer precise self-monitoring and indirect decision-support through effective tools for data tracking and data visualization. The findings of mobile diabetes interventions suggest that well-designed mobile tools with decision-support features have the potential to enhance self-management outcomes. mHealth solutions to the self-management of type 1 diabetes shall support the individualization of daily care of diabetes by providing patients with data-driven personalized feedback, being continuously adapted to their lifestyle and daily activities. In this direction, IBM and Medtronic developed the Sugar. IQ with Watson Cognitive App which is able to detect important patterns and trends in diabetes data and offer real-time and personalized guidance to people with diabetes.

The application of advanced predictive data analytics can lead to more efficient treatment recommendations grounded entirely on the knowledge present in the data. First, real-time acquisition and access to biological (e.g., blood glucose, interstitial glucose), physiological (e.g., heart rate, energy expenditure, galvanic skin response), and behavioral self-monitoring data (e.g., lifestyle, diet), making use of wearable wireless biosensors and physiological sensors, can provide an accurate picture of an individual's physical and emotional context. On this basis, adaptive machine-learning and dynamic data-mining techniques should be employed aiming at learning the short-term effect of therapy and overall patient's context (e.g., meals, physical activity, stress) on glucose concentration, and identifying established patterns in self-monitoring long-term data trajectories. More specifically, sequential (or recursive) learning algorithms with the inherent ability to represent the time-varying behavior of the underlying system will allow for a better representation of spatial and temporal input−output dependencies.

As is the case with AP systems, mobile cognitive systems in type 1 diabetes shall employ a modular architectural approach allowing the hierarchical integration of diverse components starting from functionalities supporting daily disease self-monitoring (e.g., visualization of patient's context) to functionalities assuring patient's safety in real-time (e.g., hypo- or hyperglycemia predictive alerts). Anticipatory mobile computing provides an ideal basis for identifying the modules of a mobile diabetes application [72]. Anticipatory mobile computing exploits mobile sensing and machine learning for intelligent reasoning based on past, present and anticipated context, aiming to devise sensible actionable decisions able to affect the future state of the end-user. Context sensing, context modeling and prediction and intelligent actionable feedback are the core components of the mobile anticipatory approach (Fig. 9.2).

9.2.1 Context Sensing

The advances in sensing, wearable and mobile computing technologies have enabled the monitoring of personal health- and lifestyle-related information on a more ubiquitous level.

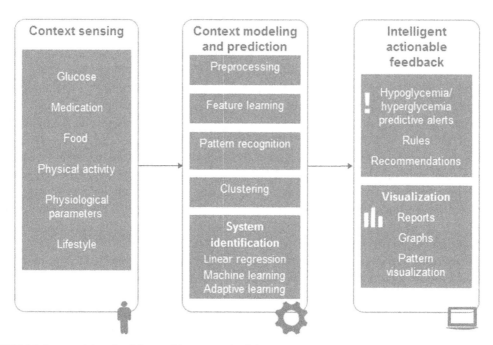

FIGURE 9.2 Core modules of mobile cognitive systems in diabetes.

Table 9.3   Types and Sources of Diabetes Data

Type	Parameter(s)	Measurement Method
Biological data	Glucose concentration	CGM system, blood glucose meter
Physiological data	Heart rate, heart rate variability (HRV), and other cardiovascular features	Wristband (Photoplethysmography sensor, PPG)
	Galvanic skin response (GSR)	Wristband (GSR sensor)
Emotional data	Stress	Wristband (PPG sensor, GSR sensor)
	Sympathetic nervous system activity	Wristband (GSR sensor)
	Excitement	Wristband (GSR sensor)
Behavioral data	Physical activity	Wristband (Accelerometer)
	Sleeping patterns	Wristband (Accelerometer)
	Nutritional habits	Specially designed electronic diary

Context monitoring consists in the collection of health, behavioral, and physiological data linked to daily diabetes management (Table 9.3). Advanced unobtrusive sensor technology and connected objects allow large collection of data from the user's everyday environment in a seamless and pervasive manner. Besides CGM, noninvasive IoT sensors can be used to acquire multiparametric behavioral and physiological data (e.g., physical activities, sleeping patterns, heart rate). A number of simple and more advanced examples of mHealth applications for type 1 diabetes have included leading health (e.g., glucometers, blood pressure monitors) and lifestyle tracking devices (e.g., wireless smart activity and sleep trackers) into their monitoring system. Self-monitoring of health-related behaviors and emotions (e.g., food intake, stress) constitutes a most challenging issue, with relative information being commonly entered manually through different levels of abstractions. Nevertheless, unobtrusive precise sensing methods are critical to the realization of pervasive information acquisition in m-health systems and long-term user engagement, especially in the care of chronic diseases.

9.2.2 Context Modeling and Prediction

Multimodal dynamic traces of patient's context enable prediction of short-term glycemic dynamics by contemporary adaptive data-driven techniques. Modality and feature selection as well as unsupervised/supervised machine-learning methods and mechanistic diabetes models can be effectively combined to construct multiscale models of an individual's glycemic state.

First, context modeling aims at inferring high-level concepts, describing the psychosocial and physical health as well as behavioral context of people with type 1 diabetes, based on sensed data. Quantizing the data space such that principles of competitive learning can be applied as well as defining and learning the most informative modes of the input signals constitute critical procedures. Sequential personal data may be explored for similarities (static data analysis). In particular, unsupervised learning (i.e., clustering) may identify groups of data with similar characteristics, in accordance with the defined feature space. In addition, cooccurrence and dynamic relationships into sequential longitudinal health and lifestyle data may be treated in the context of dynamic pattern and process mining. Toward the development of a novel adaptive framework to the dynamic identification of the glucose system, the defined feature space can be searched for interesting regularities or temporal relationships in observed data either for one individual or for groups of individuals.

Second, online machine-learning techniques in tandem with nonlinear system identification and prediction enable the short-term prediction of subcutaneous glucose concentration. In addition, physiological models aiming at assessing the kinetics of exogenous materials (i.e., subcutaneously administered insulin, glucose ingestion) in the glucose-insulin system, ranging from pure compartmental models to more complex mechanistic models can be exploited. On the basis of a well-defined set of individual features, the potential of time series and nonparametric machine-learning algorithms to: (1) identify and predict the short-term metabolic dynamics and (2) generalize adequately in nonstationary conditions, need to be investigated. Parameterized models from linear systems theory can be investigated by assuming that the examined system is linear and time-invariant. Nonlinearity can be addressed in the context of adaptive machine-learning algorithms. In addition, both univariate and multivariate input models can be investigated aiming at capturing the implicit or explicit effect of an individual's contextual information on its metabolic status. The synergy, at the input level, of physiological models and data-driven glucose predictive models should be thoroughly investigated. In particular, physiological models describing the absorption kinetics of different subcutaneously administered insulin formulations and the time course of the rate of appearance of ingested glucose into plasma, postulated as systems of ordinary or partial differential equations or systems of integral equations, can be used.

On top of these, feature evaluation algorithms, ranging from pure statistical to data-driven approaches and considering the nature of the data to be analyzed (e.g., stationarity, stochasticity), can be examined in order to assess the discriminative or predictive capacity of the feature space with respect to glucose prediction. Special emphasis should be given to context sensitive algorithms able to capture linear or nonlinear relationships between input and output signals, without relying upon strict assumptions, and specially designed for multivariate time series data. Moreover, a comprehensive preprocessing procedure has to be applied in order to assure a high-quality adequately synchronized dataset with data heterogeneities being abstracted.

Well-established approaches to the estimation of the generalization error of the prediction model, balancing the bias and the variance, are required. The expected generalization performance of the computational model is typically evaluated on observed input−output data using well-established statistical measures and approaches estimating the accuracy of forecast methods. The evaluation of the model in the hypoglycemic range has to be performed in both a sample- and an event-based mode, aiming at assessing whether an impeding event is truly preventable. In adaptive learning, the convergence behavior of the learning algorithm should be evaluated together with the time and space complexity, aiming at a real-time predictive model.

9.2.3 Intelligent Actionable Feedback

Anticipatory decision logic based on action-reward learning (e.g., reinforcement learning, latent learning) reinforces actions maximizing the reward from the environment (action value) and, in parallel, leading to favorable outcomes (action effect). To this end, predictive models of the effect of an action on the short- and long-term glucose dynamics, that is the expectation of a future state, can be developed in order to produce customizable recommendations that explain the intrapatient and interpatient variability.

9.2.4 Human−Machine Interaction

Human−machine interaction, closing the loop between actionable feedback and context sensing, should be built upon tangible as well as attentive user interface principles. Through the intuitive and efficient visualization of sensed quantities and estimated statistics and the automatic identification of trends over time, individuals will be better informed on their condition, which, in turn, can increase their self-efficacy and trigger decision making. An assortment of effective visualization tools, designed to facilitate the review of the overall, current or historical, health (e.g., blood pressure, weight) and lifestyle patterns (e.g., carbohydrate intake, calories burned, distance traveled), can be provided. In addition, the ability to sense and predict the context of the people with type 1 diabetes can serve as a basis for interaction adaptation and seamless integration with their daily routine resulting in a more responsive user behavior.

References

[1] Cryer PE. The barrier of hypoglycemia in diabetes. Diabetes 2008;57(12):3169−76.

[2] American Diabetes, A. Diagnosis and classification of diabetes mellitus. Diabetes Care 2014;37(Suppl 1): S81−90.

[3] Norgaard K, et al. Routine sensor-augmented pump therapy in type 1 diabetes: the INTERPRET study. Diabetes Technol Ther 2013;15(4):273−80.

[4] Bergenstal RM, et al. Effectiveness of sensor-augmented insulin-pump therapy in type 1 diabetes. N Engl J Med 2010;363(4):311−20.

[5] Rodbard D. Continuous glucose monitoring: a review of successes, challenges, and opportunities. Diabetes Technol Ther 2016;18(Suppl 2):S3−13.

[6] Facchinetti A. Continuous glucose monitoring sensors: past, present and future algorithmic challenges. Sensors (Basel) 2016;16(12).

[7] Thabit H, Hovorka R. Coming of age: the artificial pancreas for type 1 diabetes. Diabetologia 2016;59 (9):1795−805.

[8] Kropff J, DeVries JH. Continuous glucose monitoring, future products, and update on worldwide artificial pancreas projects. Diabetes Technol Ther 2016;18(Suppl 2):S253−63.

[9] Bequette BW. Hypoglycemia prevention using low glucose suspend systems. In: Marmarelis V, Mitsis G, editors. Data-driven modeling for diabetes: diagnosis and treatment. Berlin, Heidelberg: Springer Berlin Heidelberg; 2014. p. 73−89.

[10] Howsmon D, Bequette BW. Hypo- and hyperglycemic alarms: devices and algorithms. J Diabetes Sci Technol 2015;9(5):1126−37.

[11] Turksoy K, et al. Multivariable adaptive closed-loop control of an artificial pancreas without meal and activity announcement. Diabetes Technol Ther 2013;15(5):386−400.

[12] Turksoy K, et al. Real-time insulin bolusing for unannounced meals with artificial pancreas. Control Eng Pract 2017;59:159−64.

[13] Doyle 3rd FJ, et al. Closed-loop artificial pancreas systems: engineering the algorithms. Diabetes Care 2014;37(5):1191−7.

[14] Zarkogianni K, et al. A review of emerging technologies for the management of diabetes mellitus. IEEE Trans Biomed Eng 2015;62(12):2735−49.

[15] Anthimopoulos M, et al. Computer vision-based carbohydrate estimation for type 1 patients with diabetes using smartphones. J Diabetes Sci Technol 2015;9(3):507−15.

[16] Bally L, et al. Carbohydrate estimation supported by the GoCARB system in individuals with type 1 diabetes: a randomized prospective pilot study. Diabetes Care 2017;40(2):e6−7.

[17] Herrero P, et al. A bio-inspired glucose controller based on pancreatic beta-cell physiology. J Diabetes Sci Technol 2012;6(3):606−16.

[18] Bergenstal RM, et al. Safety of a hybrid closed-loop insulin delivery system in patients with type 1 diabetes. JAMA 2016;316(13):1407−8.

[19] Breton M, et al. Fully integrated artificial pancreas in type 1 diabetes: modular closed-loop glucose control maintains near normoglycemia. Diabetes 2012;61(9):2230−7.

[20] Patek SD, et al. Modular closed-loop control of diabetes. IEEE Trans Biomed Eng 2012;59(11):2986−99.

[21] Weisman A, et al. Effect of artificial pancreas systems on glycaemic control in patients with type 1 diabetes: a systematic review and meta-analysis of outpatient randomised controlled trials. Lancet Diabetes Endocrinol 2017;5(7):501−12.

[22] El-Khatib FH, et al. Home use of a bihormonal bionic pancreas versus insulin pump therapy in adults with type 1 diabetes: a multicentre randomised crossover trial. Lancet 2017;389(10067):369−80.

[23] Steil GM, et al. Feasibility of automating insulin delivery for the treatment of type 1 diabetes. Diabetes 2006;55(12):3344−50.

[24] Ly TT, et al. Day and night closed-loop control using the integrated Medtronic hybrid closed-loop system in type 1 diabetes at diabetes camp. Diabetes Care 2015.

[25] Steil GM, et al. The effect of insulin feedback on closed loop glucose control. J Clin Endocrinol Metab 2011;96(5):1402−8.

[26] Bequette BW. A critical assessment of algorithms and challenges in the development of a closed-loop artificial pancreas. Diabetes Technol Ther 2005;7(1):28−47.

[27] Hovorka R, et al. Nonlinear model predictive control of glucose concentration in subjects with type 1 diabetes. Physiol Meas 2004;25(4):905−20.

[28] Hovorka R. Closed-loop insulin delivery: from bench to clinical practice. Nat Rev Endocrinol 2011;7 (7):385−95.

[29] Dassau E, et al. Adjustment of open-loop settings to improve closed-loop results in type 1 diabetes: a multicenter randomized trial. J Clin Endocrinol Metab 2015;100(10):3878−86.

[30] Del Favero S, et al. Multicenter outpatient dinner/overnight reduction of hypoglycemia and increased time of glucose in target with a wearable artificial pancreas using modular model predictive control in adults with type 1 diabetes. Diabetes Obes Metab 2015;17(5):468−76.

[31] Russell SJ, et al. Outpatient glycemic control with a bionic pancreas in type 1 diabetes. N Engl J Med 2014;371(4):313−25.

[32] Thabit H, et al. Home use of an artificial beta cell in type 1 diabetes. N Engl J Med 2015;373 (22):2129−40.

[33] Renard E, et al. Day-and-night closed-loop glucose control in patients with type 1 diabetes under free-living conditions: results of a single-arm 1-month experience compared with a previously reported feasibility study of evening and night at home. Diabetes Care 2016;39(7):1151−60.

[34] Grosman B, et al. Zone model predictive control: a strategy to minimize hyper- and hypoglycemic events. J Diabetes Sci Technol 2010;4(4):961−75.

[35] Forlenza GP, et al. Application of zone model predictive control artificial pancreas during extended use of infusion set and sensor: a randomized crossover-controlled home-use trial. Diabetes Care 2017.

[36] Huyett LM, et al. Outpatient closed-loop control with unannounced moderate exercise in adolescents using zone model predictive control. Diabetes Technol Ther 2017;19(6):331−9.

[37] Turksoy K, Cinar A. Adaptive control of artificial pancreas systems − a review. J Healthc Eng 2014;5 (1):1−22.

[38] Turksoy K, et al. Multivariable adaptive identification and control for artificial pancreas systems. IEEE Trans Biomed Eng 2014;61(3):883−91.

[39] Nimri R, et al. Closing the loop. Diabetes Technol Ther 2017;19(S1):S27−41.

[40] Rodbard D. Continuous glucose monitoring: a review of recent studies demonstrating improved glycemic outcomes. Diabetes Technol Ther 2017;19(S3):S25−37.

[41] Bally L, Thabit H, Hovorka R. Closed-loop for type 1 diabetes—an introduction and appraisal for the generalist. BMC Med 2017;15:14.

[42] Christiansen SC, et al. A review of the current challenges associated with the development of an artificial pancreas by a double subcutaneous approach. Diabetes Ther 2017;8(3):489−506.

[43] Pinsker JE, et al. Randomized crossover comparison of personalized MPC and PID control algorithms for the artificial pancreas. Diabetes Care 2016;39(7):1135−42.

[44] Brown SA, et al. Multinight "bedside" closed-loop control for patients with type 1 diabetes. Diabetes Technol Ther 2015;17(3):203−9.

[45] Hughes CS, et al. Hypoglycemia prevention via pump attenuation and red-yellow-green "traffic" lights using continuous glucose monitoring and insulin pump data. J Diabetes Sci Technol 2010;4 (5):1146−55.

[46] Toffanin C, et al. Artificial pancreas: model predictive control design from clinical experience. J Diabetes Sci Technol 2013;7(6):1470−83.

[47] Thabit H, et al. Home use of closed-loop insulin delivery for overnight glucose control in adults with type 1 diabetes: a 4-week, multicentre, randomised crossover study. Lancet Diabetes Endocrinol 2014;2 (9):701−9.

[48] Kropff J, et al. 2 Month evening and night closed-loop glucose control in patients with type 1 diabetes under free-living conditions: a randomised crossover trial. Lancet Diabetes Endocrinol 2015;3 (12):939−47.

[49] Ly TT, et al. Overnight glucose control with an automated, unified safety system in children and adolescents with type 1 diabetes at diabetes camp. Diabetes Care 2014;37(8):2310−16.

[50] Ly TT, et al. Automated overnight closed-loop control using a proportional-integral-derivative algorithm with insulin feedback in children and adolescents with type 1 diabetes at diabetes camp. Diabetes Technol Ther 2016;18(6):377−84.

[51] Nimri R, et al. MD-logic overnight control for 6 weeks of home use in patients with type 1 diabetes: randomized crossover trial. Diabetes Care 2014;37(11):3025−32.

[52] Phillip M, et al. Nocturnal glucose control with an artificial pancreas at a diabetes camp. N Engl J Med 2013;368(9):824−33.

[53] Sharifi A, et al. Glycemia, treatment satisfaction, cognition, and sleep quality in adults and adolescents with type 1 diabetes when using a closed-loop system overnight versus sensor-augmented pump with low-glucose suspend function: a randomized crossover study. Diabetes Technol Ther 2016;18 (12):772−83.

[54] Stewart ZA, et al. Closed-loop insulin delivery during pregnancy in women with type 1 diabetes. N Engl J Med 2016;375(7):644−54.

[55] Anderson SM, et al. Multinational home use of closed-loop control is safe and effective. Diabetes Care 2016;39(7):1143−50.

[56] Bally L, et al. Day-and-night glycaemic control with closed-loop insulin delivery versus conventional insulin pump therapy in free-living adults with well controlled type 1 diabetes: an open-label, randomised, crossover study. Lancet Diabetes Endocrinol 2017;5(4):261−70.

[57] Grosman B, et al. Hybrid closed-loop insulin delivery in type 1 diabetes during supervised outpatient conditions. J Diabetes Sci Technol 2016;10(3):708−13.

[58] de Bock MI, et al. Feasibility of outpatient 24-hour closed-loop insulin delivery. Diabetes Care 2015;38 (11):e186−7.

[59] de Bock M, et al. Exploration of the performance of a hybrid closed loop insulin delivery algorithm that includes insulin delivery limits designed to protect against hypoglycemia. J Diabetes Sci Technol 2017;11 (1):68−73.

[60] Del Favero S, et al. Randomized summer camp crossover trial in 5- to 9-year-old children: outpatient wearable artificial pancreas is feasible and safe. Diabetes Care 2016;39(7):1180−5.

[61] Garg SK, et al. Glucose outcomes with the in-home use of a hybrid closed-loop insulin delivery system in adolescents and adults with type 1 diabetes. Diabetes Technol Ther 2017;19(3):155−63.

[62] Kovatchev BP, et al. Safety of outpatient closed-loop control: first randomized crossover trials of a wearable artificial pancreas. Diabetes Care 2014;37(7):1789−96.

[63] Kovatchev B, et al. Feasibility of long-term closed-loop control: a multicenter 6-month trial of 24/7 automated insulin delivery. Diabetes Technol Ther 2017;19(1):18–24.

[64] Leelarathna L, et al. Day and night home closed-loop insulin delivery in adults with type 1 diabetes: three-center randomized crossover study. Diabetes Care 2014;37(7):1931–7.

[65] Russell SJ, et al. Day and night glycaemic control with a bionic pancreas versus conventional insulin pump therapy in preadolescent children with type 1 diabetes: a randomised crossover trial. Lancet Diabetes Endocrinol. 4(3):2016, 233–243.

[66] Tauschmann M, et al. Day-and-night hybrid closed-loop insulin delivery in adolescents with type 1 diabetes: a free-living, randomized clinical trial. Diabetes Care 2016;39(7):1168–74.

[67] Tauschmann M, et al. Home use of day-and-night hybrid closed-loop insulin delivery in suboptimally controlled adolescents with type 1 diabetes: a 3-week, free-living, randomized crossover trial. Diabetes Care 2016;39(11):2019–25.

[68] Georga E, et al. Wearable systems and mobile applications for diabetes disease management. Health Technol 2014;1–12.

[69] Pejovic V, Musolesi M. Anticipatory mobile computing: a survey of the state of the art and research challenges. ACM Comput Surv 2015;47(3):1–29.

10 ⸬⸬

Conclusions and Future Trends

10.1 Big Data and Precision Medicine

Big-data technologies and precision medicine are tightly linked with the former providing the means for the realization of the latter. The term big data tends to encompass both large scale, streaming, highly variate, and of variable veracity data, as they are characterized by the 4Vs (i.e., volume, velocity, variety, and veracity), as well as high-throughput data analytics able to cope with big data. According to the National Institutes of Health (NIH) definition, precision medicine advocates that prognosis, diagnosis, and therapeutics of a disease should be driven by precise knowledge on an individual's genetics, environment, and lifestyle. Nowadays, the advances in omics technologies, bio- and physiological sensors, and medical imaging technologies coupled with the increasing adoption of electronic health records (EHRs) lead to an unprecedented volume and variety of longitudinal patient-specific data [1]. In parallel, advances in bioinformatics, data mining, machine learning, and overall cognitive computing on top of contemporary cloud databases and data integration services strengthen the hypothesis that these data can be translated into actionable knowledge [2]. To this end, the NIH Precision Medicine Initiative, aiming at providing the scientific evidence needed to deliver precision medicine, launched a new era in cohort studies for disease prevention, diagnosis and treatment [3]. In particular, at least 1 million participants are planned to be enrolled by the end of 2019 providing genetic, biological, behavioral (i.e., diet, lifestyle), and EHR data.

Genome wide association studies (GWAS), linking the human genome to phenotypic characteristics, and, more recently, the advent of omics technologies (e.g., proteomics, metabolomics, lipidomics, transcriptomics) have enabled the development of holistic computational modeling approaches of complex biological systems, what is defined as systems biology. In addition, metagenomics and particularly gut microbiomics may provide new insights into the microbiome−human host interplay with respect to the onset and progression of a disease [4]. The integration of omics data with EHRs as well as mobile health (mHealth) data will complement the molecular signature of an individual with his/her exposome and overall phenotype, enabling analyzing their interconnections [5−7]. In particular, the ubiquity of mHealth devices and accompanying cloud services facilitated continuous monitoring and collection of health, behavioral, emotional, and environmental information under free-living conditions.

Online interactive distributed machine-learning constitutes the forefront of big-data analytics [8]. Bioinformatics offers robust tools for analyzing the structure and function of the entire genome, whereas dynamic modeling of temporal omics data is expected to be addressed by advanced ensemble methods of statistically rigorous and computationally scalable machine-learning algorithms (e.g., continuous time Bayesian networks, deep-learning)

Personalized Predictive Modeling in Type 1 Diabetes. DOI: http://dx.doi.org/10.1016/B978-0-12-804831-3.00010-8

[9,10]. Moreover, EHRs consist of asynchronously acquired, usually unstructured, multivariate data, which representation in an interval-based format enables the extraction of predictive temporal patterns [11,12].

10.2 Toward Precision Diabetes Medicine

Knowledge of the human genome sequence has contributed significantly to our understanding of the pathogenesis and the underlying molecular mechanisms of both types 1 and 2 diabetes [13–16]. The HLA class II alleles account almost for 50% of the genetic susceptibility to Type 1 diabetes, whereas GWAS explain a lower proportion of type 2 diabetes heritability. Meyer et al. find no apparent way for precision medicine to permeate insulin therapy of type 1 diabetes and they locate its role mainly in (1) identifying effective preventive interventions targeting genetically susceptible individuals (characterized as primary prevention) and (2) understanding the immune mediators and propagators of β-cell destruction in individuals with islet autoimmunity (characterized as secondary prevention) [13]. To this end, the Environmental Determinants of Diabetes in the Young (TEDDY) multicenter study has already provided significant insight into the genetic-environmental associations triggering the development of islet autoimmunity or promoting type 1 diabetes progression in genetically at risk children (≤5 years) [17–19]. Recently, TEDDY study provided evidence of clear differences in the initiation of autoimmunity (insulin autoantibodies, GAD antibodies) according to genetic factors (e.g., presence of SNPs rs689 [INS], rs2476601 [PTPN22], rs2292239 [ERBB3], rs3184504 [SH2B3], rs3757247 [BACH2]), and environmental exposures (i.e., sex, family history, HLA, country, probiotics at age 28 days, weight at age 12 months) in infants with HLA-DR high-risk genotypes followed-up until 6 years of age [18]. On the other hand, Meyer et al. postulate that type 2 diabetes pharmacological interventions are more likely to benefit from the inclusion of precise knowledge on an individual's genotype and on predictive biomarkers of secondary complications; however, they acknowledge the lack of robust scientific evidence at present which would guide drug regulation. As a first step toward type 2 diabetes therapy individualization, the GRADE comparative effectiveness long-term study of commonly used glycemia-lowering medications (i.e., sulfonylurea, DPP-4 inhibitor, GLP-1 receptor agonist, insulin) when combined with metformin, having enrolled ∼5000 participants, assesses the differences in study outcomes by race/ethnicity, sex, age, diabetes duration, weight, body mass index, HbA1c, and measures of insulin sensitivity, insulin secretion, and the glucose disposal index [20].

The NIH Precision Medicine Initiative in tandem with other linked precision medicine activities (e.g., the National Heart, Lung and Blood Institute Trans-Omics for Precision Medicine [TOPMed] Program), supporting the collection of longitudinal multivariate data (genome, proteome metabolome, microbiome, exposome, and phenome) from large population cohorts, will enable the development of systems biology approaches to elucidating the underlying pathophysiological mechanisms of diabetes onset and progression and the identification of new biomarkers of diabetes-related vascular complications [3,15,21–23]. Data mining of daily longitudinal self-monitoring data (e.g., continuous glucose monitoring, physical activity, stress) along with EHR data is an additional valuable asset, which has the potential to explain both the short-term and long-term glycemic status of an individual and facilitate the evaluation of the glycemic effectiveness of a specific intervention [24−28]. In addition, the consequent finer stratification of people with type 1 or type 2 diabetes per se, possibly defining new diabetes subtypes, could provide opportunities for more effective personalized therapeutic schemes as well as for new hypotheses about disease pathogenesis and medical care which could be tested at different stages of disease progression [3,15,21−23]. A paradigm is the Integrated Human Microbiome Project (iHMP) aiming at identifying physiological changes in microbiome−host omics temporal profiles during healthy and stress conditions [4]. The diabetes-associated iHMP exemplar substudy tests the individual effect of stress [i.e., medical illness, physical injury/pain, major or minor operation, major life changes (birth, death, divorce, marriage, and change of home or job)] on the human microbiome, metabolome, and epigenome, as well as its common effect on the host and the microbiome based on 3-year longitudinal observation of ∼60 individuals at risk for developing type 2 diabetes. Multiomic analysis, including whole metagenome shotgun and meta-transcriptome sequencing, host whole genome/transcriptome sequencing, cytokine and autoantibody profiles, metabolome profiles, and standard clinical lab tests and surveys of behavioral and psychosocial information (e.g., physical activity, food intake, stress), lay the foundation for analyzing the biological properties of the human microbiome and host during the onset and progression of type 2 diabetes.

10.3 Precise Predictive Modeling of Glycemic Dynamics

Physiological or data-driven computational models of the glucose metabolism have the potential to advance therapeutic procedures and technological solutions for controlling diabetes, by enabling the accurate identification or prediction of the response of multiple system characteristic parameters to various stimuli. Particularly, multiparametric multiscale predictive modeling of glucose concentration trajectory may result in tighter short-term glycemic control, minimizing the risk of hypoglycemia, and prevent the long-term vascular complications of diabetes.

The problem of identification and prediction of short-term glycemic dynamics in type 1 diabetes has been largely studied on the basis of time series and machine-learning principles, with glucose models' generalization performance now being demonstrated in small-scale observational studies conducted in real-life conditions. On the one hand, parameterized models from linear systems theory assume that the examined glucose system is linear and time-invariant, and on the other, nonlinearity is treated by machine-learning models (neural networks, kernel-based methods, ensemble models). In addition, dynamic adaptive learning of the glucose system is considered an integral component of modern modeling schemes. In this context, both univariate (i.e., autoregressive glucose models) and multivariate (e.g., meals, insulin therapy, physical activities, stress) input models have been studied, whereas the input level is where the synergy between physiological models and data-driven glucose predictive models lies in. The generalization capability of existing approaches, as it has been estimated on real and in silico data, is promising; however, no consensus has been reached on feature learning and model identification and validation.

Advancements in big-data technologies and cognitive computing will shift research in diabetes toward precise predictive, potentially preventive, models being built upon novel multisensor, multisource and multiprocess information fusion schemes. An exemplar study by Zeevi et al. effectively integrated information on meal content (e.g., carbohydrates, macronutrients, micronutrients), behavior (e.g., physical activity, diet, sleep), blood tests (e.g., HbA1c, HDL), subcutaneous glucose concentration, anthropometrics (e.g., waist-to-hip ratio, body mass index), and gut microbiome into a gradient boosting regression model of postprandial glycemic response (quantified as the incremental area under the glucose curve) trained and evaluated on a cohort of $n = 800$ and $n = 100$ individuals, respectively, with prediabetes or type 2 diabetes [29]. In addition, by postprocessing model's output through partial dependence plots, Zeevi et al. confirmed the contribution of conventional features (e.g., carbohydrates, fat-to-carbohydrate ratio, dietary fibers) to postprandial glycemic excursions and elucidated the beneficial (e.g., *Eubacterium rectale*) or nonbeneficial role (e.g., *Parabacteroides distasonis*, KEGG module of cell-division transport system [M00256], *Bacteroides thetaiotaomicron*) of microbiome-based features. A subsequent dietary intervention ($n = 26$), which employed the predictive model, resulted in significantly improved glycemic outcomes accompanied by consistent beneficial alterations in gut microbiome composition, which indicates the feasibility of diet personalization in the context of diabetes management. Contemporary computational prediction models of short-term glycemic dynamics in the context of type 1 diabetes should cope with the challenges posed by four essential Vs of big data (i.e., volume, velocity, variety, and veracity) and, given the chronic and progressive nature of diabetes, combine adaptive unsupervised or supervised learning algorithms [30].

Fig. 10.1 depicts a conceptual architecture for glucose predictive models integrating three information analysis levels such that available diabetes big data are excellently exploited. Having addressed dataset quality issues, the effective specification of the input space, mainly via dimensionality reduction and feature learning techniques, forms the basis for the subsequent data mining and modeling process. Unsupervised exploratory cluster analysis can provide an initial high-level representation of the input space, portraying innate similarities among patients, which, in turn, can augment the glucose system identification and prediction process; for instance, allowing for the construction of different models depending on the group a patient is assigned to. Clustering approaches, such as k-means, expectation maximization clustering, hierarchical agglomerative clustering, have to be investigated toward identifying groups of patients with similar characteristics or behaviors, in accordance with the defined feature space, or organizing patients into a hierarchy of clusters as a first level toward patient stratification. In addition to cluster analysis, pattern recognition analysis has been emerging as a means toward precise self-management as well as medical care of diabetes, and in this direction, association analysis enables mining significant cooccurrence or

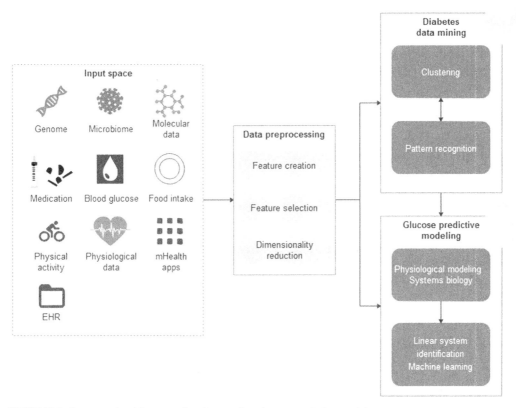

FIGURE 10.1 Conceptual architecture of an integrative glucose predictive model.

dynamic relationships in cross-sectional or longitudinal multimodal diabetes data, respectively. Dynamic data mining of health, lifestyle, and psychosocial patterns from personal health record (PHR) and EHR diabetes data is expected to enhance reasoning and quantification of the effect one patient's phenotype on his/her metabolic status and may drive glucose predictions. To this end, continuous time Bayesian networks are considered particularly expressive model structures with regard to stochastic processes which evolve continuously over time and are well suited for extracting potentially causal interactions between omics and phenotypic diabetes data over different time granularities [31−33]. Subsequently, predictive modeling, as a dynamic component, has to be built upon adaptive linear or nonlinear regression solutions balancing the trade-off among accuracy, interpretability and time and space complexity. Well-defined machine-learning techniques featuring the universal approximation property and convexity and being capable of solving recursively nonlinear prediction problems has to be extensively evaluated with respect to their ability to capture the temporal dynamics of the glucose system. In addition, interactive machine-learning approaches, relying on reinforcement learning, preference learning, and active learning, could yield more transparent (white- or glass-box) models [34]. Finally, data-driven models can be harmonically combined with mechanistic models of diabetes by either complementing their input space or refining their functionality.

Overall, both architecture and internal algorithms should be methodically specified toward precise patient-specific glucose modeling. Precision medicine initiatives, systems biology and big-data technologies give rise to multiscale computer-modeling approaches integrating information from EHR, PHR and omics data and considering, in parallel, the different time-scales and forms of nonlinearities characterizing the input−output dynamics of the glucose system. Advancing short-term glucose predictive modeling will inspire and contribute to more personalized, predictive, preventive and participatory (P4 medicine) diabetes care interventions.

References

[1] Sagner M, et al. The P4 health spectrum—a predictive, preventive, personalized and participatory continuum for promoting healthspan. Prog Cardiovasc Dis 2017;59(5):506−21.

[2] Huang BE, Mulyasasmita W, Rajagopal G. The path from big data to precision medicine. Expert Rev Precision Med Drug Dev 2016;1(2):129−43.

[3] Fradkin JE, Hanlon MC, Rodgers GP. NIH precision medicine initiative: implications for diabetes research. Diabetes Care 2016;39(7):1080−4.

[4] Integrative, H.M.P.R.N.C. The Integrative Human Microbiome Project: dynamic analysis of microbiome−host omics profiles during periods of human health and disease. Cell Host Microbe 2014;16(3):276−89.

[5] Martin Sanchez F, et al. Exposome informatics: considerations for the design of future biomedical research information systems. J Am Med Inform Assoc: JAMIA 2014;21(3):386−90.

[6] Manrai AK, et al. Informatics and data analytics to support exposome-based discovery for public health. Annu Rev Public Health 2017;38(1):279−94.

[7] Vineis P, et al. The exposome in practice: design of the EXPOsOMICS project. Int J Hyg Environ Health 2017;220(2):142−51.

[8] Zhou L, et al. Machine learning on big data: opportunities and challenges. Neurocomputing 2017;237:350−61.

[9] Liang Y, Kelemen A. Dynamic modeling and network approaches for omics time course data: overview of computational approaches and applications. Brief Bioinform 2017; [Epub ahead of print].

[10] Liang Y, Kelemen A. Computational dynamic approaches for temporal omics data with applications to systems medicine. BioData Min 2017;10:20.

[11] Batal I, et al. A temporal pattern mining approach for classifying electronic health record data. ACM Trans Intell Syst Technol 2013;4(4):1−22.

[12] Chen YC, Peng WC, Lee SY. Mining temporal patterns in time interval-based data. IEEE Trans Knowl Data Eng 2015;27(12):3318−31.

[13] Meyer RJ. Precision medicine, diabetes, and the U.S. Food and Drug Administration. Diabetes Care 2016;39(11):1874−8.

[14] Floyd JS, Psaty BM. The application of genomics in diabetes: barriers to discovery and implementation. Diabetes Care 2016;39(11):1858−69.

[15] Pearson ER. Personalized medicine in diabetes: the role of 'omics' and biomarkers. Diabet Med 2016;33 (6):712−17.

[16] Zarkogianni K, et al. A review of emerging technologies for the management of diabetes mellitus. IEEE Trans Biomed Eng 2015;62(12):2735−49.

[17] Group TS. The Environmental Determinants of Diabetes in the Young (TEDDY) Study. Ann N Y Acad Sci 2008;1150:1−13.

[18] Krischer JP, et al. Genetic and environmental interactions modify the risk of diabetes-related autoimmunity by 6 years of age: the TEDDY study. Diabetes Care 2017;40(9):1194−202.

[19] Krischer JP, et al. The 6 year incidence of diabetes-associated autoantibodies in genetically at-risk children: the TEDDY study. Diabetologia 2015;58(5):980−7.

[20] Nathan DM, et al. Rationale and design of the glycemia reduction approaches in diabetes: a comparative effectiveness study (GRADE). Diabetes Care 2013;36(8):2254−61.

[21] Florez JC. Precision medicine in diabetes: is it time? Diabetes Care 2016;39(7):1085−8.

[22] Klonoff DC. Precision medicine for managing diabetes. J Diabetes Sci Technol 2015;9(1):3−7.

[23] Rich SS, Cefalu WT. The impact of precision medicine in diabetes: a multidimensional perspective. Diabetes Care 2016;39(11):1854−7.

[24] Heintzman ND. A digital ecosystem of diabetes data and technology: services, systems, and tools enabled by wearables, sensors, and apps. J Diabetes Sci Technol 2015;10(1):35−41.

[25] Cichosz SL, Johansen MD, Hejlesen O. Toward big data analytics: review of predictive models in management of diabetes and its complications. J Diabetes Sci Technol 2015;10(1):27−34.

[26] Bellazzi R, et al. Big data technologies: new opportunities for diabetes management. J Diabetes Sci Technol 2015;9(5):1119−25.

[27] Dagliati A, et al. Integration of administrative, clinical, and environmental data to support the management of type 2 diabetes mellitus: from satellites to clinical care. J Diabetes Sci Technol 2015;10(1):19−26.

[28] Zarkogianni K, et al. Comparative assessment of glucose prediction models for patients with type 1 diabetes mellitus applying sensors for glucose and physical activity monitoring. Med Biol Eng Comput 2015;53(12):1333−43.

[29] Zeevi D, et al. Personalized nutrition by prediction of glycemic responses. Cell 2015;163(5):1079−94.

[30] Kavakiotis I, et al. Machine learning and data mining methods in diabetes research. Comput Struct Biotechnol J 2017;15:104−16.

[31] Acerbi E, et al. Continuous time Bayesian networks identify Prdm1 as a negative regulator of TH17 cell differentiation in humans. Sci Rep 2016;6:23128.

[32] Nodelman U, Shelton CR, Koller D. Learning continuous time Bayesian networks. Proceedings of the nineteenth conference on Uncertainty in Artificial Intelligence. Acapulco, Mexico: Morgan Kaufmann Publishers Inc; 2003. p. 451−8.

[33] Nodelman U, Shelton CR, Koller D. Continuous time Bayesian networks. Proceedings of the eighteenth conference on uncertainty in artificial intelligence. Alberta, Canada: Morgan Kaufmann Publishers Inc; 2002. p. 378−87.

[34] Holzinger A. Interactive machine learning for health informatics: when do we need the human-in-the-loop? Brain Inform 2016;3(2):119−31.

Index

Note: Page numbers followed by "*f*" and "*t*" refer to figures and tables, respectively.